Management of Extracranial Cerebrovascular Disease

WITH 38 CONTRIBUTORS

Management of Extracranial Cerebrovascular Disease

EDITORS

Keith D. Calligaro, MD
Chief, Section of Vascular Surgery
Pennsylvania Hospital
Associate Professor of Surgery
Thomas Jefferson University
Philadelphia, Pennsylvania

Dominic A. DeLaurentis, MD
Section of Vascular Surgery
Pennsylvania Hospital
Professor of Surgery
University of Pennsylvania School of Medicine
Philadelphia, Pennsylvania

William H. Baker, MD
Head, Section of Peripheral Vascular Surgery
Foster G. McGaw Hospital
Professor of Surgery
Stritch School of Medicine, Loyola University
Chicago, Illinois

Lippincott - Raven
PUBLISHERS
Philadelphia • New York

Acquisitions Editor: Lisa McAllister
Developmental Editor: Emilie Linkins
Senior Production Editor: Virginia Barishek
Production Service: Caslon, Inc.
Compositor: The Composing Room of Michigan, Inc.
Prepress: Jay's Publishers Services, Inc.
Color Separator: Fidelity Color
Insert Printer: The Sheridan Press
Printer/Binder: Maple Press
Cover Designer: Becky Baxendell

Library of Congress Cataloging-in-Publication Data

Management of extracranial cerebrovascular disease / editors, Keith D. Calligaro, Dominic A. DeLaurentis, William H. Baker ; with 38 contributors.
p. cm.
Includes bibliographical references and index.
ISBN 0-397-51655-X
1. Cerebrovascular disease. 2. Carotid artery thrombosis—Complications. 3. Aorta—Diseases—Complications. I. Calligaro, Keith D., 1956– . II. DeLaurentis, Dominic A. III. Baker, William Henry, 1937– .
[DNLM: 1. Carotid Artery Diseases—surgery. 2. Aortic Diseases—surgery. WL 355 M2652 1996]
RC388.5.M355 1996
616.8′1—dc20
DNLM/DLC
For Library of Congress 96-33256
CIP

Care has been taken to confirm the accuracy of the information presented and to describe generally accepted practices. However, the authors, editors, and publisher are not responsible for errors or omissions or for any consequences from application of the information in this book and make no warranty, express or implied, with respect to the contents of the publication.

The authors, editors and publisher have exerted every effort to ensure that drug selection and dosage set forth in this text are in accordance with current recommendations and practice at the time of publication. However, in view of ongoing research, changes in government regulations, and the constant flow of information relating to drug therapy and drug reactions, the reader is urged to check the package insert for each drug for any change in indications and dosage and for added warnings and precautions. This is particularly important when the recommended agent is a new or infrequently employed drug.

Some drugs and medical devices presented in this publication have Food and Drug Administration (FDA) clearance for limited use in restricted research settings. It is the responsibility of the health care provider to ascertain the FDA status of each drug or device planned for use in their clinical practice.

9 8 7 6 5 4 3 2 1

Dedicated to our wives
Ina Lee, Molly, and Ann
for their patience, support, and understanding

Contributors

Mark A. Adelman, MD
Assistant Professor of Surgery
New York University School of Medicine
Attending Surgeon
New York University Hospital
Manhattan Veterans Administration Hospital
Bellevue Hospital
530 First Avenue
New York, New York 10016

William H. Baker, MD
Professor and Chief
Division of Peripheral Vascular Surgery
Loyola University Medical Center
Chief, Division of Peripheral Vascular Surgery
Foster G. McGaw Hospital
Loyola University Medical Center
2160 South First Avenue
Maywood, Illinois 60153

Bruce J. Brener, MD
Chief, Division of Vascular Surgery
Newark Beth Israel Medical Center
Clinical Professor of Surgery
University of Medicine and Dentistry of New Jersey-Newark
201 Lyons Avenue
Newark, New Jersey 07112

David C. Brewster, MD
Clinical Professor of Surgery
Massachusetts General Hospital
Harvard Medical School
One Hawthorne Place, Suite 111
Boston, Massachusetts 02114

Donald K. Brief, MD
Clinical Professor of Surgery
University of Medicine and Dentistry of New Jersey—Newark
Chairman, Department of Surgery
Newark Beth Israel Medical Center
201 Lyons Avenue
Newark, New Jersey 07112

Richard P. Cambria, MD
Associate Professor of Surgery
Harvard Medical School
Division of Vascular Surgery
Massachusetts General Hospital
15 Parkman Street
Boston, Massachusetts 02114

Elliot L. Chaikof, MD, PhD
Assistant Professor of Surgery
Emory University School of Medicine
Box M-11
1364 Clifton Road, NE
Atlanta, Georgia 30322

Anthony J. Comerota, MD
Professor of Surgery
Department of Surgery
Temple University School of Medicine
Broad and Ontario Streets
Philadelphia, Pennsylvania 19140

Joseph S. Coselli, MD
Professor of Surgery
Baylor College of Medicine
Attending Surgeon
The Methodist Hospital
6560 Fannin, Suite 1144
Houston, Texas 77030

William H. Edwards, Sr., MD
The H. William Scott, Jr., Professor of Surgery Emeritus
Vanderbilt University School of Medicine
Medical Director
Departments of General and Vascular Surgery
St. Thomas Hospital
50 Concord Park East
Nashville, Tennessee 37205

David E. Eisenbud, MD
Attending Surgeon
Newark Beth Israel Medical Center
201 Lyons Avenue
Newark, New Jersey 07112

John G. Ferguson, MD
Director of Clinical Epidemiology and Medical Informatics
Memphis Vascular Research Foundation
910 Madison Avenue, Suite 710
Memphis, Tennessee 38103

Robert D. G. Ferguson, MD
Director, Memphis Vascular Research Foundation
Chief, Interventional Neuroradiology
Baptist Memorial Hospital
930 Madison Avenue, Suite 364
Memphis, Tennessee 38103

Gary Giangola, MD
Assistant Professor of Surgery
New York University Medical Center
Attending Surgeon
Tisch Hospital of New York University
Bellevue Hospital
Chief, Division of Vascular Surgery
Manhattan Veterans Administration Medical Center
530 First Avenue, Suite 7U
New York, New York 10016

Mark S. Gold, MD
Assistant Professor of Anesthesiology
Director of Vascular Anesthesia
New York University Medical Center
530 First Avenue
New York, New York 10016

Robert J. Goldenkranz, MD
Associate Professor of Surgery
University of Medicine and Dentistry of New Jersey Medical School
Newark, New Jersey
Director of General Surgery
Newark Beth Israel Medical Center
225 Millburn Avenue, Suite 104B
Millburn, New Jersey 07041

Richard M. Green, MD
Department of Surgery
The University of Rochester
601 Elmwood Avenue
Rochester, New York 14642

Steven M. Hertz, MD
Associate Director
Division of Vascular Surgery
Attending, Vascular Surgery
Director, Noninvasive Vascular Laboratory
Newark Beth Israel Medical Center
201 Lyons Avenue
Newark, New Jersey 07112

Robert W. Hobson II, MD
Professor of Surgery
Chief, Section of Vascular Surgery
University of Medicine and Dentistry of New Jersey Medical School
185 South Orange Avenue, MSB G-532
Newark, New Jersey 07103

Jan Huston, MD
Director, Division of Laparoscopic Surgery
Department of Surgery
Newark Beth Israel Medical Center
201 Lyons Avenue
Newark, New Jersey 07112

Glenn R. Jacobowitz, MD
Fellow in Vascular Surgery
New York University Medical Center
530 First Avenue, Suite 6F
New York, New York 10016

Mira L. Katz, MLA
Research Instructor of Surgery
Temple University School of Medicine

Chief Technologist, Vascular Laboratory
Temple University Hospital
Broad and Ontario Streets
Philadelphia, Pennsylvania 19140

Christopher J. Kwolek, MD
Assistant Professor of Surgery
University of Kentucky
Staff Surgeon
Department of Surgery
Section of Vascular Surgery
University of Kentucky—Chandler Medical Center
800 Rose Street, Room C-218
Lexington, Kentucky 40536-0084

Patrick J. Lamparello, MD
Associate Professor of Surgery
New York University School of Medicine
Associate Attending Surgeon
Tisch Hospital of New York University
530 First Avenue, Suite 6F
New York, New York 10016

Michel S. Makaroun, MD
Associate Professor
Department of Surgery
University of Pittsburgh School of Medicine
A-1011 UPMC
200 Lothrop Street
Pittsburgh, Pennsylvania 15213

Mark D. Morasch, MD
Chief Resident, Department of Surgery
Loyola University Medical Center
2160 South First Avenue
Maywood, Illinois 60153

Monica S. O'Brien-Irr, MS, RN
Clinical Nurse Specialist/Nurse Practitioner
Department of Surgery
Millard Fillmore Hospital
3 Gates Circle
Buffalo, New York 14209

Kenneth Ouriel, MD
Associate Professor of Surgery
Department of Surgery
The University of Rochester
601 Elmwood Avenue
Rochester, New York 14642

Victor Parsonnet, MD
Clinical Professor of Surgery
University of Medicine and Denistry of New Jersey
Director of Surgical Research
Medical Director of Pacemaker Center
Newark Beth Israel Medical Center
201 Lyons Avenue
Newark, New Jersey 07112

Bruce A. Perler, MD
Associate Professor of Surgery
The Johns Hopkins University School of Medicine
Attending Vascular Surgeon
Director of the Vascular Diagnostic Laboratory
The Johns Hopkins Hospital
600 North Wolfe Street, Blalock 685
Baltimore, Maryland 21287-4685

Luiz F. Poli de Figueiredo, MD, PhD
Visiting Assistant Professor
Department of Anesthesiology
The University of Texas Medical Branch at Galveston
503 Clinical Sciences, G-49
Galveston, Texas 77555-0749

Peter N. Purcell, MD
Fellow, Vascular Surgery
Division of Vascular Surgery
Massachusetts General Hospital
15 Parkman Street
Boston, Massachusetts 02114

John J. Ricotta, MD
Professor of Surgery
Director, Division of Vascular Surgery
State University of New York at Buffalo
Millard Fillmore Hospital
Department of Surgery
3 Gates Circle
Buffalo, New York 14209

Thomas S. Riles, MD
Professor of Surgery
Director, Division of Vascular Surgery

Department of Surgery
New York University Medical Center
530 First Avenue
New York, New York 10016

Robert B. Smith III, MD
Professor of Surgery
Head, General Vascular Surgery
Department of Surgery, Room H-122
Emory University School of Medicine
1364 Clifton Road, NE
Atlanta, Georgia 30322

D. Eugene Strandness, Jr., MD
Professor, Department of Surgery
University of Washington School of Medicine
University of Washington Medical Center
Department of Surgery, Box 356410
Seattle, Washington 98195-6410

Marshall W. Webster, MD
Professor and Vice Chairman
Department of Surgery
University of Pittsburgh School of Medicine
Chief, Section of Vascular Surgery and Wound Healing
University of Pittsburgh Medical Center
A-1011 UPMC
200 Lothrop Street
Pittsburgh, Pennsylvania 15213

Howard Yonas, MD
Professor, Department of Neurological Surgery
Professor, Radiology
Chief, Cerebrovascular Surgery
University of Pittsburgh Medical Center
Presbyterian University Hospital
200 Lothrop Street, Suite B-400
Pittsburgh, Pennsylvania 15235

Preface

Few subjects in vascular surgery have been as controversial as the use of carotid endarterectomy to prevent stroke. After the first carotid endarterectomy was performed in the 1950s, the number of these operations increased until they reached a peak in the mid-1980s. However, harsh criticisms by some members of the medical community resulted in a decrease in the number of these operations. Many neurologists believed that the operation was associated with prohibitively high morbidity and mortality rates, and indeed at some medical centers these suspicions were supported by analysis of surgical outcome. Recent prospective, randomized, multicenter trials have answered many controversial questions regarding treatment of carotid artery disease and have helped to justify performance of these operations under appropriate circumstance.

In an effort to provide an up-to-date perspective and analysis of these and other reports, this book attempts to provide a comprehensive review of current knowledge concerning management of extracranial cerebrovascular disease. We address cost issues, perioperative management, indications for surgical intervention, and results of surgical and other interventional procedures for treating patients with extracranial cerebrovascular disease due to carotid artery and aortic arch pathology. Some of the most respected national and international authorities in the field have contributed their experiences and recommendations concerning this subject. The editors wish to sincerely thank them for their efforts. We also want to thank Lisa McAllister of Lippincott–Raven Publishers for her tireless efforts and interest in this project. Our hope is that this book will serve not only as a useful reference for all physicians caring for these patients but also as a practical guide for the vascular surgeon and neurologist faced with treating patients with extracranial cerebrovascular disease.

Keith D. Calligaro, MD
Dominic A. DeLaurentis, MD
William H. Baker, MD

Contents

Part III
Surgical Technique of the Aortic Arch and the Extracranial Arteries

PART I

Basic Concepts and Perioperative Assessment of Patients Undergoing Carotid Artery Surgery

Management of Extracranial Cerebrovascular Disease, edited by Keith D. Calligaro et al.
Lippincott-Raven Publishers, Philadelphia © 1997.

1

Cost Concerns in Carotid Surgery

John J. Ricotta, Monica S. O'Brien-Irr

In the past decade four prospective randomized studies have established the efficacy of carotid endarterectomy (CEA) in the management of both symptomatic[1,2] and asymptomatic[3,4] high-grade bifurcation stenoses. With this question settled, much of the recent discussion about CEA has shifted to its effective (i.e., "cost-effective") application. Clinical practice has evolved toward reduced hospitalization, outpatient evaluation, and disciplined use of diagnostic studies. This chapter focuses on these and other factors as they pertain to carotid endarterectomy and evaluates their medical and financial consequences.

Management of patients who undergo carotid endarterectomy can be broken down into 3 phases for the purposes of a financial analysis: (1) preoperative diagnostic evaluation (2) in-hospital management, and (3) postoperative follow-up. While most analyses have focused on the second (in-hospital) phase because it is the most easily controlled (and regulated), the arrival of capitation clearly implies that all 3 areas require close scrutiny and control. For simplicity, each is discussed separately here.

PREOPERATIVE EVALUATION

The identification of patients who may benefit from carotid endarterectomy depends on two factors: the identification of prior cerebral ischemic events and the accurate identification of surgically significant carotid stenosis. A history of ocular or cerebral ischemia (stroke, transient ischemic attack (TIA), or amaurosis fugax) greatly increases the likelihood of a subsequent stroke in patients with stenoses >70% diameter.[1,2] This remains the most firmly established indication for carotid endarterectomy.[5] Focal neurologic symptoms can usually be identified by a thorough history and neurologic examination. The second factor in this equation is percent diameter stenosis. The North American Symptomatic Carotid Endarterectomy Trial (NASCET)[1] and European Carotid Surgery Trial (ECST)[2] have shown that stenoses >70% diameter reduction by angiogram are best treated surgically, while the Asymptomatic Carotid Atherosclerosis Study (ACAS)[3] and the Veteran's Affairs (VA)[4] asymptomatic trial have shown a benefit for surgery in those patients for stenoses that causes as little as 60%[3] or even 50%[4] diameter reduction. While stenosis was determined angiographically in all four studies, ACAS did show that ultrasound was able to serve as an alternate measure of stenosis in carefully validated laboratories.[6] Furthermore, the finding in ACAS that morbidity of angiography (1.3%) was equivalent to that of surgery,[3] has led many centers to question the use of routine angiography, particularly in asymptomatic patients.

The preceding discussion is directly relevant to the routine evaluation of patients with cerebrovascular disease. The first two questions to be considered are the efficacy of routine brain imaging (computed tomography [CT] or magnetic resonance imaging [MRI]) and the use of routine preoperative angiography. Routine neurologic evaluation but *not* routine brain imaging has been used as standard of care by a recent consensus panel of the American Heart Association.[5] The rationale for this recommendation is the desire to confirm the clinical diagnosis of ischemic stroke, identify silent stroke, or exclude other intracranial pathology such as hemorrhage, tumor, or aneurysm. Numerous studies have documented an imperfect correlation between clinical presentation and brain imaging. Approximately 20–30% of patients with a clear history or physical findings of stroke will have a normal brain scan, while about a third of neurologically normal TIA patients and a fifth of patients with asymptomatic high-grade stenosis will have evidence of prior infarction on CT or MRI.[7–9] For the most part, therapeutic decisions are made on the basis of clinical classification rather than CT findings, particularly in patients with hemispheric symptoms of cerebral ischemia. One must therefore question the clinical value of routine preoperative CT scanning in these patients. An argument has been made that the clinically asymptomatic patient with silent cerebral infarction may represent a subgroup[10] at high risk for subsequent stroke and that imaging is therefore justified in asymptomatic patients. This approach remains speculative at present, would result in a 20% yield, at most, and may deny potential benefits of CEA to patients without evidence of CT infarction. In the face of the safety and proven efficacy of endarterectomy for severe stenosis, this position is not currently tenable.

Two other arguments for preoperative CT or MR scans can be made: (1) to identify other pathology and (2) to determine perioperative risk. While the presence of alternative pathology (*i.e.*, aneurysm, tumor, hemorrhage) is a legitimate concern in someone with a fixed neurologic deficit, it would be exceedingly unusual in patients with transient deficits, amaurosis fugax, or asymptomatic stenoses. It is likely that the occurrence of unsuspected clinically significant CT findings in these groups would be <5% and perhaps in the range of 1–2%.[11,12] Similarly, there is ample data to show that the presence or absence of infarction on CT scan does not correlate with perioperative morbidity or mortality within clinical classes.[7] In the face of these data, routine preoperative brain imaging is hard to justify.

The same arguments apply to angiography. Arch and selective cut-film angiograms were the gold standard for evaluation of carotid stenosis for years. More recently, these have been replaced by digital subtraction studies in an effort to reduce dye load and neurologic complications. The resulting images, however, often preclude accurate measurement of stenosis and are plagued by artifact from plaque calcification, compounding the problem of determining plaque stenosis. Clinical decisions are now often made by combining duplex and angiographic information, or on duplex alone.

Several studies have documented measurement variations of ±10% with cut-film angiography suggesting this "gold standard" is, in fact, tarnished.[15,16] Since 1984, numerous papers have appeared suggesting that endarterectomy without angiography is a reasonable approach.[14,15,17] The recent results of the ACAS trial documented 1.3% morbidity from angiography (equivalent to that of surgery) and have lent further support to this position.[3] The ACAS trials also showed that excellent (>94%) specificity could be achieved using noninvasive studies to determine surgical stenosis, although criterion were machine specific.[6]

While routine angiography is unnecessary in a setting where duplex is highly accurate, it may provide useful information in several settings. Patients with diffuse multi-vessel disease and those in which significant proximal or intracranial disease is suspected are likely to benefit from angiography. Our experience suggests that proximal disease can be identified by physical examination or duplex evaluation and is present in 10% or less of CEA candidates.[17] Clinically significant intracranial disease is even less common (<5% of cases[18]) and is only important in cases of moderate (<70% diameter) bifurcation stenosis. Thus, the role of angiography can be markedly restricted.

Magnetic resonance angiography (MRA) has been proposed as an alternative to conventional angiography.[19,20,21] While it has less morbidity than conventional angiography and is less costly, significant problems with the accurate quantification of stenosis exist in the current systems. In fact, while several studies report equivalence or even superiority of MRA compared to angiography, in a recent three-way comparison by Pan et al,[20] duplex ultrasound was the most accurate method for quantifying carotid bifurcation stenosis. At present, MRA remains a potentially useful but imperfect technique.

Other diagnostic studies to be considered in patients with cerebrovascular ischemia include transcranial doppler (TCD) and transesophageal echocardiography (TEE). TCD has been shown to detect transient particulate emboli in the intracranial vessels,[22,23] while TEE has increased the awareness of thoracic aortic atherosclerosis as a cause of stroke.[24,25] Although both of these technologies may be useful in selected patients, they are likely to be of little clinical consequence in the patient with a surgically accessible severe carotid bifurcation stenosis and are not part of the routine preoperative evaluation of such patients.

The final area of preoperative evaluation involves cardiac screening. About 30–40% of patients with carotid stenosis have significant coronary atherosclerosis.[26] Love et al suggest a significant number (33%) have abnormal stress testing in the absence of symptoms.[27] This seems to be a compelling argument for screening these patients with stress echocardiography or nuclear cardiology testing. However, the cardiac morbidity after CEA is low in several large reported experiences.[28–30] Kirschner et al reported cardiac related death in 0.2% patients and non fatal MI in 2% of 1,035 CEA's performed over a 2-year period in Rochester, NY.[30] While this undoubtedly underestimates the incidence of subclinical cardiac ischemia, it probably accurately reflects the rate of clinically important events. Many large series of unselected CEA patients report mortality rates <5%.[28–32] In the face of these data, it is

TABLE 1-1. *Charges for preoperative studies in Buffalo, NY.*

Carotid Angiogram (arch & selective views)	$2,600.00
CT with contrast	$555.50
MRI	$760.00
Duplex Ultrasound	$250.00
Transcranial Doppler	$175.00
Transesophageal Echocardiogram	$1,800.00
Persantine Thallium Scan	$1,355.00

difficult to recommend screening to reduce perioperative mortality. However, myocardial infarction remains the leading cause of late death after CEA. Whether or not cardiac screening can reduce *late* CEA mortality remains to be proven.

Financial Considerations of Preoperative Evaluation

There are significant financial implications that result from the extent of preoperative evaluation. Charges for the various preoperative studies in our own area are listed in Table 1-1. It is apparent that carotid angiography and nuclear cardiology stress testing are the most expensive preoperative diagnostic studies and, in fact, may exceed surgeon's fees for endarterectomy. Each time angiography and preoperative MR or CT scans are avoided a $3,000–3,400 charge reduction is achieved. This totals almost half of the Medicare DRG reimbursement for CEA in our area ($7,039).

Recommendations for Preoperative Evaluation

In the face of a validated noninvasive laboratory, preoperative routine angiography is not indicated. Angiography should be reserved for patients with multi-vessel or suspected proximal arch-vessel disease. Preoperative angiography should not be routinely performed for asymptomatic stenoses since overall efficacy of CEA in this group of patients is dependent on eliminating any source of morbidity (*i.e.*, angiography). Angiography may be indicated in symptomatic patients with borderline stenosis on duplex; asymptomatic patients with such lesions should be followed by ultrasound without operation, reserving surgery for lesion progression. Using these guidelines, we estimate that only 10–20% of patients will need angiography. Brain imaging should be reserved for patients with fixed neurologic deficits or those with a confusing clinical picture. Patients with amaurosis fugax, transient ischemia, or asymptomatic stenosis do not require routine brain imaging before CEA. We estimate that only 30–40% of all CEA patients (depending on referral and practice patterns) will need brain imaging using these guidelines. TCD and TEE are not used as part of routine preoperative evaluation. Currently, stress testing for CEA patients is used only rarely in patients with a high risk clinical profile (<5% of our CEA patients).

INPATIENT MANAGEMENT

While it would seem that physicians have the most control over inpatient costs, these are in fact not as significant an economic issue as preoperative evaluation. Relevant factors affecting inpatient costs include length of stay, use of the intensive care unit (ICU) resources, and operating room charges. Of these three parameters, ICU utilization is by far the most significant.

Same-day admission for carotid endarterectomy has become a standard of care. This is facilitated by outpatient evaluation, particularly if angiography is not required. The duration of postoperative stay has become the subject of much debate. Several articles have suggested that discharge within 24 hours after CEA can be safely accomplished in 60–70% of patients.[33,34] While this is undoubtedly possible, the proportion of such patients will depend on the age and comorbidities of the operative group, as well as their home support system and their proximity to medical care. For the last several years we have planned to discharge patients within 48 hours after elective CEA. During this time period, our average postoperative length of stay has been 3.6 days with 50% of patients sent home within 48 hours of surgery. It is likely that this can be shortened further since the majority (97%) of complications occur within 24 hours of operation.[35] The one complication likely to be missed with this approach is luxury perfusion syndrome, which usually occurs 3–7 days after surgery.[36] This is characteristically seen after relief of a very severe bifurcation stenosis and associated with hemicranial headache and hypertension. The pathophysiology of increased cerebral blood flow can be documented by Xenon or TCD.[37,38] This phenomenon can have disastrous results and, when suspected, patients should remain in the hospital until it subsides. We continue to see this problem in some form, in 1–3% of our patients.

In 1991, we first suggested selective use of the ICU following carotid endarterectomy.[35] This position was based on a retrospective review of ICU services by a randomly selected group of 73 patients undergoing CEA. We found that only 18% of patients used services unique to the ICU and that the majority of these patients manifested their need for such services within 8 hours of surgery. These findings were confirmed by others[39,40] and have led us to the selective use of the ICU following CEA. Over the last 4 years, we adopted a policy of admitting all CEA patients to a step-down unit (intermediate surgical care unit) rather than to an ICU unless problems occurred intraoperatively or during the 2–3 hour observation period in the recovery room. Our results with this policy are shown in Table 1-2. Our ICU admissions dropped to 25%, the majority were admitted for monitoring because of significant cardiac history or for blood pressure control. It is likely that 88% of these patients could be adequately monitored in a cardiac step-down unit where telemetry is available.

Choice of anesthetic agent needs to be discussed in relation to hospital charges. Since the anesthetic charges depend on the duration of service rather than the type of anesthesia, no direct effect of anesthetic technique on cost is likely. However, anesthetic technique can indirectly affect cost if it influences intraoperative monitoring and postoperative care. Two recent studies suggest that early discharge after CEA can

TABLE 1-2. *Results of policy of selective use of ICU*

Disposition	N	%	ICU Services
Intermediate Surgical Care Unit	51	75	0
ICU	17	25	8
Total	68		8 (11.8%)

N = 68.

be achieved with both regional or general anesthetic techniques.[33,34] It is our experience, however, that regional anesthesia often results in a smooth intraoperative and postoperative hemodynamic course. The use of cervical block with anesthesia monitoring eliminates much of the fluctuations in blood pressure associated with induction of or emergence from anesthesia. It is our strong bias that this has allowed us to limit our use of vasoactive agents for blood pressure control and reduce the number of admissions to the ICU. Data from Lipsett et al[41] suggest that extensive hemodynamic monitoring and complex anesthetic techniques are associated with a significantly higher rate of vasoactive infusions and need for ICU monitoring than we and others have experienced.[35,39] An additional benefit of regional anesthesia is freedom from need for intraoperative monitoring such as EEG or TCD.

Regional anesthesia is not for all patients, however. A skillful anesthesiologist, a calm patient, and a willing surgeon are prerequisites for success. Surgery under regional anesthesia undoubtedly takes somewhat longer on average than that performed using a general anesthetic. The increased operating time may balance any economic benefit from decreased need for cerebral monitoring. We are enthusiastic about regional anesthesia and use it in 90% of our patients. Nonetheless, in cases where the patient is reluctant, the lesion is likely to be technically difficult (reoperation, thick neck, high lesion), or the anesthesiologist is uncomfortable, we do not hesitate to use general technique.

Financial Considerations of Inpatient Management

The major financial consideration involves reducing use of the ICU and length of hospital stay. Current inpatient charges are summarized in Table 1-3. Using regional anesthesia allows us to avoid EEG monitoring in those cases (saving $325/case) although probably at a somewhat increased operating room cost. Major monetary advantage comes from the selective use of the ICU, saving $600/day in charges. While

TABLE 1-3. *Current inpatient charges*

Anesthesia	$720
EEG	$325
ICU bed/day	$1,000
Hospital bed/day	$400

we currently keep patients for 2 days after surgery, reducing this to 1 day would save an additional $400.

Recommendations for Inpatient Management

Patients should be admitted to the ICU on a selective basis after a period of observation in the recovery room of 3–4 hours. This policy will result in the most significant cost savings. Undoubtedly, some patients can be discharged within 24 hours of CEA and most are ready to be discharged within 48 hours. One must look carefully for luxury perfusion, particularly in patients with severe stenosis, and close follow-up is needed in patients if early discharge is planned.

Anesthetic technique should be individualized, but both surgeon and anesthesiologist should be open to cervical block. This is particularly true if it can be shown to decrease the need for perioperative vasoactive drugs.

POSTOPERATIVE FOLLOW-UP

This area is often overlooked in discussions on cost of carotid endarterectomy. The major issues of concern are the detection of clinically significant restenosis and the monitoring of contralateral disease progression. The problem of recurrent or residual stenosis remains an area of controversy. In 1982 Zierler and Strandness identified "recurrent stenosis" in >20% of patients after CEA.[42] These lesions, identified by serial duplex examinations, were often asymptomatic and "regressed" in a significant number of cases. The hemodynamic phenomenon described by these authors and confirmed by others, undoubtedly represent a combination of thrombus deposition, post-surgical changes, and vessel-wall remodelling.

The incidence of clinical symptomatic recurrent stenosis is remarkably constant at 2–5% in most large published series.[43–45] Some of these lesions, particularly those proximal to the endarterectomy, undoubtedly represent residual common carotid disease and are associated with symptom recurrence. Lesions that develop within 18–24 months of surgery are usually fibrous hyperplasia, while lesions which present >3–4 years after surgery are usually atherosclerotic recurrent disease. Early lesions, even when severe, often remain asymptomatic.[43] While Mackey et al have shown that it is safe to re-operate on early and late lesions, it is not clear that this is always necessary.[46] Our policy has been to re-operate on large proximal plaque that represents residual disease, and plaque that recurs after 3 years and is associated with a severe stenosis. Anecdotally, we have seen one early stenosis in a vein graft interposition, due to fibrosis at a valve site. Based on analogy with peripheral bypasses, we elected to repair this.

The problem of contralateral stenosis also needs to be addressed in follow-up since this is a legitimate reason for follow-up carotid studies. In our own experience with 494 patients, 61 had bilateral surgical lesions at the time of initial presentation and underwent staged bilateral CEA within 6 months. Of the remaining patients, contralateral CEA on the basis of symptoms or progression to severe stenosis occurred in 26 of 397 patients (1.6%/yr). The low annual incidence of recurrent stenosis and contralateral progression raises serious questions about the cost effectiveness of routine follow-up duplex surveillance.

Financial Considerations of Postoperative Follow-Up

While duplex scanning remains low risk and relatively inexpensive, it is reimbursed at $225–500/study. A protocol of biannual scanning, as recently suggested by Ouriel and Green,[47] would cost $450–1,000/year to implement with a yield of 2%/year after the first year. Biannual scanning would likely detect new significant contralateral lesions at the rate of <2%/year.

Recommendations for Postoperative Follow-Up

Postoperative duplex scanning is indicated 1–3 months after surgery to identify residual disease and quantify the degree of stenosis in the contralateral artery. This is particularly important if duplex alone is used preoperatively. A follow-up scan may be justifiable at 12, 18, and 24 months to identify recurrent stenoses. If the 2-year scan shows no recurrent stenosis, examination at 24–36 month intervals is probably sufficient. Annual phone follow-up to identify recurrent symptoms is appropriate.

Significant contralateral disease should be identified and treated by staged endarterectomy. Subsequent contralateral disease will be detected on 12-, 18-, and 24-month studies. After 24 months, patients with no contralateral stenosis require follow-up at 24-month intervals (for recurrent disease), while those with moderate (30–50%) degrees of stenosis may need annual or even semiannual evaluation, based on degree of stenosis.

SUMMARY

Maximizing the cost effectiveness of CEA requires close attention to preoperative evaluation, in-hospital care, and postoperative follow-up. Table 1-4 lists the potential cost savings of a strategy such as the one outlined in this chapter. Such a strategy contains the following features:

1. Restrict angiography to cases with extensive disease and equivocal duplex results in symptomatic patients (≈5% total)
2. Restrict CT scans to patients with fixed neurologic deficits (≈35% total)
3. Restrict cardiac imaging to high risk patients (10% total)
4. Restrict ICU to patients who truly need ICU services (≈15% total)
5. Limit length-of-stay to 48 hours postoperatively in 90% of patients and 24 hours postoperatively in 45% of patients
6. Limit duplex follow-up to 3, 12, 18, 24 months, then biannual in 85% of patients

TABLE 1-4. *Changing strategies of care—Financial implications*

Current strategy	Cost/case	Proposed strategy	Cost/case
Routine angiography	$2,600.00	Selective angiography (15%)	$390.00
Routine CT scan	$555.50	Selective CT scan (34%)	$188.90
Routine cardiac screening	$750.00	Selective cardiac screening (10%)	$75.00
One day ICU stay	$1,000.00	Selective ICU stay (15%)	$150.00
Two-day floor stay	$800.00	One day floor stay (45%)	$620.00
Semiannual duplex (12 tests/6 yr)	$3,000.00	Modified duplex follow-up (6 tests/6 yrs)*	$1,500.00
Totals	$8,705.50		$2923.90

*Add $500 for 8 duplex/6 yr; add $1,000 for 10 duplex/6 yr.

This type of approach will allow surgeons to continue to offer the medical benefits of CEA to appropriate surgical candidates in an era of increasing cost containment.

REFERENCES

1. North American Symptomatic Carotid Endarterectomy Trial (NASCET). Beneficial effect of carotid endarterectomy in symptomatic patients with high-grade carotid stenosis. N Engl J Med 1991; 325:445–453
2. European Carotid Surgery Trial (ECST). Interim results for symptomatic patients with severe (70–99%) or with mild (0–29%) carotid stenosis. Lancet 1991;337:1235–1243
3. Asymptomatic Carotid Atherosclerosis Study (ACAS). Endarterectomy of asymptomatic carotid artery stenosis. JAMA 1995;273:1421–1428
4. Hobson RW, Weiss DG, Fields WS, et al and the Veterans Affairs (VA) Cooperative Study Group: Efficacy of carotid endarterectomy for asymptomatic carotid stenosis. N Engl J Med 1993;328:221–227
5. Moore WS, Barnett HJM, Beebe HG, Bernstein EF, Brener BJ, Brott T, Caplan LR, Day A, Goldstone J, Hobson RW, Kempczinski RF, Matchar DB, Mayberg MR, Nicolaides AN, Norris JW, Ricotta JJ, Robertson JT, Rutherford RB, Thomas D, Toole JF, Trout HH, Wiebers DO: Guidelines for carotid endarterectomy. Circulation 1995;91(2):566–579
6. Howard G, Chamless LE, Baker WH, Ricotta JJ, Jones AM, O'Leary D, Howard VJ, Elliott TJ, Lefkowitz DS, Toole JF: A multicenter validation study of Doppler ultrasound versus angiography. J Cerebrovascular Disease 1991;1:166–173
7. Street DL, O'Brien MS, Ricotta JJ, Ekholm SE, Ouriel K, Green RM, DeWeese JA: Observations on cerebral computed tomography in patients having carotid endarterectomy. J Vasc Surg 1988; 7:798–801
8. Brott T, Tomsick T, Feinberg W, et al for the asymptomatic carotid atherosclerosis study investigators: Baseline silent cerebral infarction in the asymptomatic carotid atherosclerosis study. Stroke 1994;25:1122–1129
9. Norris JW, Zhu CZ: Silent stroke and carotid stenosis. Stroke 1992;23:483–484
10. Zukowski AJ, Nicolaides AN, Lewis RT, et al: The correlation between carotid plaque ulceration and cerebral infarction seen on CT scan. J Vasc Surg 1984;1:782–286
11. Schuler JJ, Flanigan DP, Lim LT, Kiefer T, Williams LR, Behrend AJ: The effect of carotid siphon stenosis on stroke rate, death and relief of symptoms following elective carotid endarterectomy. Surgery 1982;92:1058–1067
12. Dipple DW, Vermeulen M, Braakman R, Habbema JD: Transient ischemic attacks, carotid stenosis and an incidental intracranial aneurysm. A decision analysis. Neurosurg 1994;34:449–457
13. Chervu A, Moore WS: Carotid endarterectomy without angiography. Ann Vasc Surg 1994;8:296–302
14. Hill JC, Cabonneau K, Balida PK, et al: Safe extracranial vascular evaluation and surgery without preoperative arteriography. Ann Vasc Surg 1990;77:388–390

15. Chikos PM, Fisher LD, Hirsch JH, Harley DK, Thiele BL, Strandness DE: Observer variability in evaluating extracranial carotid artery stenosis. Stroke 1983;14:885–892
16. Ricotta JJ, Bryan FA, Bond MG, Kurtz A, O'Leary D, Raines JK, Berson AS, Clouse ME: Multicenter validation study of real time (B-mode) ultrasound, arteriography and pathology: J Vasc Surg 1987; 6:512
17. Ricotta JJ, Holen J, Schenk E, et al: Is routine angiography necessary prior to carotid endarterectomy? J Vasc Surg 1984;1(1):96
18. Akers DL, Bell WH, Kerstein MD: Does intracranial dye study contribute to evaluation of carotid artery disease? Am J Surg 1988;156:87–90
19. DeMarco JK, Nesbit GM, Wesbey GE, Richardson D: Prospective evaluation of extracranial carotid stenosis: MR angiography with maximum intensity projections and multiplanar reformations compared with conventional angiography. AJR 1994;163:1205–1212
20. Pan XM, Saloner D, Reilly LM, Bowersox JC, Murray SP, Anderson CM, Gooding GA, Rapp JH: Assessment of carotid artery stenosis by ultrasonography conventional angiography: Correlation with exvivo measurement of plaque stenosis. J Vasc Surg 1995;21:82–89
21. Stock KW, Radue EW, Jacob AL, Bao XS, Steinbrich W: Intracranial arteries: Prospective blinded comparative study of MR angiography and DSA in 50 patients. Radiology 1995;1295:451–456
22. Valton L, Larrue V, Arrue P, Geraud G, Bes A: Asymptomatic cerebral embolic signals in patients with carotid stenosis. Correlation with appearance of plaque ulceration on angiography. Stroke 1995; 26:813–815
23. Siebler M, Kleinschmidt A, Sitzer M, Steinmetz H, Freund HJ: Cerebral microembolism in symptomatic and asymptomatic high grade internal carotid artery stenosis. Neurology 1994;44:615–623
24. Joffe II, Jacobs LE, Lampert C, Kotler MN: Atherosclerotic disease of the aortic arch and the risk of ischemic stroke. N Engl J Med 1995;332:1237–1238
25. Jones EJ, Kalman JM, Calafiore P, Tonkin AM, Donnan GA: Proximal aorta atheroma. An independent risk factor for cerebral ischemia. Stroke 1995;26:218–224
26. Hertzer NR, Young JR, Bevan EG, et al: Coronary angiography in 506 patients with extracranial cerebrovascular disease. Arch Int Med 1985;145:280–288
27. Love BB, Grover-McKay M, Biller J, Rezdik, McKay CR: Coronary artery disease and cardiac events with asymptomatic and symptomatic cerebrovascular disease. Stroke 1992;23:939–945
28. Callow AD, Mackey WC: Long-term follow-up of surgically managed carotid bifurcation atherosclerosis. Ann Surg 1989;210:308–316
29. McCrory DC, Goldstein LB, Samsa GP, Oddone EZ, Landsman PB, Moore WS, Matchar DB: Predicting complications of carotid endarterectomy. Stroke 1993;24:1285–1291
30. Kirshner DL, O'Brien MS, Ricotta JJ: Risk factors in a community experience with carotid endarterectomy. J Vasc Surg 1989;10:178–186
31. Green RM, Messick WJ, Ricotta JJ, et al: Benefits, shortcomings and costs of EEG monitoring. Ann Surg 1985;201:785
32. Riles TS, Imparato AM, Jacobowitz GR, et al: The cause of perioperative stroke after carotid endarterectomy. J Vasc Surg 1994;19:206–214
33. Friedman SG, Tortolani AJ: Reduced length of stay following carotid endarterectomy under general anesthesia. Am J Surg 1995;170:235–236
34. Collier PE: Are one-day admissions for carotid endarterectomy feasible? Am J Surg 1995; 170:140–143
35. O'Brien MS, Ricotta JJ: Conserving resources after carotid endarterectomy, selective use of the intensive care unit. J Vasc Surg 1991;14:796–802
36. Kieburtz K, Ricotta JJ, Moxely RT III: Seizures following carotid endarterectomy. Arch Neur 1990;47:568–570
37. Sbarigia E, Speziale F, Giannoni MF, et al: Post carotid endarterectomy hyperperfusion syndrome: Preliminary observations for identifying at risk patients by transcranial Doppler sonography and acetazolamide test. Eur J Vasc Surg 1993;7:252–256
38. Schroeder T, Sillesen J, Sorensen O, et al: Cerebral hyperperfusion following carotid endarterectomy. J Neurosurg 1987;66:824–829
39. Hoyle RM, Jenkins JM, Edwards WH Sr, Edwards WH Jr, Martin RS III, Mulherin JL. Case management in cerebral revascularization. J Vasc Surg 1994;20:396–402
40. Kraiss LW, Kilberg L, Critch S, Johansen KH: Short-stay carotid endarterectomy is safe and cost effective. Am J Surg 1995;169:512–515

41. Lipsett PA, Tierney S, Gordon TA, Perler BA: Carotid endarterectomy. Is the intensive care unit necessary? J Vasc Surg 1994;20:403–410
42. Zierler RE, Bandyk DF, Thiele BL, Strandness DE. Carotid artery stenosis following endarterectomy. Arch Surg 1982;117:1408–1415
43. Ricotta JJ, O'Brien MS, DeWeese JA: Natural history of recurrent and residual stenosis following carotid endarterectomy: Implications for postoperative surveillance and surgical management. Surgery 1992;112:656
44. Mattos MA, Shamma AR, Rossi N, et al: Is duplex follow-up cost effective in the first year after carotid endarterectomy? Am J Surg 1988;156:91–95
45. Nitzberg RS, Mackey WC, Prendiville E, et al: Long-term follow-up of patients operated on for recurrent carotid stenosis. J Vasc Surg 1991;12:121–127
46. Mackey WD, O'Donnell TF, Jr: The management of recurrent carotid stenosis: Should asymptomatic lesions be treated surgically? J Vasc Surg (in press)
47. Ouriel K, Green RM: Appropriate frequency of carotid duplex testing following carotid endarterectomy. Am J Surg 1995;170:144–147

Management of Extracranial Cerebrovascular Disease, edited by Keith D. Calligaro et al.
Lippincott-Raven Publishers, Philadelphia © 1997.

2

Cerebral Blood Flow Reactivity as an Aid in Carotid Artery Surgery

Marshall W. Webster, Howard Yonas, Michel S. Makaroun

The risk of stroke is high among patients with symptomatic carotid artery occlusive disease (CAOD). In the North American Symptomatic Carotid Endarterectomy Trial (NASCET) there was a cumulative risk of ipsilateral stroke of 26% at 2 years in unoperated patients with ≥70% diameter stenosis who were not operated on but who received best medical therapy.[1] Equally intriguing is that 74% of the patients in NASCET did not suffer a stroke during that time interval and it remains unclear which additional risk factors, other than the degree of stenosis, account for the development of cerebral infarction in any particular patient. The ability to further stratify patients with hemodynamically significant CAOD into very high or low risk groups would be an important clinical advantage.

It has long been recognized that CAOD may produce stroke either on an atheroembolic or ischemic hemodynamic basis, but it is often impossible to determine the etiology once cerebral infarction has occurred. Since the early 1950s there has been a focus on embolic events as the primary explanation for most cerebral ischemic events and surprisingly modest attention has been paid to the effect of CAOD on intracranial hemodynamics in individual patients and the correlation of those hemodynamic consequences with the risk of irreversible cerebral ischemia.[2–4]

The development and validation of stable xenon computed tomography (Xe/CT) cerebral blood flow (CBF) mapping has offered a valuable and easily accessible technique for measuring CBF.[5,6] A hardware and software package for performing Xe/CT CBF mapping is now available for most CT scanners.

Normal mixed cortical CBF (averaged gray and white matter) is approximately 50–55 mL/100 gm of brain tissue/min.[7] This baseline value may be very variable, and may be low due to either decreased supply (obstructed flow) or reduced metabolic demand. Because compromised cerebral arterial inflow is usually associated with maximum vasodilatation (reduction of resistance), the CBF response to a vasodilatory challenge should provide a better assessment of the vascular reserve or *reactivity.* Acetazolamide (ACZ) (Diamox®) induces maximal cerebral vasodilatation secondary to tissue acidosis.[8] The normal response to ACZ infusion is a significant (20–40%) increase in CBF in all vascular territories. Cerebral blood flow may change little in areas of baseline vasodilatation with moderate collateral compromise, or CBF may actually drop in territories that have a severe compromise of collaterals. This drop in CBF represents a true hemodynamic "steal" phenomenon. Although generally well tolerated, ACZ may be contraindicated in patients with cardiovascular instability, renal or hepatic insufficiency, or in patients with a history of allergy to sulfa drugs.

CBF may be measured using the stable Xe/CT CBF technique described by Gur and colleagues.[5] Baseline flow values may be obtained first and the study then repeated after a 20-minute wash-out period, following the intravenous administration of 1 gm ACZ.

Serial CT scanning is performed at two predesignated levels during the cerebral uptake phase of stable Xenon gas, which the patient breathes at a concentration of 33% for 4.5 minutes. Stable (nonradioactive) Xenon gas has an atomic number of 54, is radiodense, lipid soluble, and rapidly and freely diffuses across the blood–brain barrier. Using equations based on the Fick principle, as modified by Kety,[9] CBF is calculated and reported for each voxel (1x1x10 mm) based on the rate of change of CT density and the concurrent arterial curve obtained directly from the end tidal measurement of xenon concentration by thermoconductivity. Contiguous 2-cm diameter circular regions of interest (ROI) are placed around the cortical mantle on each of the two levels on the CT scan. An ROI encompasses approximately 314 voxels. The CBF values for each vascular territory corresponding to the anterior, middle, and posterior cerebral artery distribution are calculated by averaging the 3 to 6 ROIs in each territory on each level. The change in CBF following the administration of ACZ is computed for each of the 12 vascular territories per study. Territories that include more than 50% infarction demonstrated on a CT scan are excluded from analysis.

To further assess whether cerebral reactivity is a discrete risk factor for the development of stroke we have retrospectively reviewed the records of patients with symptomatic CAOD who have undergone Xe/CT CBF mapping, before and after ACZ, at the University of Pittsburgh Medical Center. In compliance with our Institutional Review Board guidelines, the initial individual patient contact and consent was obtained by a mailed request. All patients had symptoms of transient ischemic attacks (TIAs) or moderate nondisabling stroke and either an ipsilateral carotid artery stenosis greater than 70% or complete occlusion of the internal carotid artery confirmed by angiography. Patients were contacted immediately after consent if the CBF study had been completed more than 6 months previously, otherwise they were contacted 6 months following the CBF study. Subsequent follow-up was obtained at 6-month intervals. Patients were excluded because of inadequate follow-up or technically poor studies. Patients who underwent cerebrovascular operations prior to completion of at least 12 months follow-up were also excluded.

We identified 95 patients who were followed at least 12 months or until the onset of a new stroke or cerebrovascular reconstruction more than 12 months following the CBF determination. New strokes were confirmed with a CT scan without contrast enhancement as compared to initial CT studies. Patients who suffered persistent hemispheric neurologic deficits were also classified as having had a new stroke. Of the 95 patients who qualified for the study, 31 patients had ipsilateral carotid stenosis of

≥70%, and 64 patients had total carotid occlusion. Patient follow-up ranged from 0 to 62 months with a mean of 19.6 months.

Patients were stratified into two groups of vascular reactivity based on the CBF response to ACZ. Group I (43 patients) had either an increase in flow or no more than a 5% decrease in any vascular territory following ACZ challenge. Group II (52 patients) had a decrease in CBF of more than 5% in one or more vascular territory following the vasodilatory challenge. The most hemodynamically compromised non-infarcted vascular territory was chosen to determine group classification.

Although the use of a 5% decrease as a breakpoint is somewhat arbitrary, it is based on the recognition that failure to augment after a vasodilatory challenge is an abnormal response. Allowing for a 5% variance in CBF values makes this group of patients (Group II) a clearly physiologically abnormal group.

In this group of 95 patients, 16 developed a documented new stroke during follow-up at a mean of 8 months following CBF measurement. Twelve (75%) of these strokes were ipsilateral to the region of least reactivity.

When stratified based on the reactivity we found that in Group I (normal reactivity) only one of 43 patients (2.3%) developed a new stroke but 15 of 52 patients (28.9%) developed a stroke in Group II ($p = .0005$). In those patients with total carotid occlusion, 10 of 38 (26%) in Group II and none of 26 (0%) in Group I had a new stroke ($p = .003$). In those patients with ≥70% stenosis 5 of 14 (36%) in Group II and only 1 of 17 (6%) in Group I experienced a stroke ($p = .067$). Figure 2-1 depicts the CBF studies in all 95 patients, and illustrates the clustering of new strokes among the patients with poor vascular reactivity. All data points above the identity line represent patients in whom there was good reactivity with flow increases following ACZ challenge and a very low incidence of cerebral infarction.

Groups I and II were similar in age, gender, past history of TIA or stroke and the presence of occlusion or stenosis. Baseline CBF was also similar between Groups I and II, with the response to ACZ the only difference. Fourteen of 16 (87.5%) strokes occurred in patients with a baseline flow of ≥30 cc/100 gm of brain tissue/min (a level within the normal range) and 4 of 16 strokes occurred in patients with >50 cc/100 gm of brain tissue/min.

Age, gender, past history of TIA or stroke and the degree of carotid stenosis were not significantly associated with the occurrence of a new stroke.

Owing to its relatively high metabolic rate and inability to store energy, the brain is critically dependent on adequate CBF to maintain metabolic needs. There are multiple mechanisms for maintaining energy supplies despite severe occlusive disease and these mechanisms include autoregulation and increased oxygen extraction.

The effect of CAOD on global or regional intracranial hemodynamics is variable depending on multiple factors including the patency of communicating arteries.[10] Although embolic events may be a common cause of cerebral infarction, the independent or synergistic effect of compromised hemodynamics on intensifying the associated ischemia is poorly defined.

Currently available methods for assessing cerebral circulation include noninvasive testing, which does yield useful information such as flow velocity in the extracranial

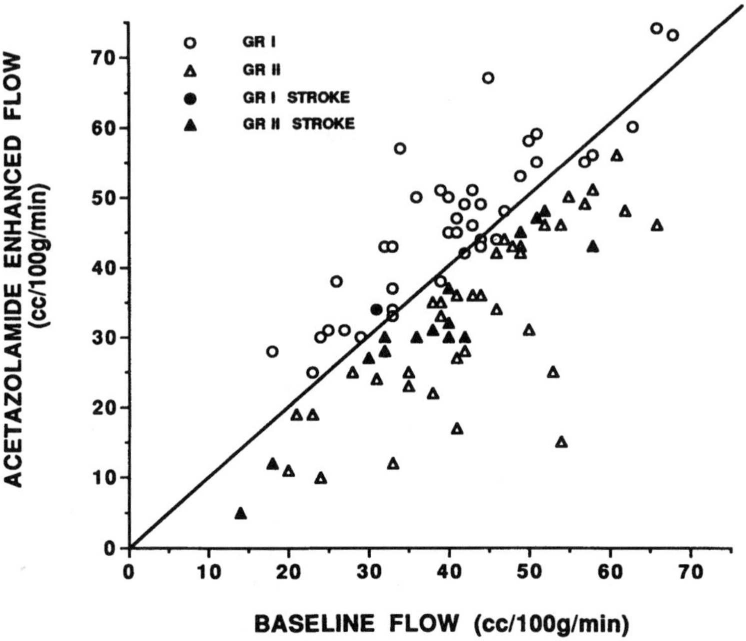

FIG. 2-1. CBF values in cc/100 g/min for each of the 95 patients depicted before and after ACZ challenge in the territory of least reactivity. Points above (to the left) of the line represent patients who had no drop in CBF. Points below (to the right) of the line represent patients with a decrease in CBF in one or more territories. Patients who sustained a stroke are depicted with a closed symbol. Patients who remain asymptomatic are depicted with open symbols.

(Duplex scanning) or intracranial (transcranial Doppler) circulation, and the measurement of ocular blood pressure (oculoplethysmography).[11,12] Angiographically defined anatomic information provides limited direct and indirect physiologic data such as cross-filling, the patency of communicating arteries, and circulation time.

Oculoplethysmography (OPG) may be an indication of compromised cerebral reserves or collateral blood flow. Gee et al[13] compared preoperative and postoperative opthalmobrachial indices in 516 patients with severe carotid stenosis undergoing carotid endarterectomy and found that 39% had limited collateral compensation. When collateral flow was inadequate there was a greater element of compensatory central hypertension. We have compared Xe/CT CBF with OPG pressures and noted that a normal OPG pressure suggests that a given patient is unlikely to have compromised CBF, and in that light it may serve as a screening test.

Positron emission tomography (PET) studies have shown that impaired perfusion pressure leads to vasodilatation and reduced cerebrovascular resistance with an associated increase in cerebral blood volume (CBV). CBF remains normal (PET type I).[7,10] With further compromise, when maximal cerebral blood volume is reached,

CBF becomes pressure dependent and normal metabolism is maintained by increasing the oxygen extraction fraction (PET type II). This group of patients has diminished CBF and depends on the collateral network for oxygen delivery. The response to vasodilatory stimuli is exhausted and some will show a decrease in local CBF, a "steal" phenomenon that has been associated with a dependence on leptomeningeal collaterals.[14,15]

The ability to measure directly CBF and its response to a vasodilatory challenge should offer valuable information regarding the net effect of extracranial and intracranial occlusive disease on regional cerebral vascular beds that have complex and variable collateral circulation and highly developed autoregulatory controls. Stable Xe/CT is easily available, cost effective, reproducible, quantitative, and provides for accurate anatomic correlation. Other modalities of obtaining similar information suffer from providing only qualitative data (SPECT), or poor resolution and no anatomic reference (^{133}Xe/CBF) or from having limited availability and considerable expense (PET). Transcranial Doppler combined with ACZ challenge may prove to be a sensitive method of examining CBF reserves in the future.

During the past decade stable Xe/CT CBF mapping has been performed on more than 9,000 patients in our hospital, including studies for many clinical diagnoses other than cerebrovascular disease. Substantial clinical experience has demonstrated that the majority of patients with cerebrovascular disease have normal baseline CBF and normal reserves or reactivity. Currently the request for CBF mapping in any specific patient is a clinical decision made by the attending physician and is usually reserved for those patients in whom CBF is likely to be abnormal based on our past experience. This accounts, in part, for the relatively high number of abnormal (Group II) patients in our retrospective review. We do not believe that this random selection of patients for analysis influences the basic finding that those patients who have reduced reactivity are at substantial risk for stroke. Cerebral blood flow is most likely to be compromised in patients with multiple extracranial arterial occluded or stenotic segments as determined by non-invasive testing such as carotid duplex scanning or transcranial Doppler evaluation. Angiographic patterns of occlusion including absent communicating arteries may suggest a relatively isolated vascular territory or hemisphere. Smith et al[16] have recently correlated Xe/CT CBF and collateral flow patterns. As noted, a substantial discrepancy in ocular blood pressure may suggest inadequate collateral blood flow.

The decision to stratify patients into two groups on the basis of no less than a 5% decrease in flow following vasodilatory challenge is arbitrary. In a previous report of the first 68 patients, we used a different grouping system that also took into consideration the baseline CBF.[17] With more patients and longer follow-up, several new strokes have appeared in patients with normal baseline values for CBF, highlighting the predictive value of ACZ response as a single indicator. Thus the stratification was modified for but remains artificial. While Group I contains all the patients with a normal response of flow augmentation in all territories, it also includes patients with mildly abnormal reactivity. Group II patients clearly represent the most severely compromised but are heterogeneous with some having more than one territory with over

5% reduction in CBF following ACZ. This explains why some of the strokes were not in the index territory, but ipsilateral in adjacent areas. The only stroke in Group I was in the contralateral hemisphere, suggesting further that it was not hemodynamic in nature. Our analysis is still evolving and we hope to refine the classification with further experience to better define risk groups.

A highly predictive classification system based on vascular reactivity could become very important in selecting patients for revascularization in some controversial areas, such as patients with asymptomatic carotid stenosis or those who may benefit from extracranial–intracranial (EC–IC) bypass for total internal carotid occlusion. The EC–IC bypass study, which found no advantage to cerebral revascularization, was conducted without evaluation or stratification based upon any assessment of CBF status.[17]

Other means of stratifying patients for the relative risk of stroke are potentially important. These include rheologic factors such as viscosity (hematocrit, fibrinogen levels) and systemic blood pressure and cardiac arrhythmias. These potential stratifiers could be included in decision making in the future. We do not mean to imply that patients with symptoms who have >70% carotid stenosis, normal CBF, and a normal response to vasodilatation challenge should not undergo carotid endarterectomy. Our current understanding of cerebrovascular disease would suggest that thromboembolic complications of carotid stenosis may occur in the absence of preexisting CBF abnormality.

Our conclusion is that patients with symptomatic CAOD who have significantly compromised CBF vasoreactivity, even with normal baseline CBF, are at substantial risk for stroke. Compromised CBF reserves are an important determinant of ischemic infarction, probably regardless of whether the final event is precipitated by embolic or hemodynamic factors. New strategies for stroke prevention may include less aggressive management of hypertension and more aggressive cerebral revascularization in selected patients.

Further information is clearly needed regarding the causation of stroke. We believe that the mere presence of single or multiple vessel occlusive disease is an inadequate indicator alone of the risk of stroke.[19] A greater understanding of the many factors which may ultimately influence the natural history of cerebrovascular disease is necessary to reduce the incidence of stroke but at the same time reduce the morbidity and mortality of potentially unnecessary interventions.

REFERENCES

1. North American Symptomatic Carotid Endarterectomy Trial (NASCET). Beneficial effect of carotid endarterectomy in symptomatic patients with high grade carotid stenosis. N Engl J Med 1991;325:445–453
2. Kleiser B, Widder B. Course of carotid artery occlusion with impaired cerebrovascular reactivity. Stroke 1992;23:171–174
3. Rogers RL, Meyer JS, Mortel KF. Additional predisposing risk factors for atherothrombotic cerebrovascular disease among treated hypertensive volunteers. Stroke 1987;18:335–341
4. Norris JW, Krajewski A, Bornstein NM. The clinical role of the cerebral collateral circulation in carotid occlusion. J Vasc Surg 1990;12:113–118

5. Gur D, Good WF, Wolfson SK Jr, Yonas H, Shabason L. In vivo mapping of local cerebral blood flow by xenon-enhanced computed tomography. Science 1982;215:1267–1268
6. Yonas H, Darby JM, Marks EC, Durham SR, Maxwell C. CBF measured by Xe-CT: approach to analysis and normal values. J Cereb Blood Flow Metab 1991;11:716–725
7. Powers WJ, Grubb RL Jr, Raichle ME. Clinical results of extracranial–intracranial bypass surgery in patients with hemodynamic cerebrovascular disease. J Neurosurg 1989;70:61–67
8. Vortsrup S. Tomographic cerebral blood flow measurements in patients with ischemic cerebrovascular disease and evaluation of the vasodilatory capacity by the acetazolamide test. Acta Neur Scand 1988;77(114):5–48
9. Kety SS. Theory and applications of the exchange of inert gas at the lungs and tissues. Pharmacol Rev 1951;3:1–41
10. Powers WJ, Press GA, Grubb RL, Jr. The effect of hemodynamically significant carotid artery disease on the hemodynamic status of the cerebral circulation. Ann Intern Med 1987;106:27–34
11. Ringelstein EB, Sievers C, Ecker S, et al. Noninvasive assessment of CO_2-induced cerebral vasomotor response in normal individuals and patients with internal carotid artery occlusions. Stroke 1988; 19:963–969
12. Schneider PA, Rossman ME, Bernstein EF, Ringelstein EB, Otis SM. Noninvasive assessment of cerebral collateral blood supply through the opthalmic artery. Stroke 1991;2:31–36
13. Gee W, Lucke JF, Madden AE. Collateral compensation of severe carotid stenosis. Eur J Vasc Surg 1989;3:297–301
14. Kanno I, Uemura K, Higano S, et al. Oxygen extraction fraction at maximally vasodilated tissue in the ischemic brain estimated from the regional CO_2 responsiveness measured by positron emission tomography. J Cereb Blood Flow Metab 1988;8:227–235
15. Vorstrup S, Brun B, Lassen NA. Evaluation of the cerebral vasodilatory capacity by the acetazolamide test before EC–IC bypass surgery in patients with occlusion of the internal carotid artery. Stroke 1986;17:1291–1298
16. Smith HA, Thompson-Dobkin J, Yonas H, Flint E. Correlation of xenon-enhanced computed tomography-defined cerebral blood flow reactivity and collateral flow patterns. Stroke 1994;25:1784–1787
17. Yonas H, Smith HA, Durham SR, Pentheny SL, Johnson DW. Increased stroke risk predicted by compromised cerebral blood flow reactivity. J Neurosurg 1993;79:483–489
18. EC/IC Bypass Study Group. Failure of extracranial–intracranial arterial bypass to reduce the risk of ischemic stroke: results of an international randomized trial. N Engl J Med 1985;313:1191–1200
19. Webster MW, Makaroun MS, Steed DL, Smith HA, Johnson DW, Yonas H. Compromised cerebral blood flow reactivity is a predictor of stroke in patients with symptomatic carotid artery occlusive disease. J Vasc Surg 1995;21:338–345

Management of Extracranial Cerebrovascular Disease, edited by Keith D. Calligaro et al.
Lippincott-Raven Publishers, Philadelphia © 1997.

3

Can Carotid Surgery Be Performed Safely Without Preoperative Arteriography?

D. Eugene Strandness, Jr.

Several innovative changes in the evaluation of carotid artery disease comprise the subject of this chapter. Arteriography is the principal and time-tested method of evaluating patients prior to any form of intervention. It provides not only anatomic information for the surgeon but also an element of intellectual comfort that is difficult to quantify. We were all trained to examine the images obtained by this method and from that information develop treatment plans for the patient. How has this changed and why?

The trend in questioning the role of arteriography began with the introduction of noninvasive methods to evaluate vascular disease. We began to realize that the functional information was in many cases more important than the anatomic data in deciding a course of action. The first change that took place without a murmur of dissent was eliminating arteriography as a diagnostic method of choice except in special circumstances; arteriography could be reserved for those cases in which intervention was planned. Arteriography of extra- and intracranial circulation was performed to obtain specific information, summarized as follows:

Are there lesions at the level of the aortic arch?
Is there disease in the carotid bulb?
What is the degree of stenosis?
What is the length of the lesion? Is there ulceration?
Is there disease in the carotid siphon?
Is there intracranial disease that may compromise outcome?
What is the status of the collateral circulation? Is there cross filling? What is the source of the collateral blood supply?

This is an impressive list given the fact that only "complete" arteriographic studies can provide all of this information. Having been trained in an environment that emphasized this approach makes it difficult to even question the option of using an alternative method prior to intervention. This would require further data and the development of methods that would provide the essential information. There can be little doubt that it was the development of ultrasonic duplex scanning that began to change many of our ideas in this area.[1–4] The field has matured enough that we can began to ask the questions that could never have been raised in the past.

The extracranial circulation is unique in that, usually, a single operation can be used to treat the vast majority of patients with atherosclerosis. This is, of course, carotid endarterectomy, which now has become accepted as the treatment of choice for patients with specific presenting complaints and degrees of stenosis.[5–8] The other very important fact to keep in mind is that when disease is found in the carotid bulb, it is usually well localized to this region. While there can be exceptions to this, the operation is designed to remove the atheroma from the bulb, restoring cerebral blood flow to normal levels.

REQUIREMENTS FOR ELIMINATING ARTERIOGRAPHY

Before considering the details of preoperative testing, it *must be shown* that performing a carotid endarterectomy without a preoperative arteriogram does not result in greater morbidity and mortality. The acceptable rates of complications would appear to have been established for both symptomatic and asymptomatic patients. In the North American Symptomatic Carotid Endarterectomy Trial (NASCET), the combined morbidity and mortality rate was 5%.[5] In the Asymptomatic Carotid Artery Surgery Trial (ACAS), it was 2.1%.[8] Since these will undoubtedly be accepted as the gold standard, they must be matched if we are to propose an alternative approach to the preoperative work-up of these patients.

What information can be obtained by duplex scanning alone or in conjunction with transcranial Doppler testing (TCD)?[4,9–13]

The carotid bulb can be examined in detail; the location and extent of the atheroma can be ascertained

It is possible to examine the flow patterns low in the common carotid artery to detect lesions at the level of the aortic arch

Lesions in the siphon can be suspected by the flow patterns in the distal internal carotid at the time of duplex scanning. If flow goes to zero at end-diastole, there has to be either a distal occlusion or very high-grade stenosis present

TCD can be used to verify the presence of lesions in the siphon

TCD has also been shown to be helpful for the detection of high-grade lesions in the middle cerebral artery

The intracranial collateral pathways can be studied in detail by the use of TCD

Siphon lesions can be seen even in neonates. When found at this time in life they appear to be intimal cushions. To what extent they persist into adult life is unknown. If the lesions seen in adults are truly secondary to atherosclerosis, they have the smooth arteriographic appearance of fibrous plaques, which are not the source of emboli unless they degenerate to become a complicated lesion. The clinical studies that have been done of the role of the carotid siphon lesions have concluded that they do not contribute to the outcome of patients with carotid bifurcation disease.[14] There is a rare exception when the siphon lesions are so tight that they impair delivery of blood to that hemisphere.

Given the above, it may be concluded that both duplex scanning and TCD are needed before proceeding with endarterectomy. This is not yet the case, since the role of TCD has not yet been completely defined and most of the information currently obtained is rarely of value in decision making. This is not because TCD is not accurate. The problem is that TCD findings have not been useful in deciding when a carotid endarterectomy should or should not be done. For example, middle cerebral artery lesions are not common. If a middle cerebral artery stenosis were found in the presence of a high-grade stenosis of the internal carotid artery, it would still be necessary to repair the carotid artery. This would eliminate the risk of either further embolization or thrombosis with total occlusion of the internal carotid artery. The stroke rate with occlusion of the internal carotid artery is in the range of 25% with an additional 15% sustaining a transient ischemic attack with the occlusion.[15,16]

What about magnetic resonance arteriography (MRA)? This new and innovative method is currently being tested and can in some instances provide useful confirmation of the ultrasound findings.[17–19] However, problems do remain and include signal drop-out in areas of high-grade stenosis, making it difficult to grade the degree of narrowing. In addition, we have found that somewhere between 10 and 20% of our patients are unable to enter the magnet due to claustrophobia. While preliminary sedation might reduce this number, this would complicate the procedure and in many cases delay its performance.

IMPACT OF CLINICAL TRIALS

There is little doubt that the four large clinical trials will have an impact on the role of carotid surgery, but they have also resulted in severe confusion as to which categories of stenosis are significant clinically. In addition, the methods of evaluating the extent of carotid stenosis will have to be modified. The results of these trials can be summarized as follows:

1. The VA asymptomatic trial found that a >50% diameter reducing stenosis should be treated surgically[7]
2. The NASCET study in symptomatic patients found a >70% stenosis was best treated by endarterectomy[5]
3. The ECST reached similar conclusions to NASCET, but the method of arteriographic measurement was different[6]
4. The ACAS study found a significant reduction in stroke events in those patients with a >60% diameter, reducing lesion of the internal carotid artery for those in the surgical arm of the trial[8]

While on the surface these trials have provided ready answers to many clinical questions, they have also raised new questions from a diagnostic standpoint. NASCET and ECST used entirely different methods of measuring the degree of stenosis. In NASCET, the internal carotid artery distal to the bulb was the "normal" reference artery. In ECST, all of the measurements were made from the bulb itself. This means that a 50% diameter reduction in a patient in the ECST would be a 0% stenosis in NASCET! While the differences tend to decrease with the higher degree of stenosis, a problem does exist that must be taken into account.

To make things even more confusing, the ACAS trial found a 60% cut-off point for surgery, while the VA asymptomatic trial found that a 50% diameter reduction was significant.[7,8] In ACAS, the cut-off point of 60% was apparently decided upon prior to the trial, each center being required to develop a "machine specific" cut-off point for a 60% diameter reduction. In this trial, a wide variety of machines were used, many of which were obsolete at the time the trial was being conducted. The arteriographic method of assessment in ACAS and the VA trials was similar to the method used in NASCET.

SOLUTIONS TO THE DIAGNOSTIC DILEMMA

There are several solutions to the problems posed by the differing degrees of stenosis used or arrived at in the clinical trials. Each could develop their own endpoints for each degree of narrowing. This would be time consuming and not in the reach of most laboratories. Our own solution to this problem is to continue to use our standard study methods and categories of disease but utilize the velocity data already being obtained to set cut-off points that would identify the lesions of interest.

Over the years we have developed the following categories of disease that we have compared to arteriography:[9]

Normal-boundary layer separation in the carotid bulb with no disease seen on B-mode imaging

1–15% stenosis. This was distinguished by minimal spectral broadening alone during diastole. We now combine this category with the normals since this is not always easy to recognize and is highly dependent on examination method and interpretation

16–49% stenosis. Disease is seen in the bulb but is not sufficient to increase the peak systolic velocity above 125 cm/sec. There is also associated spectral broadening seen during the entire pulse cycle

50–79% stenosis. The peak systolic velocity is >125 cm/sec with an end-diastolic velocity <140 cm/sec. There is associated spectral broadening

80–99% stenosis. In this case, the end-diastolic velocity is >140 cm/sec as before occlusion. There is no detectable flow in the internal carotid artery

It can be seen that this categorization is of use for only the 50% cut-off point arrived at in the VA asymptomatic trial. If we are to use the cut-off points of >70% for symptomatic patients (NASCET) and 60% for asymptomatic patients (ACAS), we will have to modify our study or develop new algorithms for these degrees of narrowing. We have conducted two studies in conjunction with the Oregon group to satisfy these requirements.[20,21]

A total of 353 patent internal carotid arteries were in the study. All of the patients in the study had arteriography performed within 30 days of the ultrasonic duplex scan. There was one internal carotid artery that could not insonated secondary to heavy calcification leaving 352 arteries for comparison. The data were from four vascular laboratories. Three from the University of Oregon system and one from the University of Washington. The studies were done with both an Acuson 128 and an ATL Ultramark 9 duplex scanners. All studies were done with an angle of 60 degrees to the long axis of the artery. The data collected included the peak systolic and end-diastolic velocities from the common carotid artery and at the site of greatest narrowing in the bulb. The arteriograms were by either intraarterial digital subtraction or conventional cut-film methods with at least two views of the bulb. The diameter of the residual lumen at the site of narrowing and the diameter of the distal internal carotid artery was measured using 2.5X loop magnification and engineering calipers. A single examiner made the measurements. He was blinded to the results of the duplex scan results.

To assess the best cut-off points for both 60 and 70% diameter reducing stenoses, receiver operator curves were generated for peak systolic velocities and end-diastolic velocities. From this sensitivity, specificity, positive predictive value, negative predictive value and overall accuracy were calculated.

For the 70–99% stenosis category, a peak systolic velocity at the site of narrowing divided by the peak systolic velocity in the common carotid of >4.0 gave a sensitivity of 90%, a specificity of 90%, a positive predictive value of 86%, a negative predictive value of 94% with an overall accuracy of 90%.[20] For the >60% diameter reducing lesions, a similar ratio was calculated to provide the optimal cut-off point for detecting this endpoint. For this algorithm, it is possible to use either the peak systolic velocity and end-diastolic velocity values at the site of narrowing or the ratio as described in (1). A peak systolic velocity of 260 cm/sec and an end-diastolic velocity of 70 cm/sec or greater predicted the presence of a >60% diameter reducing lesion with a sensitivity of 84%, specificity of 94%, a positive predictive value of 92%, a negative predictive value of 88% and an overall accuracy of 90%. Similar results can be obtained using the peak systolic velocity at the site of the stenosis divided by that from the common carotid artery. For a ratio of 3.2:3.5 similar results[21] will be obtained.

DISCUSSION

While much of the debate over the role of carotid endarterectomy has been settled, new disputes are bound to arise over the diagnostic screening methods that will be used and how patients will be selected for operation. While there may be some disagreement, it is clear to this author that arteriography cannot and must not be used as a screening test for either the symptomatic or asymptomatic patients. It is simply too costly and too dangerous to be used in this manner.[19,22] One of the unfortunate aspects of the NASCET study was their conclusion that ultrasound was not accurate enough to be used to screen patients who might be candidates for operation. This view must not be accepted for the several reasons. Much of the information that follows was derived from my serving on the Data Monitoring Committee (DMC) for NASCET. Since I have written about this experience, I feel that it is appropriate to review this in some detail.

The NASCET protocol included a baseline ultrasound study and follow-up studies at regular intervals. There was to be quality control of the ultrasound studies but this was never followed through by the NASCET investigators. The DMC was assured that information on the quality-control issue would be provided but this was not the case. We never received such information. In fact we found out during the course of the study that they had made no attempt to conduct a serious quality control program. The DMC did not meet for a total period of 30 months so we did not have an opportunity to review any of the results in that time interval.

In spite of this, NASCET chose and continues to maintain that ultrasound is not a suitable screening test.[23] The implications of this stand are horrendous. Before considering these, we must answer the question of the accuracy of ultrasound screening for the detection and assessment of carotid artery disease. Our own studies, which went through four phases, compared standard cut-film studies of three views of the bulb against duplex scanning. In conjunction with the Oregon group we have developed algorithms that can be used to classify those degrees of narrowing that are of clinical relevance. However, these studies and results were obtained by laboratories that were experienced with the methods. What about ultrasound in general in this country and Canada?

It must be kept in mind that since its introduction, duplex scanning has undergone numerous technological improvements and innovations that were not available when the clinical trials were initiated. The variety of methods that NASCET and ACAS used involved diverse and, in some cases, obsolete equipment. ACAS attempted to get around this issue by making each center develop "machine-specific" criteria for the detection of a >60% diameter reducing stenosis.

If we are to use duplex scanning for both screening and prior to carotid endarterectomy, we must be certain that our laboratories are sufficiently competent and accurate to warrant such an approach. A major step in this direction was the establishment of the Intersocietal Commission for the Voluntary Accreditation of Vascular Laboratories (ISCVAL). This independent group sponsored by all of the major medical societies in this country is an important step in ensuring that standards have been established for laboratories. This process, which is exhaustive, is an important step in ensuring that testing for carotid bifurcation disease can be as accurate as possible.

What about the issue of no preoperative arteriography? I believe that this is feasible but very dependent upon the laboratory, its experience and accuracy in predicting the degree of stenosis. All of the current evidence suggests that the approach will not lead to an increase in neurological complications and will provide a large saving in costs and complications related to arteriography.[24–28] In considering this approach, it is also important to take into account the variability associated with the interpretation of carotid arteriograms. We examined this issue in 1983 and while the variability (intra- and interobserver) varies depending upon the degree of disease, it is reasonable to expect that any estimate for the range of lesions of surgical interest is in the range of ±20%.[29]

One may assume that the discussion can end with everyone agreeing on some of the basic points relating to the role of arteriography and ultrasound as screening methods. However, the arguments continue, now concerning how to measure the degree of stenosis by arteriography. NASCET, VAH, and ACAS studies used the distal internal carotid artery as the reference vessel. However, the ECST used the carotid bulb. This has led to considerable debate because with the NASCET method it is possible to have a negative degree of stenosis for those lesions in the bulb that do not extend beyond the limits of the bulb. Thus, a 50% diameter reducing stenosis by the ECST method would be a 0% stenosis according to NASCET.

The argument continues with recent studies from European and NASCET investigators.[30–32] European investigators now recommend using the common carotid artery as the reference artery, while NASCET investigators continue to defend their method. Even the clinical trial enthusiasts cannot agree on the best method. It is remarkable that they concentrate more on the details of each method than on the variability associated with any single measurement.

Usually, a 50% diameter reducing stenosis is not considered to be a precise measurement by arteriography. It could actually be greater or less than that, depending on several factors that may be impossible to determine from the study itself. Most surgeons feel that the degree-of-stenosis measurement is only an estimate—patient presentation plays a very important role in decision making. For example, I consider a 50% diameter reducing lesion in a symptomatic patient warrants serious consideration for operation. On the other hand, a similar degree of narrowing in an asymptomatic patient may dictate a conservative course. It is clear that this debate will rage on while ultrasound will continue to be used as the screening method and, in selected cases, the only study prior to endarterectomy.

REFERENCES

1. Strandness DE, Jr: Duplex Scanning in Vascular Disorders (2nd ed.). New York: Raven Press, 1993
2. Barber FE, Baker DW, Nation AWC, et al. Ultrasonic duplex echo Doppler scanner. IEEE Trans Biomed Eng 1974;21:109–113
3. Barber FE, Baker DW, Strandness DE, Jr. Duplex scanner II for simultaneous imaging of artery tissues and flow. Ultrasonics Symposium Proc IEEE 1974;74CH0896-ISU
4. Langlois YE, Roederer GO, Chan ATW, Phillips DJ, Beach KW, Martin D, Chikos PW, Strandness DE, Jr. Evaluating carotid artery disease: the concordance between pulsed Doppler/spectrum analysis and angiography. Ultrasound Med Biol 1983;9:51–63
5. North American Symptomatic Carotid Endarterectomy Trial. Beneficial effect of carotid endarterectomy in symptomatic patients with high-grade carotid stenosis. N Engl J Med 1991;325:445–463
6. European carotid surgery trialists' collaborative group. MRC European carotid surgery trial. Interim results for symptomatic patients with severe (70–99%) or with mild (0–29%) stenosis. Lancet 1991; 337:1235–1243
7. Hobson RW, Weiss DG, Fields WS, et al. Efficacy of carotid endarterectomy for asymptomatic carotid stenosis. N Engl J Med 1993;328:221–227
8. Clinical Advisory. Carotid endarterectomy for patients with asymptomatic carotid artery stenosis. Stroke 1994;25:2523–2524

9. Strandness DE, Jr. Extracranial arterial disease. In Strandness DE, Jr (ed). Duplex scanning in vascular disorders. New York, Raven Press, 1993:113–157
10. Schregel W. Relevance of transcranial Doppler sonography. Infusionsther Transfusionsmed 1993; 20:267–271
11. Röther J, Schwartz A, Wentz KU, Rautenberg W, Hennerici M. Middle cerebral artery stenoses: Assessment by magnetic resonance angiography and transcranial Doppler ultrasound. Cerebrovasc Dis 1994;4:273–279
12. Giller CA, Mathews D, Walker B, Purdy P, Roseland AM. Prediction of tolerance to carotid artery occlusion using transcranial Doppler ultrasound. J Neurosurg 1994;81:15–19
13. Becker G, Lindner A, Hofmann E, Bogdahn U. Contribution of transcranial color-coded real-time sonography to the etiopathogenetic classification of middle cerebral artery stenosis. J Clin Ultrasound 1994;22:471–477
14. Roederer GO, Langlois YE, Chan RTW, Chikos PM, Strandness DE, Jr. Is siphon disease important in predicting the outcome of carotid endarterectomy? Arch Surg 1983;118:1177–1181
15. Nicholls SC, Kohler TR, Bergelin RO, Primozich JF, Lawrence RL, Strandness DE, Jr. Carotid artery occlusion, natural history. J Vasc Surg 1986;4:479–485
16. Nicholls SC, Bergelin RO, Strandness DE, Jr. Neurological sequelae of unilateral carotid occlusion, immediate and late. J Vasc Surg 1989;10:542–548
17. Turnipseed WD, Kennell TW, Turski PA, Acher CW, Hoch JR. Magnetic resonance angiography and duplex imaging: Noninvasive tests for selecting symptomatic carotid endarterectomy candidates. Surgery 1993;114:643–649
18. Mittl RL, Jr., Broderick M, Carpenter JP, Goldberg HI, Listerud J, Mishkin MM, Berkowitz HD, Atlas SW. Blinded-reader comparison of magnetic resonance angiography and duplex ultrasonography for carotid artery bifurcation stenosis. Stroke 1994;25:4–10
19. Riles TS, Eidelman EM, Litt AW, Pinto RS, Olford F, Thoe Schwartzenberg GWS. Comparison of magnetic resonance arteriography, conventional arteriography and duplex scanning. Stroke 1992; 23:333–341
20. Moneta GL, Edwards JM, Chitwood RW, Taylor LM, Lee RW, Cummings CA, Porter JM. Correlation of North American Symptomatic Carotid Endarterectomy Trial (NASCET) angiographic definition of 70% to 99% internal carotid artery stenosis with duplex scanning. J Vasc Surg 1993;17:152–160
21. Edwards JM, Moneta GL, Papanicolaou G, Hatsukami T, Strandness DE, Jr, Porter JM. Duplex ultrasound criteria for determining ≥50% and ≥60% internal carotid stenosis: implications for screening examinations. J Vasc Surg 1994 (submitted)
22. Davies KN, Humphrey PR. Complications of cerebral angiography in patients with symptomatic carotid territory ischaemia screened by carotid ultrasound. J Neurol Neurosurg Psychiatry 1993;56:967–972
23. Haynes RB, Taylor DW, Sackett DL, Fox A, Barnett HJM. Poor performance of Doppler detecting high-grade carotid stenosis. Clin Res 1992;40:184A(abstract)
24. Dawson DL, Zierler RE, Kohler TR. Role of arteriography in the preoperative evaluation of carotid artery disease. Am J Surg 1991;161:619–624
25. Moore WS, Ziomek S, Quinones-Baldrich WJ, Machleder HI, Bussuttil RW, Baker EW. Can clinical evaluation and noninvasive testing substitute for arteriography in the evaluation of carotid artery disease? Ann Surg 1988;208:91–94
26. Ricotta JJ, Holen J, Schenk E, et al. Is routine arteriography necessary prior to carotid endarterectomy? J Vasc Surg 1984;1:96–102
27. Dawson DL, Zierler RE, Strandness DE, Jr, Clowes AW, Kohler TR. The role of duplex scanning and arteriography before carotid endarterectomy: A prospective study. J Vasc Surg 1993;18:673–683
28. Cartier R, Cartier P, Fontaine A. Carotid endarterectomy without angiography. The reliability of Doppler ultrasonography and duplex assessment in preoperative assessment. Can J Surg 1993; 36:411–416
29. Chikos PM, Fisher LD, Hirsch JH, Harley JD, Thiele BL, Strandness DE, Jr. Observer variability in evaluating extracranial arterial stenosis. Stroke 1983;14:885–892
30. Rothwell PM, Gibson RJ, Slattery J, Sellar RJ, Warlow CP. Equivalence of measurements of carotid stenosis: A comparison of three methods on 1001 angiograms. Stroke 1994;25:2435–2439
31. Rothwell PM, Gibson RJ, Slattery J, Warlow CP. Prognostic value and reproducibility of measurements of carotid stenosis: a comparison of three methods in 1001 angiograms. Stroke 1994; 25:2440–2444
32. Eliasziw M, Smith RF, Singh N, Holdsworth DW, Fox AJ, Barnett HJM. Further comments on the measurement of carotid stenosis from angiograms. Stroke 1994;25:2445–2449

Management of Extracranial Cerebrovascular Disease, edited by Keith D. Calligaro et al. Lippincott-Raven Publishers, Philadelphia © 1997.

4

Effectiveness of Antiplatelet Agents for Carotid Artery Disease

Kenneth Ouriel, Richard M. Green

When commencing the study of carotid artery disease, novices generally assume that cerebrovascular events occur as the result of the hemodynamic consequence of a severe carotid stenosis. Given the pathophysiology of cardiac and lower-extremity ischemic symptoms, one would naturally assume that the mechanisms underlying cerebrovascular symptoms are analagous. In fact, flow limitation at the carotid bifurcation was thought to be the etiologic mechanism of stroke well into the midportion of the twentieth century.[1] While this mechanism may play a role in a small number of cases, the vast majority of cerebral infarctions occur as a result of platelet–fibrin formation on atheromatous arterial lesions, leading to distal embolization.[2] In 1950, C. Miller Fisher and Raymond D. Adams examined the brains and cerebral vasculature of 373 patients who died of cerebral infarction.[3] Fisher and Adams concluded that nearly all of the cases were of embolic origin and that the premorbid transient clinical events in some of these patients may have occurred as a result of the temporary arrest of small emboli in medium-sized cerebral arterioles.

Thus, medical management of cerebrovascular disease must, of necessity, address the problem of platelet deposition on the irregular surface of an atherosclerotic plaque. Fortunately, cerebral infarction is preceded by transient ischemic attack or amaurosis fugax in many cases.[2,4] These heralding symptoms provide the opportunity to address the thromboembolic problem prior to the development of a devastating loss of cerebral or ophthalmic function. Antiplatelet agents have been effectively employed in this setting to decrease the complications associated with cerebrovascular thromboembolic disease.

PHYSIOLOGY OF PLATELET DEPOSITION

Healthy arteries maintain a smooth, nonthrombogenic luminal endothelial lining. The presence of an atherosclerotic plaque significantly affects the luminal surface, with elongation and cobblestoning of the endothelial cells.[5] Paradoxically, areas of frank endothelial denudation are infrequent overlying an atherosclerotic plaque, but adherence of activated leukocytes and platelets to the abnormally elongated endothelial cells is commonly observed. When plaque rupture does occur, platelet–

fibrin deposition proceeds rapidly. Platelets adhere to the damaged arterial surface, primarily as a result of the exposure of such subendothelial substrates as collagen types I and II, diabetic collagen, tissue thromboplastin, and subendothelial von Willebrand factor. Like atherogenesis, a prime determinant of platelet deposition is shear rate.[6] Shear rate is proportional to the velocity of blood flow, and inversely proportional to the third power of the lumen radius. In contrast to atherogenesis, where plaque formation develops in areas of low shear rate,[7] thrombogenesis and platelet deposition develops in areas of high shear rate.[8]

Platelet deposition can be conceptually divided into three somewhat interrelated processes; platelet adherence, platelet activation, and platelet cohesion. To understand these mechanisms, one must first understand the cell biology of the platelet. Simplified, the platelet may be envisioned as a membrane-bound cytoplasmic remnant. The nucleus and other elements of the protein-manufacturing apparatus are absent. Nevertheless, the platelet membrane is a complex structure containing a wide variety of membrane glycoprotein receptors.[9] These receptors bind to a variety of ligands, including fibrinogen, von Willebrand factor, collagen, fibronectin, and vitronectin.[10,11] Glycoprotein Ia binds collagen under conditions of low shear rate. Glycoprotein Ib binds to von Willebrand factor, especially under conditions of high shear rate.[12] Glycoprotein IIb/IIIa binds to a variety of ligands, fibrinogen, and von Willebrand factor and is unique in its ability to bind to many different ligands.[13] This property is explained by the presence of a binding site for the tripeptide arginine-glycine-aspartate, or "RGD" in the commonly employed single letter peptide sequence abbreviation scheme.[14] Glycoprotein IIb/IIIa is the most populous platelet membrane receptor, with as many as 50,000 molecules present on a single stimulated platelet.[15] Through its RDG site, fibrinogen may bind to the glycoprotein IIb/IIIa receptors of two platelets, forming a bridge between them. As this process is repeated between countless platelets and fibrinogen molecules, a platelet–fibrinogen matrix is formed, initiating the process of platelet aggregation. It is important to note that fibrinogen is the ligand with the highest concentration in the blood. Other ligands, such as von Willebrand factor, however, may substitute for fibrinogen in the formation of a platelet plug.[16] Von Willebrand factor may actually be the most important ligand under conditions of high shear rate and in patients with congenital afibrinogenemia.[17]

Once the platelet membrane receptors bind to a ligand, the process of platelet activation is initiated.[18] Calcium is discharged from the dense tubular system by the action of phospholipase on platelet membrane phosphatidylinositol. Cytoplasmic calcium levels rise and the rise in calcium acts in concert with calmodulin to activate the light chain of myosin, initiating the actin–myosin interaction and contraction of the platelet. The platelet no longer appears discoid; rather, it assumes an ameboid shape with numerous pseudopodia projecting outward.

Increased cytoplasmic calcium simultaneously stimulates arachidonic acid release from the membrane.[19] Through the catalytic actions of cyclooxygenase, the cyclic endoperoxides prostaglandin intermediaries G_2 and H_2 are generated.[20] Thromboxane synthetase converts these intermediaries to thromboxane A_2, which is released and binds to new platelet membrane receptors, amplifying the process of platelet activation through a positive feedback mechanism. The "platelet release reaction" occurs as the platelet is stimulated and releases the contents of its four types of granules (Table 4-1). Many of the compounds present in the granules are themselves potent platelet stimulators, including serotonin and adenosine diphosphate. The release of these compounds further potentiates the positive feedback loop associated with platelet activation and deposition.

Thrombin, through its attachment to a specific platelet membrane G-protein, may be the most potent platelet stimulator known.[21,22] Activation of the putative thrombin receptor causes the rapid release of calcium from the dense tubules and initiates the process of platelet activation and the release reaction. This property of thrombin accounts for the close association between coagulation (thrombin generation) and platelet deposition. This mechanism also explains the little appreciated but very powerful antiplatelet activity of heparin, mediated through its inhibition of thrombin generation.

The process of platelet–fibrin thrombus formation is now easily understood, given the principles of platelet physiology. The first step in this process is the appearance of a thrombogenic focus on the arterial luminal surface, usually from a fissure or ulceration at the site of an atherosclerotic plaque. Collagen and other subendothelial ligands are exposed to the flowing blood, and platelet membrane receptors specific for these ligands cause platelets to be deposited along the area of endothelial denudation. A carpet composed of a platelet monolayer forms rapidly, and each platelet becomes activated through the release reaction, with platelet spreading and exposure of additional membrane receptors. Fibrinogen, von Willebrand factor, and other ligands attach to the activated platelets. As new platelets attach to the spoke-like projections of the ligands, the ligands act as bridges between adjacent platelets, and the process of platelet aggregation (cohesion) is initiated.

Hemodynamic conditions and the strength of the initial platelet–subendothelial attachment and platelet–platelet cohesive forces now determine the ultimate outcome. Rapid blood flow will tend to push the platelet thrombus distally, and these shear forces will be greater with increased cross-sectional area of the thrombus. If shear forces greatly outweigh the forces binding the platelets to the subendothelium, the platelet thrombus will embolize distally at a diminutive size. Clinically, the tiny platelet embolus may go unnoticed. If the forces binding the platelet to the subendothelium outweigh the shear forces, the platelet thrombus may remain attached. In this setting, an increase in the size of the platelet thrombus may terminate in vessel occlusion. In between these two extremes lie the conditions where the forces of de-

TABLE 4-1. *The platelet granules and their contents.*

Granule	Contents
Dense granules	adenosine diphosphate, calcium, serotonin
Alpha granules	fibrinogen, von Willebrand factor, fibronectin, thrombospondin, platelet-derived growth factor, platelet factor 4, beta-thromboglobulin
Lysosomes	acid hydrolases, cathepsin D & E
Peroxisomes	catalase

tachment and adhesion are similar. In these cases, platelet thromboembolism may occur at a relatively macroscopic level, at a size where occlusion of a terminal cerebral or retinal artery may result in tissue infarction.

BIOCHEMISTRY OF ANTIPLATELET AGENTS

There exist three basic mechanisms whereby platelet inhibitors exert their effects.[20] One mechanism involves the direct inhibition of the arachidonic acid pathway. A second mechanism increases platelet cyclic adenosine monophosphate levels. A third mechanism involves the direct or indirect inhibition of thrombin.[22]

Nonsteroidal anti-inflammatory agents, the prototype being aspirin, act through inhibition of the platelet pathways involved in the formation of thromboxane A_2.[23] These agents irreversibly acetylate platelet cyclooxygenase, inhibiting the conversion of arachidonic acid to the cyclic endoperoxides, thereby decreasing the amount of substrate available for conversion by thromboxane synthetase to thromboxane A_2. These agents only partially inhibit platelet aggregation, however, and the adherence of the initial layer of platelets to exposed subendothelium continues almost unabated. This observation has implications in the formation of intimal hyperplasia, where the initial monolayer of platelets may release platelet-derived growth factor and other mitogens involved in smooth muscle cell proliferation and migration.[24]

There exist several caveats of aspirin-induced platelet inhibition that are worthy of mention. First, *platelet* cyclooxygenase inhibition is permanent and the effects of the agents last for the life of the platelet. By contrast, *endothelial cell* cyclooxygenase inhibition is temporary, since these nucleated cells are capable of synthesizing new enzyme. This observation has implications in choosing the frequency of administration of aspirin.[25,26] An infrequent dosing regimen will theoretically allow the replenishment of endothelial cell prostacylin stores prior to the entry of large quantities of new platelets with active cyclooxygenase into the circulation.

A second caveat of aspirin therapy relates to the dose–response relationship of the drug. The antiplatelet effects of aspirin can be achieved with a relatively low dose, well below 325 mg/day. In this fashion, effective antiplatelet effects may be achieved without the gastrointestinal toxicity associated with higher doses.[23] In addition, low doses may allow complete hepatic clearance of aspirin and prevent any significant entry of active agent into the systemic circulation.[27] In this scenario, no endothelial cell cyclooxygenase will be inhibited and peripheral prostacyclin production will proceed unabated. By contrast, since significant aspirin concentrations are maintained in the portal circulation, and since all platelets traverse the portal circulation on a regular basis, platelet cyclooxygenase will be inhibited and thromboxane A_2 production will diminish.[28–30]

The second group of platelet antagonists comprise those agents that increase platelet cyclic adenosine monophosphate (cAMP) levels. Dipyridamole may increase cAMP through an inhibition of phosphodiesterase, an enzyme that degrades cAMP.[31] Dipyridamole simultaneously activates adenylate cyclase through a prostacyclin-mediated mechanism on the platelet membrane, increasing the concentration of platelet cytoplasmic cAMP.[32] Finally, plasma levels of adenosine are increased through an inhibition of uptake by endothelial cells and erythrocytes. The increased plasma adenosine further enhances platelet adenylate cyclase activity. Elevation of plasma adenosine concentration is also responsible for the vasodilator effects of dipyridamole.[31] Prostaglandins E1 and I2 and the prostacyclin analogues such as Iloprost also act through an increase in platelet cAMP. Although the platelet inhibitory effects of these agents are transient (less than 30 minutes), they are of sufficient magnitude to allow cardiopulmonary bypass without heparinization.[33]

A third group of platelet-inhibiting agents are the thrombin inhibitors, principally heparin and hirudin. As mentioned, thrombin is the most potent naturally occurring platelet agonist known. Heparin, through its activation of antithrombin-III, indirectly inhibits thrombin, and eliminates thrombin's platelet stimulatory effects. Hirudin acts in a similar fashion, although its inhibition of thrombin occurs through a direct binding between the two molecules.[22] This direct mechanism along with the relatively smaller size of the hirudin molecule is responsible for its more efficient thrombin inhibition when compared to heparin.[34] Coumadin, by contrast, is a poorer antiplatelet agent, as only moderate reductions in the concentration of the vitamin K dependent clotting protein produces less significant reductions in thrombin activity.

The remaining platelet inhibitors, dextran, sulfinpyrazone, and ticlopidine, do not fall within one of the three aforementioned groups. Sulfinpyrazone, formerly used more frequently than today, acts through the incomplete and reversible inhibition of platelet cyclooxygenase. Sulfinpyrazone also blocks the platelet aggregating actions of platelet-activating factor. Ticlopidine, the newest of the clinically available antiplatelet agents, inhibits fibrinogen binding to activated platelet membrane glycoprotein receptor IIb/IIIa.[35] The clinical platelet defect associated with ticlopidine appears similar to that in patients with Glanzmann's thrombasthenia. Dextran, used with considerable frequency in the perioperative period, has an unclear mechanism of action. Dextran may interfere with the factor VIII-von Willebrand complex or, alternatively, alter platelet membrane function.[23] Our own laboratory studies did not document any increment in platelet inhibition beyond what would have been expected from the hemodilution effects of the agent alone.[6]

CLINICAL STUDIES OF ANTIPLATELET AGENTS IN CEREBROVASCULAR DISEASE

Prior to the 1970s, anticoagulation was used in the prevention of cerebral thromboembolic events. Thereafter, antiplatelet agents replaced coumadin as the mainstay of medical management, reasoning that these events occurred as a result of platelet-fibrin accumulation within a high-flow arterial setting. The first randomized prospective trial of aspirin in cerebral ischemia was reported by Fields in 1977 (Table 4-2).[36] In this study, 178 patients with carotid territory transient ischemia were assigned to aspirin or placebo and followed over a mean of 37 months. When a combined out-

TABLE 4-2. *Summary of randomized, prospective trials of antiplatelet agents in the treatment of cerebrovascular ischemic events.*

Trial	Eligibility	End point	Groups	N	Outcome	Significance
AITIA Study[36]	TIA	CVA or death, 24 mo	ASA, 650 mg bid	88	19%	
			Placebo	90	27%	p = 0.18
Canadian Study[37]	TIA	CVA or death, 24 mo	Sulfinpyrazone, 200 mg qid	115	23%	= Placebo
			ASA, 325 mg qid	98	15%	p = 0.005
			Both	102	8%	= ASA alone
			Placebo	91	19%	
French Study*[38]	TIA, CVA	CVA, 24 mo	ASA, 330 mg tid	198	7%	p = 0.05
			ASA (330 mg) + DP (75 mg) tid	202	8%	= ASA
			Placebo	204	13%	
American-Canadian Study[39]	TIA	CVA or death, 24 mo	ASA, 325 mg qid	442	8.2%	
			ASA (325 mg) + DP (75 mg) qid	448	8.6%	n.s.
CATS[43]	CVA	CVA, MI, death, 24 mo	Ticlopidine, 250 mg bid	525	18%	
			Placebo	528	25%	p = 0.006
TASS[44]	TIA, CVA	CVA or death, 24 mo	Ticlopidine, 250 mg bid	1515	10%	
			ASA, 650 mg bid	1519	12%	p = 0.048

*men only

come index of cerebral infarction, retinal infarction or death was used, a benefit was observed in favor of aspirin treatment. No significant difference was realized when the outcome measures were not grouped and were restricted to a single end point.

A second study, the Canadian Cooperative trial, was reported one year following the study of Fields.[37] This study was designed to compare aspirin, sulfinpyrazone, both or neither in the treatment of threatened stroke. Overall, 585 patients were randomized, and patient acquisition actually began one year prior to the start of the Fields' trial. In this higher powered study, aspirin reduced the risk of stroke or death by 31 percent and this benefit was most pronounced in male patients. In fact, no statistical benefit was observed in females. No benefits were realized with sulfinpyrazone alone.

The 1980s saw the performance of trials designed to compare alternative aspirin strategies, utilizing aspirin in conjunction with dipyridamole. Two important studies appeared in 1983 and 1985. The first trial, conducted in France, randomized 604 patients with cerebral atheroembolic events to aspirin, aspirin and dipyridamole, or placebo.[38] The American-Canadian Co-operative Study Group randomized 890 patients with carotid territory transient events to aspirin or aspirin and dipyridamole.[39] In both of these well-designed investigations, aspirin was beneficial in decreasing the incidence of subsequent cerebral events. Dipyridamole, however, provided no additional protection over aspirin alone.

The effect of the dose of aspirin was studied in two well-controlled trials. The Dutch TIA Trial Study Group conducted an investigation of two doses of aspirin, 30 mg/day and 283 mg/day, in the treatment of transient cerebral ischemia and minor ischemic stroke.[40] A total of 3,131 patients were randomized and followed for a mean of 2.6 years. There were no differences in the frequency of the combined end point of stroke, myocardial infarction, or death in the patients treated with the lower dose of aspirin, averaging approximately 17% in the two groups at 36 months of follow-up. There was, however, a slightly higher incidence of major and minor bleeding in the higher dose group.

A second trial, the SALT (Swedish Aspirin Low-dose Trial) Collaborative Group studied the effects of low-dose aspirin on the prevention of stroke and death after minor cerebrovascular events.[41] Overall, 1,360 patients were randomly assigned to 75 mg/day aspirin or placebo. After a mean follow-up of 32 months, an 18% reduction in the risk of stroke or death was realized in the aspirin group. Bleeding episodes were more common in the aspirin treated patients, 7.2% versus 3.2% ($p = 0.001$). The authors concluded that an aspirin dose of 75 mg/day provided satisfactory prophylaxis against subsequent stroke or death in patients with cerebrovascular ischemic events, limiting the risk of gastrointestinal bleeding associated with higher doses.

The prevention of cerebral embolic events following carotid artery surgery was the subject of a randomized, double-blind, placebo-controlled Swedish trial appearing in 1993.[42] A total of 232 patients undergoing carotid endarterectomy were randomized to placebo or 75 mg/day aspirin. Aspirin was begun the evening prior to operation and continued for 6 months. All patients were treated with dextran 40 during the first three postoperative days. There was a significantly lower incidence of strokes without complete recovery in the aspirin-treated group, 1.7% versus 9.6% at 6 months ($p = 0.01$). Mortality differences between the aspirin and placebo groups did not attain statistical significance, 3.4% and 6%, respectively ($p = 0.12$). The investigators concluded that low-dose aspirin was beneficial in preventing stroke following carotid endarterectomy.

Ticlopidine has been investigated in two large prospective studies, the Canadian-American Ticlopidine Study,[43] or "CATS," and the Ticlopidine Aspirin Stroke Study,[44] or "TASS." Patients in CATS had thromboembolic stroke and were randomized to 250 mg ticlopidine twice a day (525 patients) or placebo (528 patients) and followed for a mean of 24 months. Of note, severe neutropenia occurred in four patients receiving ticlopidine (0.8%), versus only one patient receiving placebo (0.2%). Ticlopidine was responsible for a reduction in the rate of recurrent stroke, 10.8% per year versus 15.3% per year in the placebo group for a relative risk reduction of 30 percent.

In TASS, 3,069 patients with transient or minor completed cerebrovascular events were randomized to ticlopidine (250 mg, twice daily) or aspirin (650 mg, twice daily). The frequency of stroke was decreased in the ticlopidine group, 13% versus 18% at 5 years ($p = 0.01$). A subgroup analysis revealed that this difference was independent of sex. The authors concluded that ticlopidine was more effective than aspirin in the prophylaxis against recurrent cerebrovascular events.

In summary, aspirin has been shown to be of benefit in the prevention of subsequent cerebral events in patients with prior atheroembolic ischemia. These benefits are evident at substantially lower doses than are generally employed. Ticlopidine is at least as effective as aspirin and may actually be associated with a decreased frequency of cerebrovascular events over long periods of follow-up. The benefits of sulfinpyrazone and dipyridamole are less well defined. Well controlled studies suggest that these agents offer little protection over aspirin therapy alone. Hopefully, subsequent investigative work will define the most advantageous dose and frequency of administration for aspirin. Newer antiplatelet agents, specifically the membrane receptor antagonists, hold much promise for the future, but clinical use must await the completion of basic investigation and prospective clinical trials.

REFERENCES

1. Hunt JR. The role of the carotid arteries in the causation of vascular lesion of the brain with remarks on certain features of the symptomatology. Am J Med Sci 1913;134:704
2. Dyken ML. Evaluation of cerebral ischemia: transient, focal, lateralizing, and nonhemispheric ischemic attacks. In: Bergan JJ, Yao JST (eds). Cerebrovascular insufficiency. New York: Grune & Stratton, Inc. 1983:57–68
3. Fisher CM, Adams RD. Observations on brain embolism with special reference to the mechanism of hemorrhagic infarction. J Neuropath Exp Neurol 1951;10:92
4. Hollenhorst RW. Significance of bright plaques in the retinal arterioles. Trans Am Ophthal Soc 1966;59:252
5. Burrig KF. The endothelium of advanced arteriosclerotic plaques in humans. Arterioscler Thromb 1991;11:1678–1689
6. Blebea J, Ouriel K, Zollo RA, Marder VJ. Deposition of platelets and fibrinogen on ex vivo vascular segments: dependence on shear rate. Surg Forum 1990;41:357–358

7. Zarins CK, Giddens DP, Balasubramanian K, et al. Carotid plaques localize in regions of low flow velocity and shear stress. Circulation 1981;64(suppl. IV):44
8. Ouriel K, Donayre C, Shortell CK, Cimino C, Donnelly J, Oxley D, et al. The hemodynamics of thrombus formation in arteries. J Vasc Surg 1991;14:757–62; discus.
9. Coller BS, Beer JH, Scudder LE, Steinberg MH. Collagen–platelet interactions: evidence for a direct interaction of collagen with platelet GPIa/IIa and an indirect interaction with platelet GPIIb/IIIa mediated by adhesive proteins. Blood 1989;74:182–192
10. Badimon L, Badimon JJ, Turitto VT, Vallabhajosula S, Fuster V. Platelet thrombus formation on collagen type I: a model of deep vessel injury: influence of blood rheology, von Willebrand factor, and blood coagulation. Circulation 1988;78:1431–1442
11. Mohri H, Ohkubo T. How vitronectin binds to activated glycoprotein IIb-IIIa complex and its function in platelet aggregation. Am J Clin Pathol 1991;96:605–609
12. Fressinaud E, Baruch D, Girma JP, Sakariassen KJ, Baumgartner HR, Meyer D. Von Willebrand factor-mediated platelet adhesion to collagen involves platelet membrane glycoprotein IIb-IIIa as well as glycoprotein Ib. J Lab Clin Med 1988;112:58–67
13. Coller BS, Folts JD, Smith SR, Scudder LE, Jordan R. Abolition of in vivo platelet thrombus formation in primates with monoclonal antibodies to the platelet GPIIb/IIIa receptor. Correlation with bleeding time, platelet aggregation, and blockade of GPIIb/IIIa receptors [see comments]. Circulation 1989;80:1766–1774
14. Beer JH, Springer KT, Coller BS. Immobilized Arg-Gly-Asp (RGD) peptides of varying lengths as structural probes of the platelet glycoprotein IIb/IIIa receptor. Blood 1992;79:117–128
15. Fuster V, Badimon L, Badimon JJ, Ip JH, Chesebro JH. The porcine model for the understanding of thrombogenesis and atherogenesis. Mayo Clin Proc 1991;66:818–831
16. Badimon L, Badimon JJ, Turitto VT, Fuster V. Role of von Willebrand factor in mediating platelet–vessel wall interaction at low shear rate; the importance of perfusion conditions. Blood 1989;73:961–967
17. Cho JS, Ouriel K. Thrombus formation on polytetafluoroethylene surfaces: the importance of von Willebrand factor. J Cardiovasc Surg 1995;in press
18. Scharfstein J, Loscalzo J. Molecular approaches to antithrombotic therapy. Hosp Pract 1992;May 15:41–50
19. Alonso MT, Sanchez A, Garcia-Sancho J. Arachidonic acid-induced calcium influx in human platelets: comparison with the effect of thrombin. Biochem J 1990;272:435–443
20. Mruk JS, Chesebro JH, Webster MWI. Platelet aggregation and interaction with the coagulation system: implications for antithrombotic therapy in arterial thrombosis. Cor Art Ds 1990;1:149–158
21. Seiler SM, Michel IM, Fenton JW. Involvement of the "tethered-ligand" receptor in thrombin inhibition of platelet adenylate cyclase. Biochem Biophys Res Commun 1992;182:1296–1302
22. Donayre CE, Ouriel K, Rhee RY, Shortell CK. Future alternatives to heparin: low-molecular-weight heparin and hirudin. J Vasc Surg 1992;15:675–682
23. Stein B, Fuster V, Israel DH, Cohen M, Badimon L, Badimon JJ, et al. Platelet inhibitor agents in cardiovascular disease: an update. J Am Coll Cardiol 1989;14:813–836
24. Clowes AW, Karnovsky MJ. Failure of certain antiplatelet drugs to affect myointimal thickening following arterial endothelial injury in the rat. Lab Invest 1977;36:452–464
25. De Caterina R, Boem A, Gazzetti P, Sicari R, Giannessi D, Ciabattoni G, et al. Long-term maintenance of thromboxane inhibition by two different aspirin regimens in patients with unstable angina. Thromb Res 1990;60:169–175
26. Patrono C, Ciabattoni G, Patrignani P. Clinical pharmacology of platelet cyclooxygenase inhibition. Circulation 1985;72:1177–1184
27. FitzGerald GA, Lupinetti M, Charman SA, Charman WN. Presystemic acetylation of platelets by aspirin: reduction in rate of drug delivery to improve biochemical selectivity for thromboxane A2. J Pharmacol Exp Ther 1991;259:1043–1049
28. Beving H, Eksborg S, Nordlander R, Olsson P, Olsson U. Effects on cyclo-oxygenase of low and high dose aspirin. Thromb Res 1990;59:227–235
29. Hoet B, Deckmyn H, Arnout J, Vermylen J. Pharmacological manipulation of the thromboxane pathway in blood platelets. Blood Coagul Fibrinolysis 1990;1:225–233
30. Jimenez AH, Stubbs ME, Tofler GH, Winther K, Williams GH, Muller JE. Rapidity and duration of platelet suppression by enteric-coated aspirin in healthy young men. Am J Cardiol 1992;69:258–262
31. Fitsgerald GA. Dipyridamole. N Engl J Med 1987;316:1247–1257
32. Moncada S, Korbut R. Dipyridamole and other phosphodiesterase inhibitors act as antithromboic agents by potentiating endogenous prostacyclin. Lancet 1978;1:1286–1289

33. Coppe D, Sobel M, Seavans L, et al. Preservation of platelet function and number by prostacyclin during cardiopulmonary bypass. J Thorac Cardiovasc Surg 1981;81:274–278
34. Fareed J, Walenga JM, Iyer L, Hoppensteadt D, Pifarre R. An objective perspective on recombinant hirudin: a new anticoagulant and antithrombotic agent. Blood Coagul Fibrinolysis 1991;2:135–147
35. Di Minno G, Cerbone AM, Mattioli PL. Functionally thrombasthenic state in normal platelets following the administration of ticlopidine. J Clin Invest 1985;75:328–338
36. Fields WS, Lemak NA, Frankowski RF. Controlled trial of aspirin in cerebral ischemia. Stroke 1977;8:301–314
37. The Canadian Cooperative Study Group. A randomized trial of aspirin and sulfinpyrazone in threatened stroke. N Engl J Med 1978;299:53–59
38. Bousser MG, Eschwege E, Haguenau M, et al. "AICLA" controlled trial of aspirin and dipyridamole in the secondary prevention of athero-thrombotic cerebral ischemia. Stroke 1983;14:5–14
39. The American-Canadian Co-operative Study Group. Persantine aspirin trial in cerebral ischemia. Part II: Endpoint results. Stroke 1985;16:406–415
40. The Dutch TIA Trial Study Group. A comparison of two doses of aspirin (30 mg vs. 283 mg a day) in patients after a transient ischemic attack or minor ischemic stroke. N Engl J Med 1991;325:1261–1266
41. The SALT Collaborative Group. Swedish aspirin low-dose trial (SALT) of 75 mg aspirin as secondary prophylaxis after cerebrovascular ischaemic events. Lancet 1991;338:1345–1349
42. Lindblad B, Persson NH, Takolander R, Bergqvist D. Does low-dose acetylsalicylic acid prevent stroke after carotid surgery? Stroke 1993;24:1125–1128
43. Gent M, Easton JD, Hachinski VC. The Canadian American ticlopidine study (CATS) in thromboembolic stroke. Lancet 1989;1:1215–1220
44. Hass WK, Easton JD, Adams HP, et al. A randomized trial comparing ticlopidine hydrochloride with aspirin for the prevention of stroke in high-risk patients. N Engl J Med 1989;321:501–507

Management of Extracranial Cerebrovascular Disease, edited by Keith D. Calligaro et al.
Lippincott-Raven Publishers, Philadelphia © 1997.

5

Evaluation of Cardiac Risk in Patients Undergoing Carotid Artery Surgery

Peter N. Purcell, Richard P. Cambria

In spite of advances in diagnosis, patient selection, and surgical treatment of carotid artery disease, the impact of associated coronary artery disease (CAD) remains significant. CAD is the most frequent source of early and late morbidity and mortality in patients treated with carotid endarterectomy (CEA).[1] While many patients will have undergone some form of cardiac testing before being referred for surgery, it is necessary for the surgeon to be well versed in both testing modalities and the choice of whom to test. To approach the identification of these patients rationally and cost-effectively, the clinician should realize that patients with coexistent carotid stenosis and CAD present in distinct clinical subsets, and the context of the clinical presentation will guide the desirability of testing for associated CAD. This chapter examines the incidence and impact of CAD, and the principles and goals of cardiac risk stratification (CRS) in patients with carotid artery disease. Finally, a rationale for the selective use of CRS are presented. Other chapters deal with carotid evaluation in patients who require coronary artery bypass grafting (CABG), while this chapter focuses on the evaluation of cardiac risk in CEA candidates.

INCIDENCE AND IMPACT OF CAD IN CAROTID DISEASE

In approaching the assessment of coexistent CAD in CEA candidates it is important to realize that the prevalence of CAD in these patients is significant. Herzer et al, in a prospective study of 1,000 patients with vascular disease, all of whom underwent coronary angiography, found that severe CAD was present in one third of patients presenting for CEA.[2] Some studies even indicate a linear relationship between the severity of carotid artery stenosis and the extent of CAD.[3] Urbinati et al reported silent CAD in 25% of patients with symptomatic carotid artery stenosis.[4] However, the converse is not true. The prevalence of significant carotid artery disease in patients presenting for CABG ranges from 4.5–8%, depending on the age of the prospective CABG cohort.[5] These data suggest that carotid disease may be considered a marker for CAD and should alert the clinician dealing with CEA candidates that the prevalence of CAD will be high.

The most obvious short-term impact of CAD in these patients is their increased risk of perioperative cardiac events: fatal and non-fatal myocardial infarction, arrhythmias and cardiac ischemia. The reported incidence of myocardial infarction (MI) complicating CEA is 1.5–5%.[6] While it has been felt that the risk of MI following CEA in patients with CAD was less than that for other vascular procedures, recently published data from our institution indicates that the incidence of MI's in patients undergoing carotid or aortic surgery is equivalent.[7] Perioperative MI also carries a very high mortality, up to 50% in some reports.[6,8]

The long-term impact of CAD in patients who have undergone CEA becomes clear when their late survival is examined. CAD is the primary source of late mortality in patients with carotid disease.[1,9] Cohen, in the VA Cooperative Study 167 (CEA for asymptomatic carotid disease), found an annual mortality of 9% with two thirds of all deaths being cardiac-related.[10] Urbinati found the 7-year survival of patients undergoing CEA who had silent CAD detected preoperatively to be 51%, versus 98% survival in those without silent CAD.[4] It is important to note that this high long-term morbidity and mortality occurs whether or not the patient undergoes CEA. Using the same cohort of VA cooperative study patients, Hobson found that the long-term cardiac mortality was not significantly different in medically managed versus surgically managed asymptomatic carotid stenosis.[11] The asymptomatic carotid atherosclerosis study (ACAS) recently detailed the results of a randomized prospective study of 1,659 patients with asymptomatic carotid stenosis of 60% or greater. At a median follow-up of 2.7 years, half of the combined annual mortality rate of 4% was cardiac-related.[12] Chambers and Norris, in a study of 500 asymptomatic patients with cervical bruits, found a higher risk of cardiac ischemic events than of stroke,[9] and in a separate study found an annual cardiac death rate of 6.5% in patients with severe asymptomatic carotid stenosis.[13] The late cardiac mortality of patients with cerebral ischemia even exceeds that of patients with angina pectoris.[14]

In spite of the high prevalence of CAD in these patients, however, it is important to realize that in contemporary practice CEA is accompanied by extremely low rates of perioperative morbidity. In our unit, the senior author has performed 420 CEAs in the past 8 years with combined stroke and death rates in the 1% range and a combined major and minor cardiac complication rate of 3%, consistent with ACAS data showing a perioperative morbidity and mortality of 2.7%.[12] The current safety of CEA and its urgent nature in certain patients suggest that CRS may be carried out in the early postoperative period, if necessary, in those circumstances where CEA is indicated on an urgent basis. Because of the high prevalence of CAD and the substantial incidence of late cardiac sequelae in patients presenting for CEA, careful assessment of cardiac status is indicated in these patients. CRS then serves the dual purpose of minimizing perioperative complications and clarifying the patient's late cardiac prognosis. This information will help to predict if the patient will live long enough to benefit from a prophylactic procedure. Before addressing the question of which patients should undergo testing, several general principles of CRS deserve comment.

PRINCIPLES AND GOALS OF CARDIAC RISK STRATIFICATION

An important principle of CRS is that its usefulness extends beyond simple identification of patients at risk for a perioperative event. CRS provides a longitudinal perspective of the patient's long-term cardiac risk, allows modification of that risk and therefore may influence the initial judgments about the worth of proceeding with CEA.[7,15] In fact, with the current safety of CEA and the high late cardiac death rate in this group, for many patients the longitudinal perspective afforded by CRS will be more important than its potential benefit in decreasing perioperative cardiac risk.[15,16]

Within the context of perioperative cardiac complications and their prevention, the goal of CRS is to provide a quantitative assessment of the amount of potentially jeopardized myocardium. While it is not the purpose or within the scope of this chapter to review comprehensively the modalities available for CRS, and with the perspective that the testing modality chosen by an individual clinician will vary with the particular expertise of the institution, some mention of the modalities available for CRS is appropriate.

In the past, two general types of tests have been used in CRS: assessments of ventricular function, and those techniques which define potential for perioperative myocardial ischemic injury. Prior to the availability of dipyridamole-thallium scanning (D-THAL), determination of resting ejection fraction was commonly performed to assess perioperative risk. However, while a markedly decreased ejection fraction has prognostic implications for long-term survival,[17] well-preserved ventricular function does not correlate with freedom from a perioperative cardiac event.[18,19] Tests that only provide information about preoperative resting ventricular function, therefore, are inadequate to accurately predict the presence of jeopardized myocardium; for this purpose, a functional study, such as D-THAL scanning or another stress-inducing modality, is necessary.

The earliest assessments of perioperative cardiac risk involved clinical variables only. The scoring systems originally proposed by Goldman and later modified by Detsky et al in the late 1970s remain valid.[20] However, Hertzer et al identified significant CAD in 15% of patients about to undergo vascular surgery who had no previous clinical history of CAD, a finding which emphasizes the potential for significant, albeit occult, CAD in patients who present with peripheral vascular disease and suggests an advantage to using a testing modality which can identify these patients.[2]

The rationale for ambulatory EKG monitoring is that silent ischemia, which is more common than angina, has been found to correlate with the risk of perioperative MI.[21,22] Fleisher, however, found that ambulatory EKG monitoring had a positive predictive value of 0.38 and a negative predictive value of 0.86, implying that D-THAL scanning may be a better test in patients with any of the above cardiac risk markers.[23] Further, the requirement for 24 hours or more of monitoring may impede timely evaluation of results.[16]

Finally, the stress-inducing testing modalities can be physical exercise (treadmill walking), pharmacological agents other than dipyridamole, such as adenosine and dobutamine, or actual cardiac pacing with a temporary transvenous pacing wire. After induction of myocardial stress, ischemic regions of the myocardium are identified by either EKG monitoring, wall motion analysis (performed with either surface or transesophageal echocardiography), or radionuclide assessment of regional myocardial perfusion.

Popularized by Boucher and colleagues at this institution,[24] D-THAL scanning has become our noninvasive test of choice. Its sensitivity and specificity are equal to or better than those of conventional exercise testing.[25] Instead of interpreting the test as simply positive (reversible defect) or negative (fixed defect or no defect), we use it to provide quantitative global information about: (1) the number and location of zones of potential ischemia; (2) evidence of fixed ventricular scarring due to prior infarction; and (3) dipyridamole-induced left ventricular dysfunction that may indicate global ischemia or three-vessel disease.[25,26,27] This interpretation increases the predictive value of D-THAL scanning.[24,28] In our unit, patients with indications for vascular surgery who are discovered to have single coronary territory redistribution on D-THAL are sent for the indicated operation without further cardiac intervention, whereas those with multiple zones of reversibility or reversibility suggestive of left main disease may undergo coronary angiography.

Thus, D-THAL is appropriate to address another goal of CRS, namely, identifying those patients whose CAD would, on its own merits, warrant mechanical intervention with angioplasty or CABG. The well-known coronary artery surgery study (CASS) followed over 2,000 patients who either had mild or moderate angina or were asymptomatic survivors of MI. Of this cohort, patients with left-main or three-vessel disease were identified as having a significantly improved survival with CABG.[29] An unpublished autopsy study at this institution showed that 18 of 21 patients who died of MI after vascular surgery had either left-main or three-vessel CAD, indicating that those patients who die of MI after vascular surgery are likely to have diffuse CAD that would independently warrant correction. Effective CRS can identify those patients so they may undergo coronary angiography and subsequent CABG for its demonstrated survival benefit.

Finally, it is important to consider how the clinician will react to the information gained from CRS. Although some patients will be identified as candidates for coronary angiography and intervention with CABG or balloon angioplasty, information gained from CRS need not lead to the two extremes of deferring vascular operation or full evaluation and treatment with angiography and CABG. It may be used to influence anesthetic management, the need for invasive perioperative monitoring, decisions to institute anti-ischemic medical therapy and, perhaps most important, the level of awareness afforded to the perioperative medical therapy of associated CAD. Indeed, of all potential scenarios applied to the CEA candidate, proceeding to surgery with optimal medical management of the associated CAD is the most common. In light of the purely prophylactic aim of CEA in asymptomatic carotid stenosis and the fact that the risk of de novo stroke in asymptomatic patients is 3–5% per year,[9,13] the information gained from CRS may result in deferring surgery if the patient's CAD is severe, uncorrectable, or if the patient is otherwise not a candidate for CABG.

CARDIAC RISK STRATIFICATION: A SELECTIVE APPROACH BASED ON CLINICAL PROFILING OF ASSOCIATED CAD

In deciding which patients to test, the surgeon should remember that the clinical context of the patient's carotid disease is the most important factor. Patients with a truly urgent need for CEA (*i.e.*, those with evolving stroke, crescendo or multiple transient ischemic attacks [TIAs], or truly compelling anatomy such as a 95% stenosis with an occluded contralateral carotid artery) should not undergo cardiac testing; they should proceed directly to surgery after optimization of their medical therapy, not only because of the urgent nature of their carotid disease, but because of the possibility that cardiac testing may result in transient hypotension and cerebral ischemia. Asymptomatic patients or those with lesser degrees of stenosis may be candidates for CRS.

The next issue is which patients in the asymptomatic category should undergo noninvasive testing. Some centers advocate preoperative testing for all elective CEA candidates.[8] There seems little doubt that the ready availability of noninvasive testing has resulted in its indiscriminate use and the corresponding overuse of coronary angiography in preoperative patients. Unfortunately, this strategy results in the performance of many normal tests and thus diminishes the overall positive predictive value, regardless of the test employed. With regard to D-THAL, several studies, including Baron's prospective study of 457 vascular surgery patients undergoing D-THAL scanning, have shown that routine testing of all patients without regard to clinical profiling results in low specificity and poor predictive value for perioperative cardiac events.[28] Therefore, many patients who do not require intervention will be referred for coronary angiography, which is expensive and exposes the patient to further risks. These results are not surprising since it is clear that many patients with significant CAD can safely undergo vascular surgery. A decade of experience with CRS at The Massachusetts General Hospital has convinced us that a selective approach to CRS based on clinical profiling is the best strategy for identifying those patients at risk of having significant CAD that would effect the subsequent management.

Among the first clinical scoring systems was Goldman's in 1977. In a study at The Massachusetts General Hospital, over 1,000 consecutive patients undergoing noncardiac surgery underwent multivariate analysis of a battery of clinical and laboratory variables, from which arose a preoperative cardiac risk index.[20] However, only 160 of these patients were admitted for peripheral vascular operations. The Goldman index is less accurate for estimating cardiac risk in the more homogeneous but higher-risk subset of patients with vascular disease. Other clinical scoring systems for vascular surgery patients have been developed but have generally been found to have insufficient sensitivity for prediction of cardiac events when used alone.[18,30] In order to overcome this deficiency, clinical scoring is best combined with noninvasive testing.

The clinical scoring system in use at The Massachusetts General Hospital is detailed in a series of reports from Eagle and colleagues.[31,32] In the initial study, 111 patients undergoing vascular surgery were prospectively evaluated. D-THAL scans were found to be unnecessary in a subgroup of patients felt to be at low risk on the basis of clinical factors alone (aged younger than 70 years, absence of diabetes, angina, prior MI, and congestive heart failure). This low-risk group had a negligible rate of cardiac events regardless of the result of D-THAL.[31] In a separate study,[32] intended to demonstrate the cumulative significance of increasing numbers of clinical markers of CAD, logistic regression analysis on 254 patients who underwent vascular surgery demonstrated five clinical markers of CAD—Q waves on the preoperative EKG, history of angina, history of ventricular arrhythmias, diabetes, and older than 70 years—as independent predictors of postoperative ischemic events. Thallium redistribution and ischemic EKG changes after thallium injection on D-THAL scans were also predictive of postoperative ischemia. However, greater specificity (81%) with equal sensitivity for the prediction of postoperative cardiac ischemic changes was obtained using a model combining clinical and D-THAL features than using either alone.

Interestingly, clinical factors alone could distinguish patients with very low risk (*i.e.,* those with none of the five clinical markers) and those at high risk—with three or more of the clinical markers. These high- and low-risk groups were not further distinguished by the presence or absence of thallium redistribution. The patients in the intermediate-risk group (those with one or two clinical markers) benefited most from subsequent D-THAL. Therefore, those at low risk could undergo their surgery without further noninvasive testing, and those at high risk could proceed directly to coronary angiography if further knowledge of their coronary anatomy would influence their management. Those at intermediate risk would undergo D-THAL. Paul et al applied this clinical risk index to angiographic data from Hertzer's original database of 1,000 coronary angiograms and found that a gradient of risk for severe CAD was seen with the presence of an increasing number of clinical markers. As displayed in Figure 5-1, the clinical risk index alone predicted severity of CAD quite accurately. If a "positive" coronary angiogram were defined as either (1) three-vessel CAD with ≥50% stenosis in each vessel, (2) two-vessel CAD with ≥70% stenosis of the left anterior descending artery, or (3) left main CAD with ≥50% stenosis, then the clinical index alone was accurate in predicting negative angiograms in 83% of patients clinically classified as low risk. Similarly, 77% of patients classified as high risk based on the clinical index profiling had "positive" coronary angiograms. Finally, the anatomic discrimination for those whose clinical profile was classified as "intermediate" was poor and, as noted above, it is these patients in which D-THAL imaging is most useful (Fig. 5-1).[33]

In addition to these occult markers of CAD, some patients will present with major clinical markers of CAD, such as a history of recent MI, the presence of unstable or new onset angina, and recent or poorly controlled left ventricular dysfunction. These patients will be best served by eliminating the preliminary step of performing D-THAL. If felt to be potential candidates for CABG or angioplasty prior to their CEA, they should proceed directly to coronary angiography, presuming the CEA is an "elective" intervention.

Based on these observations, an algorithm has been developed at our institution

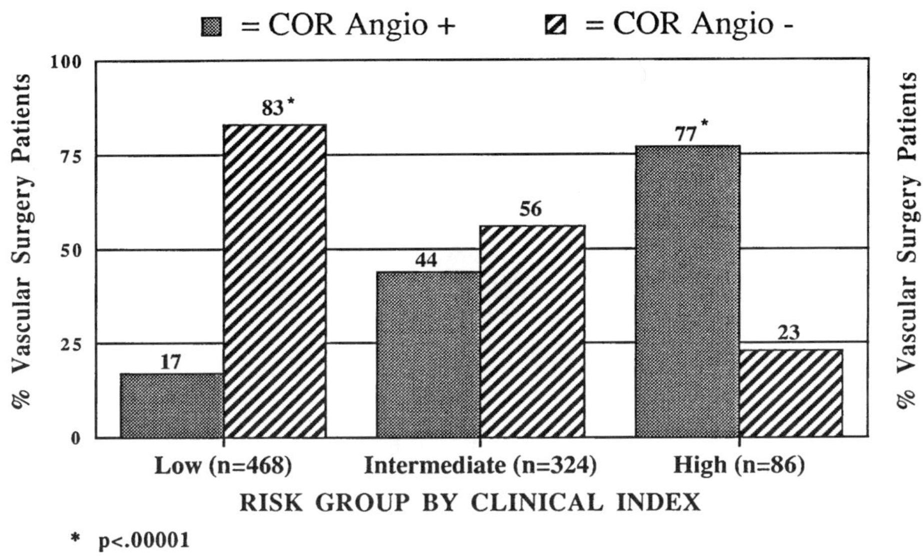

FIG. 5-1. Graph shows concordance between risk defined by clinical risk index assessment and the presence of a positive coronary angiogram in preoperative vascular surgery patients. Clinical index alone is accurate in predicting a positive or negative coronary angiogram for patients in low- and high-risk categories; it is those patients in the intermediate risk category who most benefit from testing with D-THAL.[33]

that can be applied to CEA candidates (Fig. 5-2). As previously described, patients with evolving stroke, crescendo TIAs, and truly compelling carotid anatomy proceed directly to CEA with optimal medical management of their CAD. Patients who are truly asymptomatic or have a history of remote stroke should undergo clinical evaluation. Those with none of the five clinical markers of CAD, or those who have a history of prior CABG, which appears to be protective for perioperative cardiac complications,[24] and perhaps those with only risk factors of age or diabetes mellitus alone, may proceed directly to CEA. Those with up to two clinical markers or with controlled CAD or stable left ventricular dysfunction fall into the intermediate risk category for which noninvasive testing is most beneficial. Those with three or more clinical markers may be considered high risk and proceed directly to coronary angiography if they are still felt to be candidates for CEA. Patients with no or single coronary territory redistribution on D-THAL may safely undergo CEA without coronary angiography. Those with multiple zones of redistribution should undergo coronary angiography. Patients with severe CAD on coronary angiography may undergo antecedent CABG or angioplasty if their disease is reconstructable; if it is not, reconsideration of their need for CEA is warranted.

In summary, the prevalence of CAD in patients with carotid bifurcation disease warrants awareness of the potential for perioperative and long-term cardiac morbidity and mortality. The clinical context of the carotid lesion and clinical profile with respect to CAD are the important variables in deciding the desirability and timing of

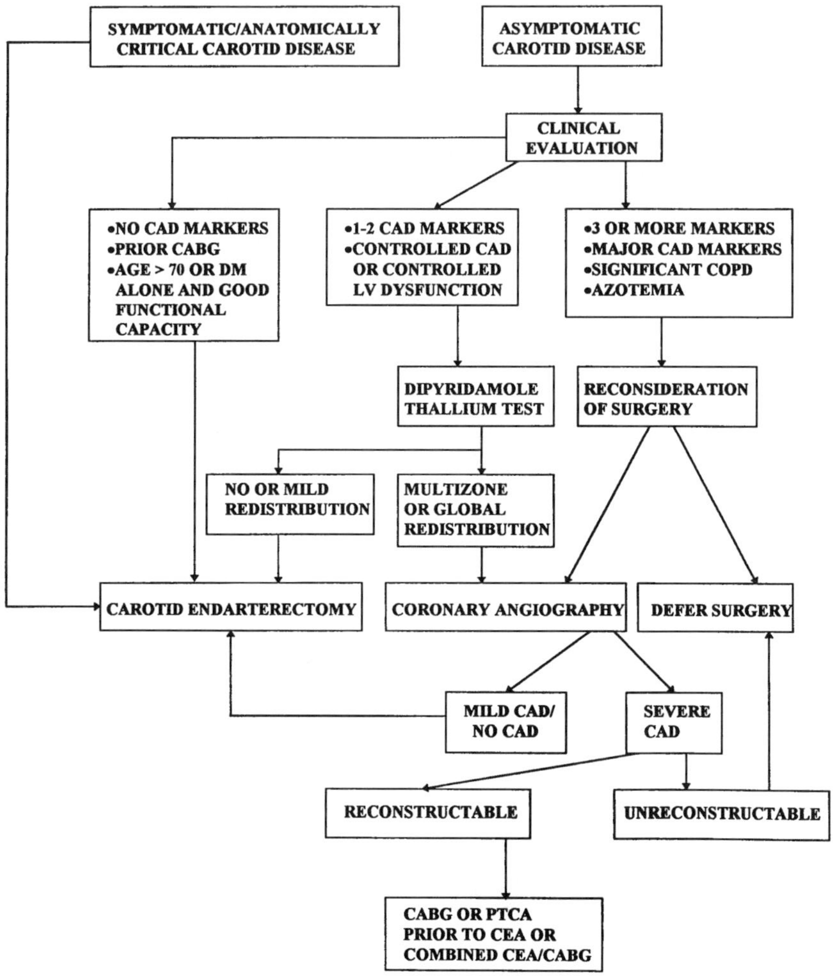

FIG. 5-2. Suggested algorithm for management of patients with carotid disease. Clinical markers of CAD are older than 70 years, diabetes, history of angina, myocardial infarction, and ventricular arrhythmias. (CAD, coronary artery disease; CABG, coronary artery bypass graft; COPD, chronic obstructive pulmonary disease)

CRS. This approach permits safe and cost-effective detection of and intervention for CAD to minimize perioperative and long-term cardiac events after CEA.

REFERENCES

1. Callow A, Mackey W. Long-term follow-up of surgically managed carotid bifurcation atherosclerosis. Ann Surg 1989;210:308

2. Hertzer NR, Beven EG, Young JR, et al. Coronary artery disease in peripheral vascular patients. A classification of 1,000 coronary angiograms and results of surgical management. Ann Surg 1984;199: 223–233
3. Wofford JL, Kahl FR, Howard GR, et al. Relation of extent of extracranial carotid artery atherosclerosis as measured by B-mode ultrasound to the extent of coronary atherosclerosis. Arterioscler Thromb 1991;11:1786
4. Urbinati S, DiPasquale G, Andreoli A, et al. Frequency and prognostic significance of silent coronary artery disease in patients with cerebral ischemia undergoing carotid endarterectomy. Am J Cardiol 1992;69:1166–1170
5. Brenner B, Brief D, Alpert J, et al. The risk of stroke in patients with asymptomatic carotid stenosis undergoing cardiac surgery: a follow-up study. J Vasc Surg 1987;5:269–279
6. Yeager R, Moneta R. Assessing cardiac risk in vascular surgical patients: current status. Perspect Vasc Surg 1989;2:18–36
7. L'Italien G, Cambria RP, Cutler B, et al. Comparative early and late cardiac morbidity among patients requiring different vascular surgery procedures. J Vasc Surg 1995;21:935–944
8. Gillespie DL, LaMorte WW, Josephs LG, et al. Characteristics of patients at risk for perioperative myocardial infarction after infrainguinal bypass surgery: an exploratory study. Ann Vasc Surg 1995;9: 155–162
9. Chambers BR and Norris JW. Outcome in patients with asymptomatic neck bruits. N Engl J Med 1986;315:860–865
10. Cohen SN, Hobson RW, Weiss DG, et al. Death associated with asymptomatic carotid artery stenosis: long-term clinical evaluation. J Vasc Surg 1993;18:1002–1011
11. Hobson RW, Weiss DG, Fields WS, et al. Efficacy of carotid endarterectomy for asymptomatic carotid stenosis. N Engl J Med 1993;328:221–227
12. Executive Committee for the Asymptomatic Carotid Atherosclerosis Study. Endarterectomy for asymptomatic carotid artery stenosis. JAMA 1995;273:1421–1428
13. Norris JW, Zhu CZ, Bornstein NM, Chambers BR. Vascular risks of asymptomatic carotid stenosis. Stroke 1991;22:1485
14. Adams HP, Jr, Kassel NF, Mazuz H. The patient with transient ischemic attacks. Is this the time for a new therapeutic approach? Stroke 1984;15:371–375
15. Cutler BS, Hendel RC, Leppo JA. Dipyridamole-thallium scintigraphy predicts perioperative and long-term survival after major vascular surgery. J Vasc Surg 1992;15:972–981
16. Pasternack PF, Grossi EA, Baumann FG, et al. Silent myocardial ischemia monitoring predicts late as well as perioperative cardiac events in patients undergoing vascular surgery. J Vasc Surg 1992;16:171–180
17. Kazmers A, Cerqueira MD, Zierler RE. The role of preoperative radionuclide ejection fraction in direct abdominal aortic aneurysm repair. J Vasc Surg 1988;8:128–136
18. Blunt JT. The role of a defined protocol for cardiac risk assessment in decreasing perioperative myocardial infarction in vascular surgery. J Vasc Surg 1992;15:626–634
19. Pasternack PF, Imparato AM, Bear G, et al. The value of radionuclide angiography as a predictor of preoperative myocardial infarction in patients undergoing abdominal aortic aneurysm resection. J Vasc Surg 1984;1:320–325
20. Goldman L, Caldera DL, Nussbaum SR, et al. Multifactorial index of cardiac risk in noncardiac surgical procedures. N Engl J Med 1977;297:845–850
21. Miller DD. Clinical risk factor analysis and electrocardiographic evaluation modalities. Sem Vasc Surg 1991;4:67–76
22. Pasternack PF, Grossi EA, Baumann F, et al. The value of silent myocardial ischemia monitoring in the prediction of perioperative myocardial infarction in patients undergoing peripheral vascular surgery. J Vasc Surg 1989;10:615–617
23. Fleischer LA, Rosenbaum SH, Nelson AH, et al. The predictive value of preoperative silent ischemia for postoperative ischemic cardiac events in vascular and nonvascular surgery patients. Am Heart J 1991;122:980
24. Boucher CA, Brewster DC, Darling RC, et al. Determination of cardiac risk by dipyridamole-thallium imaging before peripheral vascular surgery. N Engl J Med 1985;312:389–394
25. Cutler BS. Interpretation and results of intravenous dipyridamole thallium scintigraphy. Sem Vasc Surg 1991;4:83–89
26. Cambria RP, Brewster DC, Abbott WM, et al. The impact of selective use of dipyridamole-thallium scans and surgical factors on the current morbidity of aortic surgery. J Vasc Surg 1992;15:43–51

27. Lette J, Waters D, Lassonde J, et al. Multivariate clinical models and quantitative dipyridamole-thallium imaging to predict cardiac morbidity and death after vascular reconstruction. J Vasc Surg 1991;14:160–169
28. Baron JF, Mundler O, Bertrand M, et al. Dipyridamole-thallium scintigraphy and gated radionuclide angiography to assess cardiac risk before abdominal aortic surgery. N Engl J Med 1994;330:663–669
29. Chaitman BR, Ryan TJ, Kronmal RA, et al. Coronary artery surgery study (CASS): comparability of 10 year survival in randomized and randomizable patients. J Am Col Cardiol 1990;16:1071–1078
30. Cooperman M, Pflug B, Martin EW, et al. Cardiovascular risk factors in patients with peripheral vascular disease. Surgery 1978;84:505–509
31. Eagle KA, Singer DE, Brewster DC, et al. Dipyridamole-thallium scanning in patients undergoing vascular surgery. JAMA 1987;257:2185–2189
32. Eagle KA, Coley CM, Newell JB, et al. Combining clinical and thallium data optimizes preoperative assessment of cardiac risk before major surgery. Ann Intern Med 1989;110:859–66
33. Paul SD, Eagle KA, Kuntz KM, et al. Concordance of a validated clinical risk index with coronary angiography prior to vascular surgery (VAS): the Cleveland Clinic (CCF) experience. Presented at The American Heart Association 67th Scientific Sessions Meeting, November 14–17, 1994

PART II

Indications for Carotid Artery Surgery

Management of Extracranial Cerebrovascular Disease, edited by Keith D. Calligaro et al. Lippincott-Raven Publishers, Philadelphia © 1997.

6

Current Status of Carotid Endarterectomy for Asymptomatic Carotid Stenosis

Robert W. Hobson II

Asymptomatic carotid stenosis develops in patients who are, generally, 50 years of age or older, have an acknowledged increase in the incidence of coronary artery disease, hypertension, smoking, and hyperlipidemia.[1–4] Crouse et al[2] developed an ultrasonic scoring system of atherosclerotic carotid arterial wall thickening, and its increase has been documented for each decade of life after 40 years of age and for increasingly severe asymptomatic coronary artery disease. Furthermore, the association of increasingly severe internal carotid artery stenosis and a higher incidence of neurological events has been reported by several authors.[5,6] However, justification for prophylactic carotid endarterectomy in patients with asymptomatic carotid stenosis must be based on the supposition that its associated complications are less than the expected morbidity and mortality of the non-operated population. Analysis of carotid endarterectomy must consider the incidence of perioperative complications, including combined stroke and mortality (Table 6-1). In a recent review, Thompson[7] documented the low complication rates associated with operative intervention in patients with asymptomatic high-grade carotid stenosis. While these data represent clinical series of excellence, this must be contrasted with the higher complication rates reported in citywide analyses; for example, where the mortality was reported at 2.3% and the stroke rate at 5.6%.[8] Justification for prophylactic endarterectomy presupposes that the combined 30-day perioperative stroke and death rate will be less than 5% and preferably less than 3%.[9]

Despite publication of data from randomized clinical trials, surgical intervention in patients with asymptomatic carotid stenosis remains controversial. Results from two randomized clinical trials[10,11] in patients with asymptomatic carotid stenosis have been inconclusive. However, results from two recently published clinical trials, one conducted within the Veterans Administration (VA)[12] and one larger trial supervised by the National Institutes of Health (NIH)[13] demonstrated efficacy for carotid endarterectomy in management of asymptomatic carotid stenosis. The VA trial confirmed a reduction in combined neurological events of transient ischemic attack and stroke. Although stroke alone was reduced by a factor of 2:1 in the surgical group, addition of perioperative mortality resulted in the loss of statistical significance for this end point.[12] However, the NIH trial (Asymptomatic Carotid Atherosclerosis Study,

TABLE 6-1. *Morbidity and mortality of carotid endarterectomy for asymptomatic carotid disease*

Author (ref.)	Operations	Mortality	Morbidity: Transient	Morbidity: Permanent
Thompson et al[5]	167	0	2(1.2%)	2(1.2%)
Moore et al[6]	78	0	2(2.6%)	0
Hertzer et al[39]	95	1(1.1%)	–	4(4.2%)
Whitney et al[40]	279	3(1.1%)	5(1.8%)	6(2.2%)
Javid et al[41]	65	1(1.5%)	1(1.5%)	1(1.5%)
Anderson, Hobson et al[42]	120	0	2(1.7%)	0

ACAS) reached a positive conclusion regarding the benefit of carotid endarterectomy in reducing stroke alone and stroke/death in this asymptomatic population.[13]

Data from these two randomized clinical trials[12,13] now have confirmed an important role for operative intervention in significantly reducing neurological complications in patients with high-grade asymptomatic carotid stenosis in institutions reporting low surgical complication rates. This chapter reviews results from the various clinical trials and suggests a role for prophylactic carotid endarterectomy in selected patients with asymptomatic carotid stenosis.

DEFINING DEGREES OF STENOSIS

Characterizing the severity of carotid stenosis, particularly in the asymptomatic population continues to be a point of some contention.[14,15] The importance of determining the degree of stenosis relates to the threshold severity of stenosis selected by prospective randomized trials and their implications regarding patient management. The definition of clinically significant but asymptomatic carotid stenosis is usually related to the magnitude of stenosis present at the carotid bifurcation and proximal internal carotid artery. By convention, this has been defined as a 50% reduction in the luminal diameter of the artery or a 75% reduction in the cross-sectional area when accompanied by a positive noninvasive study such as ocular pneumoplethysmography (OPG)[16] or duplex scan.[17] The percentage stenosis is determined by comparing the least transverse diameter at the stenosis with the diameter of the distal uninvolved carotid artery (Fig. 6-1). This arteriographic methodology was adopted by the investigators in the VA asymptomatic trial[18] and subsequently by the ACAS investigators.[19] However, correlation between duplex scanning and the degree of stenosis as defined by the University of Washington criteria[20,21] requires modification to correlate these values with arteriographic estimates of stenosis.[22] One possible solution has been to recommend use of the 50% diameter reducing stenosis accompanied by positive OPG or duplex scan (area reducing stenosis of 75%) as the threshold lesion for intervention in symptomatic as well as asymptomatic patients.[14] However, use of rigid cut-off points is not realistic in clinical practice and should not be recommend-

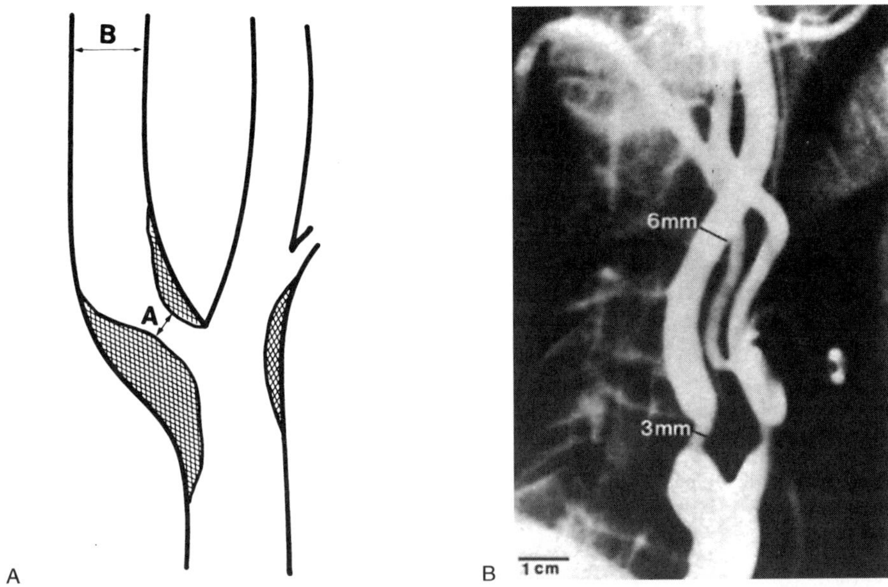

FIG. 6-1. The percentage of stenosis is calculated by dividing the least transverse diameter of the internal carotid artery at the stenosis (A), by the diameter of the distal, uninvolved artery (B). The minimum residual lumen diameter is equivalent to the least transverse diameter (A) divided by the magnification factor (MagF) of the arteriogram. The example illustrates a 50% stenosis by diameter and a minimum residual lumen diameter of 2.2 mm. (From Lynch TG, Hobson RW. Noninvasive cerebrovascular diagnostic techniques. In: Wilson SE, Veith FJ, Hobson RW, Williams RA (eds.). Vascular surgery: principles and practices. New York, McGraw Hill, 1987;105–134, with permission)

ed. To do so would eliminate some patients who might benefit from operation and needlessly subject many patients to the hazard of arteriography. Clinical data have confirmed that higher grade stenoses associated with a least transverse diameter of $\leq$ 1.0 mm at the stenosis[14,15] correlates stroke risk in symptomatic and asymptomatic patients. However, it should be emphasized that an analysis of the medical treatment groups from two randomized clinical trials[12,13] demonstrated that approximately 20% of the medical group sustained all neurological end points. Additional risk factors that must be considered in the future include ultrasonic plaque morphology, incidence of silent cerebral infarction confirmed by computed tomography (CT), status of the collateral cerebral circulation, and combination of clinical risk factors such as hypertension, coronary artery, history of smoking and peripheral vascular disease, which, when superimposed on the threshold degree of stenosis (area reducing stenosis of $\geq$ 75%), must be considered in contemplating endarterectomy. While it is incumbent on the clinical vascular surgeon to be aware of these issues, adoption of a plan to consider operative intervention in selected patients with asymptomatic carotid stenosis of 75% or more can now be recommended with confidence.

RESULTS OF RANDOMIZED CLINICAL TRIALS

During the past two years, results from randomized clinical trials on the efficacy of carotid endarterectomy in patients with asymptomatic carotid disease have been presented.[10–13] These results have been controversial at times and yet show a progression in terms of increasing numbers of patients randomized and their clinical impact on surgical practice.

Mayo Clinic Asymptomatic Carotid Endarterectomy Trial

The Mayo group[10] undertook a randomized clinical trial designed to compare the effects of carotid endarterectomy with medical management using low-dose aspirin in patients with asymptomatic carotid stenosis. Unfortunately, during a 30-month period of recruitment, only 71 randomizations were recorded and these investigators reported too few cerebral ischemic events to judge the comparative effectiveness of carotid endarterectomy versus low-dose aspirin. In addition, the trial was terminated because of a significantly higher incidence of myocardial events in the surgical group, which may have been related to absence of aspirin therapy in the patients managed by carotid endarterectomy. These investigators emphasized the importance of maintaining aspirin therapy in the surgically managed population and urged follow-up of the larger clinical trials.

CASANOVA Trial (Carotid Surgery Versus Medical Therapy in Asymptomatic Carotid Stenosis)

The CASANOVA investigators[11] suggested that this trial constituted a comparison of medical versus surgical management. However, as discussed in the authors' response[23] to an editorial review of the trial,[24] they agreed that a more appropriate understanding of the trial would be reflected in the proposed title, "Prophylactic Surgery Versus Selective Surgery for Treatment of Asymptomatic, Moderate (50–90%) Carotid Artery Stenosis." Their conclusion that no differences were observed between treatment groups, thereby negating the value of carotid endarterectomy in asymptomatic carotid stenosis, should be considered as an inappropriate judgment. This is based on several concerns regarding this particular trial. A total of 410 patients were identified as having asymptomatic stenosis in the range of 50–90%. Group A patients received carotid endarterectomy plus aspirin therapy (n=206) and Group B received aspirin therapy alone (n=204). Unfortunately, patients with stenoses ≥90% were immediately referred for operation, thereby negating the influence of surgical management on the group with perhaps the greatest likelihood of neurological events. Likewise, a number of patients in the so called "medical" group underwent operation but their outcome was not credited to carotid endarterectomy. This was based on an "intent to treat" protocol that resulted in an element of bias against surgical management. If a patient randomized to medical management showed disease progression to 90% stenosis or greater during the course of the follow-up, the patient underwent carotid endarterectomy. Of the medical group patients, 20% had carotid endarterectomy immediately after randomization (30 patients as part of the protocol for bilateral lesions and 10 in violation of the protocol) and an additional 20% had carotid endarterectomy as performed as part of the protocol during follow-up. Consequently, the CASANOVA investigators reported no significant difference in outcomes between two heterogenous treatment groups. Consistent with the trialists' final opinion, however, they recommended that further trials were necessary to resolve the question.

Veterans Affairs Trial on Asymptomatic Carotid Stenosis

A multicenter randomized clinical trial on asymptomatic carotid stenosis[12,18] was conducted at 11 Veterans Affairs Medical Centers throughout the United States to determine the efficacy of carotid endarterectomy on the combined incidence of transient ischemic attack, transient monocular blindness, and stroke in 444 adult male patients (mean age 64.5 years) with asymptomatic carotid stenosis (minimal stenosis for randomization: 50% arterial lumen diameter reduction on arteriography in the presence of a positive OPG or duplex scan, 75% area reduction). Patients were assigned randomly to optimal medical care including antiplatelet medication (aspirin) plus carotid endarterectomy (surgical group, 211 patients) or optimal medical management alone (medical group, 233 patients). All patients were followed independently by a vascular surgeon and a neurologist at each center for a mean period of 47.9 months. The combined incidence of ipsilateral neurologic events was 8% in the surgical group and 20.6% in the medical group ($p < 0.001$), relative risk (surgical group versus the medical group) of 0.38 (95% confidence interval, 0.22–0.67) (Fig. 6-2). Although the incidence of ipsilateral stroke alone was 4.7% in the surgical group and 9.4% in the medical group ($p = 0.056$), this 2:1 advantage in favor of the surgical group lost statistical significance when the 30-day operative mortality of 1.9%[12,25] was included in the analysis (Table 6-2). For those clinicians requiring significant reductions in stroke and death[26] among this group of patients, the results of the VA trial on asymptomatic carotid stenosis were not definitive and did not settle the controversy entirely. However, this randomized clinical trial was the first to confirm a reduction in neurological events in patients undergoing carotid endarterectomy for high-grade asymptomatic carotid stenosis.

Asymptomatic Carotid Atherosclerosis Study (ACAS) Trial

The ACAS trialists conducted the largest randomized clinical trial on asymptomatic carotid stenosis reported so far.[13] Acquisition of patients began in November 1987 and was completed in December 1992 with randomization of 1,662 male and female patients. This sample size is nearly four times that generated in the VA trial.

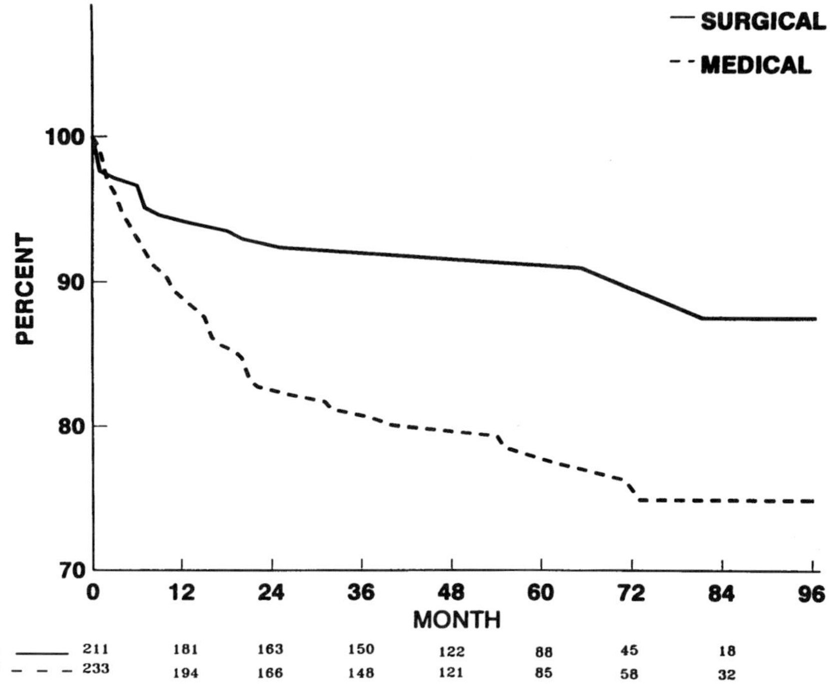

FIG. 6-2. Kaplan-Meier curves for event-free rates of first ipsilateral stroke and transient ischemic attack including transient monocular blindness. The analysis shows the time to the first event in the surgical and medical groups. The number of patients remaining event-free and in the study at the beginning of each 12-month period is shown below the graph. Comparisons between treatment groups (surgical, solid line; medical, dashed line) by the log-rank test demonstrated significant differences in favor of the surgical group ($p<0.001$). The relative risk in the surgical group as compared with the medical group was 0.38 (95% confidence interval, 0.22 to 0.67). (From Hobson, RW et al. N Engl J Med 1993;328:221–227, with permission)

While the VA trialists were able to document a reduction in TIA plus stroke after carotid endarterectomy, the ACAS trialists adjusted their statistical analysis midway during the trial to follow stroke alone in addition to the originally conceived combined neurological outcome of transient ischemic attack and stroke. On 28 September 1994 (after notification by the monitoring committee of the National Institute of

TABLE 6-2. *Incidence of ipsilateral stroke (%) and 30-day operative stroke or mortality (%) for VA[16] amd ACAS[13] trials*

	VA (n = 444)		*ACAS* (n = 1662)	
	Medical	Surgical	Medical	Surgical
Ipsilateral Stroke	9.4	4.7*	10.6	4.8**
Operative Complications	–	4.3	–	2.3

*Benefit for carotid endarterectomy, p = 0.056.
**Benefit for carotid endarterectomy, p = 0.006.

Neurological Disorders and Stroke), the ACAS Operations Center notified participating clinicians that an end point for stroke alone had reached statistical significance favoring carotid endarterectomy.[27] Using Kaplan-Meier projections at 5 years, the primary outcome of ipsilateral stroke was 5.1% for the surgical group and 11% for the medical group (Fig. 6-3). The larger sample size with its low surgical complica-

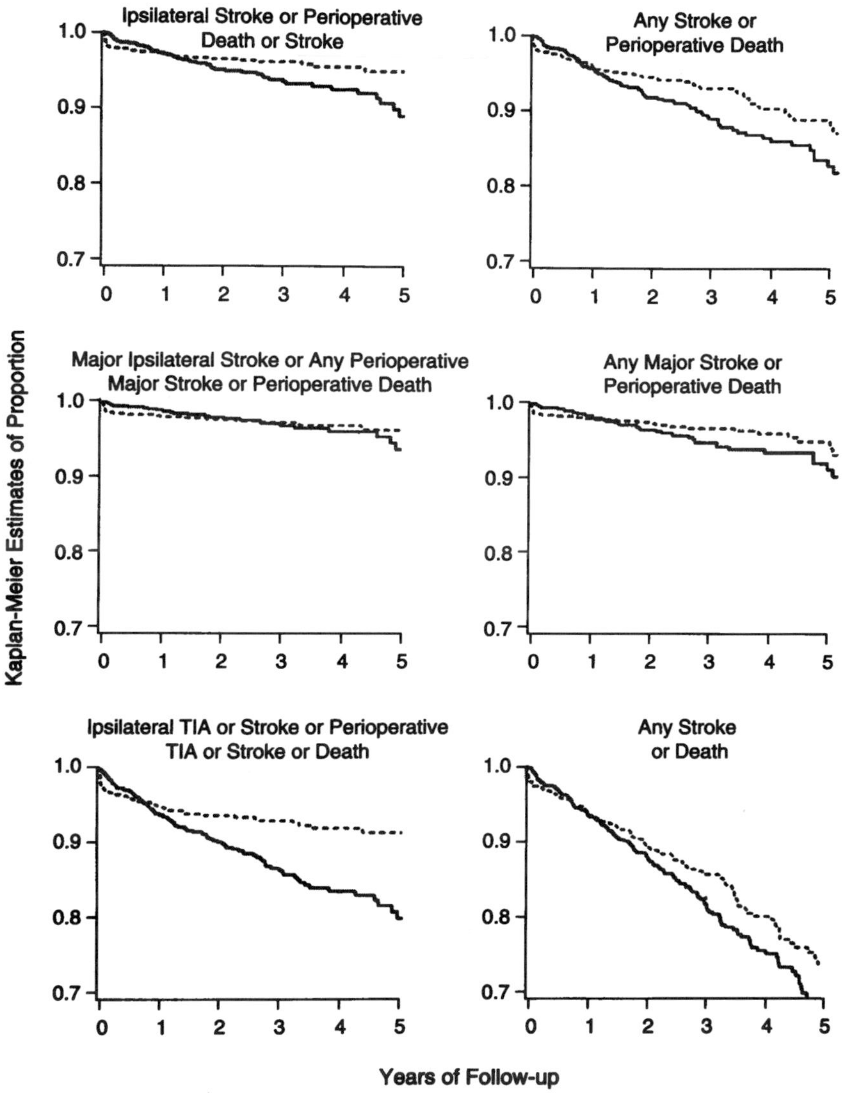

FIG. 6-3. Proportion of patients without end point at a given time during follow-up, by treatment group, using Kaplan-Meier estimation method. Solid line indicates medical patients; broken line, surgical patients; and TIA, transient ischemic attack. (From The Executive Committee for the Asymptomatic Carotid Atherosclerosis Study, JAMA 1995; 273:1421–1428, with permission)

tion rate (30-day stroke and perioperative mortality, 2.3% versus 4.7% for the VA trial) resulted in confirmation of this statistically significant reduction in stroke alone and stroke/death (p = 0.006), (Table 6-2). Differences in any major stroke or perioperative death and any stroke or death are of lesser significance. Although this represents a 53% relative risk reduction[13] in the primary end point of ipsilateral stroke, it should be noted that an absolute risk reduction of 11% in the medical group to 5.1% in the surgical group was achieved. Projected over a 5-year follow-up, this translates into an approximately 1% per year benefit, which, although significant, is a much less dramatic reduction than documented among symptomatic patients. This also presupposes confirmation of the operative complication rate reported in this trial–1.1% 30-day perioperative stroke or death with 1.2% attributed to angiography (combined 2.3% morbidity and mortality). If this track record can not be duplicated by a given institution's surgical group, use of prophylactic endarterectomy in this population indicates reassessment or referral to other groups.

European Trial on Asymptomatic Carotid Stenosis

The European trialists prepared a protocol for the randomization of patients with asymptomatic carotid stenosis.[28] Some pilot patients have been randomized and an analysis of feasibility has been completed. Patient acquisition is now underway and an important subset analysis on the influence of plaque morphology as determined by duplex scanning is included in the protocol. The complexity of reporting has been minimized in this trial's methodology and the trialists anticipate randomization of several thousand patients during the next 3–4 years.

OTHER CLINICAL ISSUES IN ASYMPTOMATIC CAROTID STENOSIS

A variety of other important issues have also been presented based on these prospective randomized trials. The influence of aspirin in patients with symptomatic carotid occlusive disease probably does have marginal benefit.[29] However, it should be emphasized that the use of antiplatelet therapy in patients with asymptomatic carotid stenosis has yet to be confirmed by randomized clinical trial. Hobson and the VA trialists,[30] however, reported a reduced incidence of combined neurological events (transient ischemic attack and stroke) in patients able to tolerate aspirin as compared with the group of patients unable to tolerate the drug. This suggests that aspirin therapy also may have a modest benefit in those patients with asymptomatic carotid stenosis who are unable to tolerate carotid endarterectomy.

Another important issue in the management of carotid asymptomatic carotid stenosis has to do with the cardiac prognosis and the incidence of significant complications in patients with and without coronary artery disease. Chimowitz and the VA group[31] reviewed the clinical data base in patients with carotid stenosis and coronary artery disease. It has been well recognized for some time that asymptomatic carotid stenosis and coronary disease are significantly correlated.[32] However, the influence of patients with and without history of coronary disease was considered important. These investigators confirmed that men with carotid stenosis and no history of coronary artery disease have a lower rate of cardiac events than men with carotid stenosis and a history of coronary artery disease. However, a subgroup of patients with carotid stenosis and no history of coronary artery disease who had coexistent intracranial occlusive disease, diabetes, or peripheral vascular disease have a risk of cardiac events similar to that of patients with a history of coronary disease. These data emphasize that absence of a history of coronary artery disease is not enough to eliminate this important risk factor in patients selected for carotid endarterectomy.[31] At the time of randomization of patients to the VA trial (1983–1987),[12] noninvasive scanning was not available for the assessment of patients with potential coronary disease. However, in our current practice we recommend the use of selective thallium scanning based on clinical criteria.[33] While it is acknowledged that use of screening tests for coronary artery disease will not reduce the currently reported low operative complication rates associated with carotid endarterectomy (see Table 6-1), these data can be used effectively in identifying patients with significant coronary disease and, if indicated, allow further work-up for possible coronary angiography, angioplasty, or bypass. In addition, these data may be used to select higher risk patients for medical management alone awaiting development of neurological symptoms before operative intervention. However, this should not be adopted as a routine justification for delay as reported strokes in one randomized trial[12] were not preceded by transient ischemic events, which confirmed the low incidence of warning neurological symptoms[34,35] in other retrospective studies.

Further analyses by Cohen et al[36] demonstrated that among adult male patients with high-grade asymptomatic carotid stenosis,[12] an overall mortality of 37% was reported at a mean follow-up of 4 years. Multivariate analysis resulted in a demonstrably greater risk for increased mortality rates in the presence of abnormal electrocardiograms, diabetes, and claudication. Patients with two or three of these risk factors were at high risk of death (Table 6-3) and may require aggressive treatment of their concurrent medical disease before considering carotid endarterectomy. In this way, risk management assessment becomes a factor in selecting patients for operative in-

TABLE 6-3*. *Mortality rate based on abnormal electrocardiography, diabetes and claudication as risk factors*

Risk group	No. of patients	Deaths (%)	Odds ratios	95% Confidence Intervals	
				Lower	Upper
No risk factors	65	14(22)	–	–	–
One risk factor	163	48(30)	1.52	0.76	3.00
Two risk factors	161	72(45)	2.95	1.51	5.75
Three risk factors	55	29(53)	4.06	1.84	8.99

*(From Cohen, SN et al. Deaths associated with asymptomatic carotid stenosis: long-term clinical evaluation. J Vasc Surg 1993; 18:1002–1011, with permission)

TABLE 6-4*. *Annual percentage rate of vascular events over period of follow-up*

Degree of stenosis	TIA	Stroke	Cardiac	Vascular deaths
<50% (mild)	1.0	1.3	2.7	1.8
50–75% (moderate)	3.0	1.3	6.6	3.3
>75% (severe)	7.2	3.3	8.3	6.5

*(From Norris JW, et al. Vascular risk of asymptomatic carotid stenosis. Stroke 1991; 22:1485, with permission).

tervention. Furthermore, recent assessment of the risk of stroke in patients with stenoses of >75%[37] suggests that this is an appropriate threshold for considering intervention. Patients with stenoses of <50% or <75% had a stroke risk of 1.3% annually, whereas those with stenosis of >75% had a combined TIA and stroke risk of 10.5% per year (Table 6-4). Cardiac event rates and vascular deaths correlated with increasing severity of asymptomatic carotid stenosis. In addition, patients with silent CT confirmed cerebral infarction were also at greater risk of subsequent stroke.[38]

CURRENT RECOMMENDATIONS

Data from randomized clinical trials have demonstrated that carotid endarterectomy combined with optimal medical management can reduce the incidence of ipsilateral neurologic outcome events,[12,13] now including stroke alone and stroke or death[13] in patients with arteriographically confirmed high-grade asymptomatic carotid stenosis. Despite the enhanced risk of transient ischemic attack and stroke for this population of patients, however, most will die as a result of coronary atherosclerosis. Consequently, care must be exercised in the selection of patients for operation. Acceptably low perioperative complication rates (see Table 6-1) should be confirmed by clinical audit at each institution before a program of operative intervention is instituted. Based on clinical criteria[33] and risk management assessments,[31,36] noninvasive testing for significant coronary artery disease is recommended. As noted above, this information may result in a non-operative decision in some patients; however, for those patients cleared of the associated risk of significant coronary artery diseases, carotid endarterectomy offers important advantages for selected individuals whose surgeons have confirmed low complication rates.

REFERENCES

1. Crouse JR, Toole JO, McKinney WM, et al. Risk factors for extracranial carotid artery atherosclerosis. Stroke 1987;16:990–996
2. Crouse JR, Harpold GH, Kahl FR, et al. Evaluation of a scoring system for extracranial carotid arteries with B-mode ultrasound. Stroke 1986;17:270–275
3. Wolf PA, Lannel WB, Sorlie P, et al. Asymptomatic carotid bruit and the risk of stroke. JAMA 1981;245:1442–1145

4. Heyman W, Wilkinson WE, Heyden S, et al. Risk of stroke in asymptomatic persons with cervical arterial bruits: a population study in Evans County, Georgia. N Engl J Med 1980;302:838–841
5. Thompson JF, Patman RD, Talking CM. Asymptomatic carotid bruit: long-term outcome in patients having endarterectomy compared with unoperated controls. Ann Surg 1978;188:308–316
6. Moore WS, Boren C, Malone JM, Goldstone J. Asymptomatic carotid stenosis: immediate and long-term results after prophylactic endarterectomy. Am J Surg 1979;138:228–233
7. Thompson JE. Carotid endarterectomy for asymptomatic carotid stenosis: an update. J Vasc Surg 1991;5:669–676
8. Brott TG, Labutta RJ, Kempczinski RF. Changing patterns in the practice of carotid endarterectomy in a large metropolitan area. JAMA 1986;255:2609–2612
9. Callow AD, Caplan LR, Correll JW, et al. Carotid endarterectomy: what is its current status? Am J Med 1988;85:835–838
10. The Mayo Asymptomatic Carotid Endarterectomy Study Group. Results of a randomized controlled trial of carotid endarterectomy for asymptomatic carotid stenosis. Mayo Clin Proc 1992;67:513–518
11. The CASANOVA Study Group. Carotid surgery versus medical therapy in asymptomatic carotid stenosis. Stroke 1991;22:1229–1235
12. Hobson RW, Weiss DG, Fields WS, Goldstone J, Moore WS, Towne JB, Wright CB, and the Veterans Affairs Cooperative Study Group. Efficacy of carotid endarterectomy for asymptomatic carotid stenosis. N Engl J Med 1993;328:221–227
13. The Executive Committee for the Asymptomatic Carotid Atherosclerosis Study. Endarterectomy for asymptomatic carotid artery stenosis. JAMA 1995;273:1421–1428
14. Hobson RW, Strandness, DE, Jr. Carotid artery stenosis: what's in the measurement? J Vasc Surg 1993;18:1069–70
15. Ackerman RH, Candia MR. Identifying clinically relevant carotid disease. Stroke 1994;25:1–3
16. Gee W, Mehigan JT, Wylie EJ. Measurement of collateral cerebral hemispheric blood pressure by ocular pneumoplethysmography. Am J Surg 1975;130:121–127
17. Blackshear WM, Jr, Phillips DJ, Thiele BL, et al. Detection of carotid occlusive disease by ultrasonic imaging and pulsed Doppler spectrum analysis. Surg 1979;86:698–706
18. A Veterans Administration Cooperative Study. Role of carotid endarterectomy in asymptomatic carotid stenosis. Stroke 1986;17:534–539
19. The Asymptomatic Carotid Atherosclerosis Study Group. Study design for randomized prospective trial of carotid endarterectomy for asymptomatic atherosclerosis. Stroke 1989;20:844–849
20. Roederer GO, Langlois YE, Jager KA, et al. The natural history of carotid arterial disease in asymptomatic patients with cervical bruits. Stroke 1984;15:605–613
21. Strandness DE, Jr. Extracranial arterial disease. In: Strandness DE, Jr (ed.) Duplex Scanning in Vascular Disorders. New York: Raven Press, 1990:90–120
22. Moneta GL, Edwards JM, Chitwood RW, et al. Correlation of North American Carotid Endarterectomy Trial (NASCET) angiographic definition of 70% to 90% internal carotid artery stenosis with duplex scanning. J Vasc Surg 1993;17:152–159
23. Diener HC: Response to Letter to the Editor. Stroke 1992;23:918
24. Solis MM, Ranval TJ, Barone GW, et al. The CASANOVA Study: immediate surgery versus delayed surgery for moderate carotid artery stenosis? (letter to the editor). Stroke 1992;23:917
25. Towne JB, Weiss DG, Hobson RW II. First phase report of cooperative Veterans Administration asymptomatic carotid stenosis study—operative morbidity and mortality. J Vasc Surg 1990;11:252–259
26. Barnett HJM, Haines SJ. Carotid endarterectomy for asymptomatic carotid stenosis. N Engl J Med 1993;328:276–279
27. ACAS Operations Center Announcement. Unpublished data, 1994
28. Halliday AW, Mansfield AO, Peto R. Medical Research Council, London. Unpublished data, 1994
29. Sze PC, Reitman D, Pincus MM, et al. Antiplatelet agents in the secondary prevention of stroke: meta-analysis of the randomized controlled trials. Stroke 1988;19:436–442
30. Hobson RW, Krupski WC, Weiss DG, et al. Influence of aspirin in the management of asymptomatic carotid artery stenosis. J Vasc Surg 1993;17:257–265
31. Chimowitz MI, Weiss DG, Cohen SL, et al. Cardiac prognosis of patients with carotid stenosis and no history of coronary artery disease. Stroke 1994;25:759–765
32. Wolf PA, Kannel WB, Sorlie P, et al. Asymptomatic carotid bruit and risk of stroke: the Framingham study. JAMA 1981;245:1442–1445
33. Eagle KA, Coley CM, Newell JB, et al. Continuing clinical and thallium data optimizes preoperative assessment of cardiac risk before major vascular surgery. Ann Intern Med 1989;110:859–866

34. Hennerici M, Hulsbomer HB, Hefter H, et al. Natural history of asymptomatic extracranial arterial disease. Brain 1987;110:777–791
35. Bogousslavsky J, Despland PA, Regli F. Asymptomatic tight stenosis of the carotid artery: long-term prognosis. Neurol 1986;36:861–863
36. Cohen SN, Hobson RW, Weiss DG, et al. Death associated with asymptomatic carotid artery stenosis: long-term clinical evaluation. J Vasc Surg 1993;18:1002–1011
37. Norris JW, Zhu CZ, Bornstein NM, et al. Vascular risks of asymptomatic carotid stenosis. Stroke 1991;22:1485–1490
38. Norris JW, Zhu CZ. Silent stroke and carotid stenosis. Stroke 1992;23:483–485
39. Hertzer NR, Flanagan RA, Beven EG, O'Hara PJ. Surgical versus nonoperative treatment of asymptomatic carotid stenosis. Ann Surg 1986;204:163–171
40. Whitney DG, Kahn EM, Estes JW, Jones CE. Carotid artery surgery without a temporary indwelling shunt. Arch Surg 1980;115:1393–1399
41. Javid H, Ostermiller WE, Hengesh JW, et al. Carotid endarterectomy for asymptomatic patients. Arch Surg 1971;102:389–391
42. Anderson RJ, Hobson RW II, Padberg FT, Jr, et al. Carotid endarterectomy for asymptomatic carotid stenosis: a ten-year experience with 120 procedures in a fellowship training program. Ann Vasc Surg 1991;5:111–115

Management of Extracranial Cerebrovascular Disease, edited by Keith D. Calligaro et al.
Lippincott-Raven Publishers, Philadelphia © 1997.

7

Operative Strategies for Combined Carotid and Coronary Disease

Steven M. Hertz, Bruce J. Brener, Donald K. Brief, Robert J. Goldenkranz, David E. Eisenbud, Jan Huston, Victor Parsonnet

The presence of simultaneous carotid and coronary atherosclerosis presents a difficult clinical challenge. Carotid endarterectomy (CEA) performed without addressing severe coronary stenosis may be associated with an increased risk of perioperative myocardial infarction (MI). Conversely, coronary artery bypass grafting (CABG) in patients with severe carotid stenosis may have an increased risk of perioperative strokc (CVA). Combining these two procedures was first described by Bernhard[1] in 1972; since that report many surgical series have been published detailing a varied experience with combined CEA/CABG. To date, there has been no clear consensus as to the appropriate usage of simultaneous and staged operative strategies in this high-risk patient group.

INCIDENCE OF SIMULTANEOUS DISEASE

The incidence of severe carotid stenosis in patients undergoing CABG varies depending on patient selection, screening protocol, and criteria utilized. The largest series of patients screened pre-CABG was published by Brener[2] from our institution. To date, over 6,000 patients have been studied; high-grade stenoses are present in approximately 5% of patients. Salasidis[3] reported that 8.5% of patients awaiting nonemergent CABG had a carotid lesion >80% by duplex scanning. Recently, Schwartz[4] noted a 22% incidence of >50% stenosis in 582 patients and a 12% incidence of >80% stenosis or occlusion. Ricotta[5] reported a 6.6% incidence of lesions greater than 75% by duplex scanning. It is clear from a review of this information that while incidence will vary by institution, many patients scheduled for elective CABG will harbor significant carotid artery stenoses. As patient selection for CABG expands to include older and sicker patients, carotid artery disease is likely to be present in even a higher proportion.

The incidence of severe coronary artery disease (CAD) in patients undergoing CEA has been studied as well. A classic paper by Hertzer[6] described the results of cardiac catheterization on 506 patients with carotid disease treated at the Cleveland Clinic. This study revealed a 35% incidence of severe coronary stenosis and occlusion. Boucher[7] noted redistribution abnormalities on cardiac thallium stress testing in 41% of patients awaiting peripheral vascular surgical repairs and demonstrated a correlation of this finding with perioperative ischemic events. Again, while the institution specific incidence will vary, a high percentage of patients with carotid disease will have significant CAD.

INCIDENCE OF ADVERSE EVENTS

Several additional facts must be established before a risk-to-benefit analysis of the various management strategies can be weighed. One important aspect of this decision revolves around the anticipated effect of proceeding with the planned procedure despite the presence of disease in the other arterial system. What effect could simultaneous disease be expected to have on the outcome of the planned primary procedure?

The occurrence of perioperative stroke, MI, and death in patients undergoing carotid endarterectomy has been well documented. Data from NASCET,[8] in which patients with coronary disease were carefully selected out, demonstrated a 1.8% risk of major or permanent stroke, a 0.9% risk of MI, and a 0.6% risk of death. In contrast, Ennix[9] reported the results of CEA in a series of over 1,500 patients. A subgroup of 77 patients with angina underwent CEA with a 15% risk of MI and a 18% risk of death. In fact it was results like this as described by Bernhard[1] in 1972 that led to his initial series of combined CEA/CABG.

The development of perioperative complications following CABG has also been thoroughly reported. Rizzo,[10] reporting the Brigham experience of over 3,000 coronary bypass procedures performed on patients without known carotid disease, showed a 1% rate of permanent stroke, 4.7% rate of MI, and a 4% rate of death. In contrast to this experience are reports of patients undergoing isolated CABG with known carotid disease. Brener[2] demonstrated a 6.3% stroke risk and a 15.7% mortality risk in this patient group. Ricotta[5] analyzed over 1,000 patients undergoing CABG, reporting a 1.6% stroke rate and a 2.3% mortality rate. In this study approximately 15% of patients screened by carotid duplex were found to have lesions creating a stenosis >50%. Logistic regression analysis showed that carotid stenosis greater than 50% was an independent risk factor to identify patients at risk for stroke from CABG.

STAGED VERSUS SIMULTANEOUS PROCEDURES

Knowledge that isolated procedures performed on patients with combined carotid and coronary disease carry increased risks have prompted a vast and varied experience in strategies of operative management. To assist in determining whether this experience could be used to draw conclusions about optimal patient care, Brener[11] performed a meta-analysis of the available reports of staged and combined operative strategies. Review of this data and other available reports is enlightening and supports many of the suspicions of previous authors.

Staged Strategy—CEA 1st, CABG 2nd

More than 15 studies provide information on the results of staged surgery in which the carotid endarterectomy was performed prior to the CABG.[1,9,12–26] The only study performed in a prospective, randomized fashion was published by Hertzer[22] in 1989. In this series from the Cleveland Clinic, the strategy of CEA first represented a small fraction of the total patients with combined disease whose cardiac disease was "stable" (24/275; 8.7%). Stroke and death rates for these patients were 4.2% and 4.2% for the two procedures cumulatively. Ruel[18] reported the largest series of 164 patients with this operative strategy, yielding a 2.4% stroke rate and a 4.9% death rate. Recently Coyle's report[25] showed a 4.4% stroke rate and a low 2.2% death rate. Curl[26] presented similar encouraging data in a carefully selected group with combined disease undergoing staged CEA followed by CABG, yielding a 3.1% stroke rate and a 3.1% death rate. As these studies were not randomized, clearly patients are preselected to undergo the particular sequence of operations chosen. This may result in a selection bias and, therefore, patients in these reports with staged performance of CEA first are likely to have less severe or less symptomatic heart disease. In addition, refinements in appropriate patient selection, improvements in preoperative, intraoperative and postoperative patient care, and better management of myocardial infarction might be expected to improve results. Despite this possible influence, Brener's meta-analysis[11] showed a high rate of MI (11.5%) and death (9.4%) when an "unprotected" CEA followed by CABG was performed. Combined stroke rate was 5.3%. These results suggest a high rate of cardiac event and death in this operative strategy, while yielding an acceptable combined stroke rate.

"Reversed" Staged Strategy—CABG 1st, CEA 2nd

Multiple studies have been published reporting "unprotected" CABG followed by CEA.[1,9,12,14,20,22] In Hertzer's report,[22] 58 patients were randomized to this "reversed" staged strategy. The combined stroke rate was 14%. The stroke rate associated with subsequent CEA decreased from 11 to 2.2% when CEA was performed more than 2 weeks after CABG. The mortality rate was 3.7%. Ennix[9] reported a far more favorable experience with a combined risk of stroke (2.4%), MI (2.4%), and death (1.2%). As in the previous strategy described, it is clear that selection bias may well have influenced results in different series. In the meta-analysis by Brener,[11] the strategy of CABG followed by CEA represented the smallest subset, comprising 213 patients out of a total 2,928 (7.3%). Overall stroke risk for both procedures was 10%. The risk of MI was 2.7% and the risk of death 3.6%. The majority of strokes occurred in the CABG perioperative period but many occurred several days following CABG.

In the Cleveland Clinic series, the stroke rate for subsequent CEA was 5 of 81 (6%), higher than their experience performing CEA in other patients.

Comparison of the two staged strategies demonstrates that in patients undergoing staged CABG followed by CEA, the overall risk of stroke appears increased. Performance of preliminary CABG in the reversed staged strategy, however, may be protective of cardiac morbidity and mortality.

Combined Repair—Simultaneous CEA and CABG

More than 20 years of experience with combined repair of the carotid and coronary vessels has been accumulated. Many reports have been published, representing over 2,300 operations.[1,2,10,12–24,27–44] Indications for simultaneous repair and conduct of the procedure varied by institution, and, therefore, results are subject to selection bias as were the alternative strategies. In the only prospective, randomized data, Hertzer[22] reported on 71 patients assigned to simultaneous repair. The stroke rate was 5.3% and the mortality rate was 5.3%. Rizzo,[10] in a series with over 100 patients, noted similar statistics, with a 6.3% risk of CVA and a 5.5% risk of death.

Others have reported better outcomes. Chang[44] showed a 1% stroke rate and a 2% mortality rate. Still other current series show far worse statistics. Coyle[25] demonstrated a 26.2% combined risk of stroke and death. Brener's meta-analysis showed a 6.2% stroke risk, 4.7% MI risk, and a 5.6% death risk for this combined strategy.[11]

COMPARISON OF MANAGEMENT STRATEGIES

Can the information presented in this chapter be used to draw meaningful comparisons among the possible strategies and, thus, aid clinical decision making? In the meta-analysis of operative strategies, the stroke risk was significantly higher in the "reversed" staged strategy (CABG 1st, CEA 2nd). Stroke risk was similar if CEA preceded CABG or was performed simultaneously. The risk of MI and death was increased in the staged strategy (CEA 1st, CABG 2nd) in comparison to the other strategies.

Based on this information, it would appear that a combined approach may be a practical solution for patients with severe carotid and coronary disease. The economic and psychologic benefits of performing one operation is another factor which should be considered.

NEED FOR A RANDOMIZED PROSPECTIVE STUDY

The findings summarized in this chapter confirm that performance of carotid endarterectomy in the presence of unaddressed severe cardiac disease may be likely to result in an unacceptable rate of cardiac morbidity and mortality. Also confirmed is the suspicion that coronary artery bypass grafting performed in the face of critical carotid stenosis may lead to an unacceptably high risk of perioperative neurologic events. A combined surgical approach may provide a safe, practical alternative in this difficult and high-risk patient group.

Conclusions drawn from the experience discussed in this chapter, however, must be taken with the knowledge that significant selection and referral bias is likely to exist in the majority of the reports discussed. It is likely that many retrospective reports fail to identify some patients who never had the second part of a planned staged procedure because of an adverse event after the first operation, thereby underreporting the true morbidity and mortality statistics. Only a carefully designed, prospective, randomized study could definitively answer the questions raised.

CONCLUSIONS

The management of patients with coronary and carotid disease is complex. The greater severity of disease in one system may make a staged approach appropriate in carefully selected patients. Patients with severe disease in both arterial areas may be best served by combined procedures.

REFERENCES

1. Bernhard VM, Johnson WD, Peterson JJ. Carotid artery stenosis: association with surgery for coronary artery disease. Arch Surg 1972;105:837–840
2. Brener BJ, Brief DK, Alpert J, Goldenkranz RJ, Parsonnet V. The risk of stroke in patients with asymptomatic carotid stenosis undergoing cardiac surgery: a follow-up study. J Vasc Surg 1987;5:269–279
3. Salasidis GC, Latter DA, Steinmetz OK, Blair J, Graham AM. Carotid artery duplex scanning in the preoperative assessment for coronary artery revascularization: the association between peripheral vascular disease, carotid artery stenosis, and stroke. J Vasc Surg 1995;21:154–162
4. Schwartz LB, Bridgman AH, Kieffer RW, Wilcox RA, McCann RL, Tawil MP, Scott SM. Asymptomatic carotid artery stenosis and stroke in patients undergoing cardiopulmonary bypass. J Vasc Surg 1995;21:146–153
5. Ricotta JJ, Faggioli GL, Castilone A, Hassett JM. Risk factors for stroke after cardiac surgery: Buffalo cardiac-cerebral study group. J Vasc Surg 1995;21:359–364
6. Hertzer NR, Young JR, Beven EG, Graor RA, O'Hara PJ, Ruschhaupt WF, deWolfe VG, Maljovec LC. Coronary angiography in 506 patients with extracranial cerebrovascular disease. Arch Intern Med 1985;145:849–852
7. Boucher CA, Brewster DC, Darling RC, Okada RD, Strauss HW, Pohost GM. Determination of cardiac risk by dipyridamole-thallium imaging before peripheral vascular surgery. N Engl J Med 1985;312:389–394
8. North American Symptomatic Carotid Endarterectomy Trial (NASCET). Beneficial effect of carotid endarterectomy in symptomatic patients with high-grade carotid stenosis. N Engl J Med 1991;325: 445–453
9. Ennix CL, Lawrie GM, Morris GC, Crawford ES, Howell JF, Reardon MJ, Weatherford SC. Improved results of carotid endarterectomy in patients with symptomatic coronary disease: an analysis of 1,546 consecutive carotid operations. Stroke 1979;10:122–125
10. Rizzo RJ, Whittemore AD, Couper GS, Donaldson MC, Aranki SF, Collins JJ, Mannick JA, Cohen LH. Combined carotid and coronary revascularization: the preferred approach to the severe vasculopath. Ann Thorac Surg 1992;54:1099–1109
11. Brener BJ, Hermans H, Eisenbud DE, et al. The management of patients requiring coronary bypass and carotid endarterectomy. Chapter in press.

12. Urschel HC, Razzuk MA, Gardner MA. Management of concomitant occlusive disease of the carotid and coronary arteries. J Thorac Cardiovasc Surg 1976;72:829–834
13. Mehigan JT, Buch WS, Pipkin ED, Fogarty TJ. A planned approach to coexistent cerebrovascular disease in coronary artery bypass candidates. Arch Surg 1977;112:1403–1409
14. Rosenthal D, Caudill DR, Lamis PA, Logan W, Stanton PE. Carotid and coronary artery disease: a rational approach. Am Surg 1984;50:233–235
15. Berkoff HA, Turnipseed WD. Patient selection and results of simultaneous coronary and carotid artery procedures. Ann Thorac Surg 1984;38:172–175
16. Ivey TD. Combined carotid and coronary disease—a conservative strategy. J Vasc Surg 1986;3:687–689
17. Babu SC, Shah PM, Singh BM, Semel L, Clauss RH, Reed GE. Coexisting carotid stenosis in patients undergoing cardiac surgery: indications and guidelines for simultaneous operations. Am J Surg 1985;150:207–211
18. Reul GJ Jr, Cooley DA, Duncan JM, et al. The effect of coronary bypass on the outcome of peripheral vascular operations in 1093 patients. J Vasc Surg 1986;3:788–798
19. Marinelli G, Turinetto B, Bombardini T, Dozza F, Pierangeli V, Pierangeli A. Surgical approach to combined carotids and coronaries lesions. Inter Angio 1987;6:393–396
20. Newman DC, Hicks RG. Combined carotid and coronary artery surgery: a review of the literature. Ann Thorac Surg 1988;45:574–581
21. Schultz RD, Sterpetti AV, Feldhaus RJ. Early and late results in patients with carotid disease undergoing myocardial revascularization. Ann Thorac Surg 1988;45:603–609
22. Hertzer NR, Loop FD, Beven EG, O'Hara PJ, Krajewski LP. Surgical staging for simultaneous coronary and carotid disease: a study including prospective randomization. J Vasc Surg 1989;9:455–463
23. Faggioli GI, Curl GR, Ricotta JJ. The role of carotid screening before coronary artery bypass. J Vasc Surg 1990;12:724–731
24. Carrel T, Stillhard G, Turina M. Combined carotid and coronary artery surgery: early and late results. Cardiology 1992;80:118–125
25. Coyle KA, Gray BC, Smith RB, et al. Morbidity and mortality associated with carotid endarterectomy: effect of adjunctive coronary revascularization. Ann Vasc Surg 1995;9:21–27
26. Curl GR, Leney GA, Castilone A, et al. Carotid endarterectomy in coronary bypass patients: the effect of timing and risk factors on outcome (abstract) presented at the 9th annual Eastern Vascular Society Meeting, Buffalo, NY, May 1995 (publication pending)
27. Okies JE, MacManus Q, Starr A. Myocardial revascularization and carotid endarterectomy: a combined approach. Ann Thorac Surg 1977;23:560–563
28. Rice PL, Pifarré R, Sullivan HJ, Montoya A, Bakhos M. Experience with simultaneous myocardial revascularization and carotid endarterectomy. J Thorac Cardiovasc Surg 1980;79:922–925
29. Schwartz RL, Garrett JR, Karp RB, Kouchoukos NT. Simultaneous myocardial revascularization and carotid endarterectomy. Circulation 1982;66(Suppl I):I-97–I-101
30. Hertzer NR, Loop FD, Taylor PC, Beven EG. Combined myocardial revascularization and carotid endarterectomy. J Thorac Cardiovasc Surg 1983;85:577–589
31. Perler BA, Burdick JF, Williams M. The safety of carotid endarterectomy at the time of coronary artery bypass surgery: analysis of results in a high-risk patient population. J Vasc Surg 1985;2:558–563
32. Dunn EJ. Concomitant cerebral and myocardial revascularization. Surg Clin North Am 1986;66:385–395
33. Lord RSA, Graham AR, Shanahan MX, Chang V, Reece AS, Farnsworth AE, Esmore DS, Spratt P. Rationale for simultaneous carotid endarterectomy and aortocoronary bypass. Ann Vasc Surg 1986;1: 201–207
34. Matar AF. Concomitant coronary and cerebral revascularization under cardiopulmonary bypass. Ann Thorac Surg 1986;44:431–435
35. Lubicz S, Kelly A, Field PL, Westlake GW, Buxton B, Connell JL, Clarebrough JK. Combined carotid and coronary surgery. Aust N Z J Surg 1987;57:593–597
36. Lusiani L, Visona A, Castellani V, Ronsisvalle G, Pagnan A, Bonanonome A, Scaldalai E, Cirillo FM, Valfre C, Gallucci V. Prospective evaluation of combined carotid and coronary surgery. Eur J Cardiothorac Surg 1987;1:16–19
37. Minami K, Gawaz M, Ohlmeier H, Vyska K, Körfer R. Management of concomitant occlusive disease of coronary and carotid arteries using cardiopulmonary bypass for both procedures. J Cardiovasc Surg 1989;30:723–728

38. Jausseran JM, Bergeron P, Reggi M, Chiche G, Serra-Rosset G, Courbier R. Single staged carotid and coronary arteries surgery: indications and results. J Cardiovasc Surg 1989;30:407–413
39. Cambria RP, Ivarsson BL, Akins CW, Moncure AC, Brewster DC, Abbott WM. Simultaneous carotid and coronary disease: safety of the combined approach. J Vasc Surg 1989;9:56–64
40. Duchateau J, Nevelsteen A, Sergeant P, Flameng W, Suy R. Combined myocardial and cerebral revascularization. J Cardiovasc Surg 1989;30:715–722
41. Pome G, Fassini L, Colucci V, et al. Combined surgical approach to coexistent carotid and coronary artery disease. J Cardiovasc Surg 1991;32:757–793
42. Weiss SJ, Sutter FP, Shannon TO, Goldman SM. Combined carotid operation and carotid endarterectomy during aortic cross-clamping. Ann Thorac Surg 1992;53:813–816
42. Vermeulen FEE, Hamerlijnck RPHM, Defauw JJAM, Ernst SMPG. Synchronous operation for ischemic cardiac and cerebrovascular disease: early results and long-term follow-up. Ann Thorac Surg 1992;53:381–390
43. Vermeulen FEE. Simultaneous extensive extracranial and coronary revascularization: long-term follow-up up to 13 years. Eur J Cardiothorac Surg 1988;2:113–123
44. Chang BB, Darling RC III, Shah DM, Paty PSK, Leather RP. Carotid endarterectomy can be safely performed with acceptable mortality and morbidity in patients requiring coronary artery bypass grafts. Am J Surg 1994;168:94–96

Management of Extracranial Cerebrovascular Disease, edited by Keith D. Calligaro et al.
Lippincott-Raven Publishers, Philadelphia © 1997.

8

How Soon Can Carotid Endarterectomy Be Safely Performed Following an Ischemic Stroke?

Mark D. Morasch, William H. Baker

Carotid endarterectomy was introduced into the therapeutic armamentarium of physicians in the 1950s. Shortly after Eascott and colleagues[1] described the first successful carotid reconstruction to treat transient hemispheric symptoms, others began exploring new indications for the procedure. As a result, in the early 1960s carotid endarterectomy was thought by many to be a panacea for both patients with transient symptoms and patients with strokes. Consequently, the operation was performed in patients with both acute and chronic stroke syndromes who, in addition, had a significant carotid stenosis or occlusion. Reports from this era were mixed but it soon became evident that the operation should not be performed in the acute setting in those patients who had a severe neurologic deficit. Today, the benefits of carotid endarterectomy in both symptomatic and asymptomatic patients with significant carotid artery stenosis have been firmly established.[2,3,4] The question of when is the best time to perform carotid endarterectomy in specific subgroups of patients, including those following mild to moderate acute ischemic stroke, remains unanswered.

THE HISTORY OF EMERGENCY SURGERY FOR ACUTE STROKE

The initial reports of early carotid endarterectomy in patients who had had acute cerebrovascular accidents were disappointing. A significant number of postoperative deaths resulting from cerebral hemorrhage were noted during the early 1960s. Bruetman et al[5] were the first to describe these catastrophic results. They reported their findings in six stroke patients who underwent acute revascularization of the ischemic hemisphere. Following revascularization in the acute phase of stroke they noted consistent post-mortem findings of significant intracerebral hemorrhage with blood in the ventricles and subarachnoid spaces. These findings were similar to the pathologic changes seen in patients who died following stroke as described by Fisher and Adams in 1951.[6]

These early reports formed the basis for the observation that the timing of surgery to reestablish normal cerebral perfusion pressure is of critical importance. Early establishment of pressure into recently infarcted brain could lead to cerebral hemorrhage. One year later, Wylie[7] described 9 patients with acute stroke; catastrophic hemorrhages developed in 5 of 9 patients during the perioperative period; 3 followed thromboendarterectomy of completely occluded internal carotid vessels while the other 2 were noted following endarterectomy of high-grade stenotic lesions. He implicated hemorrhage following destruction of a previously intact blood brain barrier as the cause. Similarly, in 1969 Rob[8] reported his results following acute revascularization of 74 occluded carotid arteries in patients with completed or progressing stroke symptoms. He reported that only 21% derived benefit with regards to symptomatology, while 29% died during the postoperative period. Similar manuscripts with similar results followed and, consequently, carotid surgery for acute stroke, particularly when associated with profound deficits, was, for the most part, abandoned.[9,10,11] It may be important to note that the majority of the early reported failures occurred in patients who were operated on in the face of profound neurologic deficits with altered sensorium. Many operations were performed to re-open totally occluded vessels and virtually all were completed many hours to days following the acute event.

In 1969 the Joint Study of Extracranial Occlusion[12] indicted early revascularization, citing a 42% mortality rate following operations on the carotid in the face of acute stroke. The group concluded that owing to the increased incidence of complications following vascular surgery performed during the first few days after an acute neurologic deficit, revascularization in this setting was contraindicated. They also concluded that complete occlusion of the internal carotid artery constituted a contraindication to carotid endarterectomy. The paucity of evidence proving benefit, the increased incidence of conversion to hemorrhagic infarct, and the high perioperative mortality rate formed the basis for these opinions. As a result, this report led to an era in which all patients with any sort of neurologic deficit had at least a 30-day waiting period between the onset of any persistent deficit and the performance of a revascularization procedure. A series of reports and editorials extending into the 1980s lended support to these recommendations, resulting in reluctance to relax these guidelines.[11,13,14,15]

It must be noted, however, that not all of these early reports were entirely condemning. Throughout the 1960s and 1970s sporadic reports of successes begged the question of whether there were subgroups of patients with acute stroke who may benefit from earlier operation. In a reappraisal of his series Rob[16] felt that in the case of embolic obstruction from a cardiac source the results of carotid thromboembolectomy were satisfactory when the condition was promptly diagnosed and treated. Following a 1971 review of 53 patients undergoing emergent carotid revascularization, Najafi et al[17] agreed that patients with profound deficits as well as patients with stroke syndrome lasting beyond a few hours were not good candidates for emergent surgery. They did, however, report that nearly half of the patients operated on following rapid assessment benefited dramatically from surgery, some with complete resolution of symptoms, and they were able to achieve a mortality rate of only 12% in this group. Meyer et al[18] added clinical support to the concept of a critical period of reversible ischemia, in which compromised neurons may be salvaged, when they reported their optimistic results following emergent carotid revascularization in 34 patients with acute carotid occlusion and profound neurologic deficits. Thirty eight percent made a dramatic recovery while their 20% mortality compared favorably with the natural history of profound stroke. While they agreed that operation should not be considered following prolonged delay, they also indicated that the absence of a middle cerebral embolus and the presence of good collateral flow permitted time for preoperative angiography, and this was the underlying basis for their success. Donaldson[19] suggested that the progression from cell injury to cell infarction is related to both the degree and duration of ischemia. In theory, carotid endarterectomy may even be expected to reverse neurologic deficit if (1) the severe carotid stenosis or occlusion were merely compromising neurologic function by decreasing blood flow to cerebral tissue and (2) damage to the brain was not yet irreparable. The single common denominator noted among these early success stories was rapid assessment and treatment, often within a few hours of the onset of symptoms, prior to the completion of the infarct.

LABORATORY OBSERVATIONS

Numerous reports have followed the initial publications by Breutman and Wylie describing intracranial hemorrhage following ipsilateral carotid endarterectomy in the face of acute stroke. These reports have certainly prompted a degree of caution among vascular surgeons, which continues today. The etiology of the conversion of "bland" to hemorrhagic infarction is not entirely understood but evidence would suggest that the pathophysiology is multifactorial. Devastating post-endarterectomy hemorrhage has been observed most commonly following revascularization and reperfusion of frankly infarcted cerebral tissue. Fatal hemorrhage has been reported to occur from hours to weeks post carotid endarterectomy and has also been noted to occur in areas of brain outside the infarcted zone.[20] Recently, similar cases of postoperative intracerebral hemorrhage have been reported in patients with no preoperative clinical or radiographic evidence of stroke[21,22] apparently related to restoration of normotensive blood flow to vessels that have lost the normal ability to autoregulate.[22] Risk factors for postendarterectomy hemorrhage have been noted to include hypertension[20,23] anticoagulation,[24] hyperperfusion syndrome, following correction of longstanding high-grade internal carotid artery stenosis[23] as well as recent stroke. Hemorrhage has variably been attributed not only to reperfusion but to uncontrolled postoperative hypertension[20] and to particulate embolization at the time of surgery.[25]

Animal studies carried out in the 1950s by Harvey and Rasmussen[26] resulted in the initial descriptions of hemorrhagic infarct and they were the first to suggest that changes in blood pressure within ischemic tissue could lead to these typical ischemic findings. Fisher and Adams[6] performed pathologic sectioning of post-mortem cadaveric specimens. They described hemorrhagic infarction following embolism as "obviously arterial" with necrotic tissue "stippled with small hemorrhages" resulting from extravasation from arterioles, capillaries, and venules. Meyer[27] induced brain tissue infarction in monkeys by clamping the middle cerebral artery. Within 2 hours a cascade of microscopic changes occurred, culminating in severe endothelial cell damage with pericapillary and periventricular hemorrhage both in and around the area of infarction. Rapid return of perfusion pressure to the area resulted in further extension and large hemorrhagic infarction. Maximal perivascular bleeding was noted between the second and fourth day following vessel occlusion.

An abundance of clinical and experimental evidence exists to suggest that not only is reperfusion of frankly infarcted tissue likely to result in hemorrhagic changes, but hemorrhage can also extend throughout the peri-infarct tissue and into adjacent normal, nonischemic brain, owing to the lost ability of local cerebral vasculature to autoregulate. In ischemic brain tissue, normal autoregulatory mechanisms responsible for resisting changes in blood flow are lost, and vessels tend to remain maximally dilated. Hachinski[28] utilized positron emission tomography (PET) to demonstrate a zone of ischemic but viable brain tissue surrounding focal infarction. Within this "ischemic penumbra" vessels appear to maximally vasodilate regardless of changes in perfusion pressure (*i.e.,* they are in a state of vasomotor paralysis).[29] When the ability for blood vessels to autoregulate is lost, blood flow becomes passively dependent on blood pressure. The combination of the loss of vasomotor tone and hypertension results in abnormally elevated perfusion pressures, which are capable of precipitating small vessel disruption and hemorrhage within and adjacent to areas of infarct. Carotid endarterectomy of a critical stenosis invariably results in increased ipsilateral blood flow and pressure. Clinically hemorrhagic infarction may occur. On the other hand, if infarction and hemorrhage do not occur, endarterectomy could theoretically salvage non-infarcted ischemic brain tissue within the ischemic penumbra as well as, potentially, prevent further ischemic damage due to recurrent embolization.

It has been suggested that the presence or absence of cerebral vasomotor reactivity can be identified and quantitated within the distribution of the ipsilateral middle cerebral artery by means of cerebral blood flow studies or by transcranial Doppler (TCD) evaluation used in concert with varying degrees of hypo- and hypercarbia or acetazolamide. Utilizing TCD measurements and CO_2 inhalation Ringelstein et al[30] were able to identify a significant reduction in vasomotor reactivity in patients with CT scan positive low-flow infarcts when compared to patients with normal CT scans. There was no difference in vasomotor reactivity between groups of patients with CT scan positive embolic stroke and patients with normal CT scans. Infusion of acetazolamide has since been found to be as sensitive as hyper- and hypocarbia and more convenient to use.[31] The ability to quantify hemispheric vasomotor reserve may help identify patients who may benefit from early carotid endarterectomy while decreasing the risk for perioperative hemorrhagic infarction. To our knowledge, this technology, while encouraging, has not been applied clinically in the acute stroke patient who is undergoing evaluation prior to early endarterectomy.

THE VALUE OF COMPUTED TOMOGRAPHY AND MAGNETIC RESONANCE IMAGING

At present computed tomography (CT) and magnetic resonance imaging (MRI) do not reliably differentiate between areas of reversible and irreversible ischemia (*i.e.,* between infarct and "ischemic penumbra"). It has been suggested that CT can delineate areas of cerebral tissue where the vascular integrity has been breached. Wing et al[32] have implied that the radiographic enhancement seen in and around areas of infarction on non-contrast CT brain scan results from loss of integrity of the blood–brain barrier. This is said to be due to loss of the normal autoregulatory mechanisms as detailed above. This implies that the presence of localized enhancement on preoperative CT scan predicts an increased risk of postoperative hemorrhagic infarction if endarterectomy proceeds in the acute setting. Ricotta et al[33] reported that the results of urgent carotid endarterectomy for acute stroke were directly related to the findings on preoperative CT scanning. When the preoperative CT scan was negative for stroke, they noted that 15 of 17 patients (88%) improved clinically, while only 1 patient deteriorated. When the CT scan was abnormal, only 5 patients (50%) improved while 4 (40%) clinically deteriorated. Little,[34] from the Cleveland Clinic, reported similar findings. Of 22 neurologically stable patients with mild deficits and normal results of a CT scan all survived operation well without permanent morbidity or mortality. Two patients with moderate, stable neurologic deficits and recent infarction on CT also had uneventful postoperative courses. Five patients were neurologically unstable preoperatively. Two patients with transient ischemic attacks and normal scans did well. Two of the 3 patients with a progressive neurologic picture and recent infarction on CT had extension of their neurologic deficit postoperatively. Thus, the patients neurologic status seems to be as important as the findings on the CT scan.

This opinion has been substantiated by numerous other investigators who report no increase in the incidence of hemorrhagic infarction following urgent carotid endarterectomy, even if the preoperative CT scan demonstrates radiologic evidence of stroke.[11,35] Most recently, Gasecki and associates reported the results from the North American Symptomatic Carotid Endarterectomy Trial (NASCET). Not only was the risk of subsequent stroke after carotid endarterectomy equal in two groups (operation less than 30 days and greater than 30 days), but there were no strokes in 17 patients operated on early who had an abnormal CT scan.[36]

MRI possesses the capability to define more precisely areas of cerebral infarction; this modality is able to identify these areas earlier than with CT. The use of MRI in the preoperative evaluation of patients with acute stroke syndromes has not yet been thoroughly investigated. The development of this modality may lead to more defined surgical criteria. At present the usefulness of MRI and CT scanning in the preoperative evaluation of the acute-stroke patient with respect to timing surgical intervention is undefined.

STROKE IN EVOLUTION

The Ad Hoc Committee to the Joint Council of the Society for Vascular Surgery and the North American Chapter of the International Society for Cardiovascular Surgery in March of 1992[37] defined stroke in evolution as a variation of acute stroke where neurologic changes begin with "one level of deficit, and in a progressive or stuttering fashion the deficit worsens." Questions regarding proper management of patients with stroke in evolution have been frequently addressed. Goldstone and Moore,[38] in 1976, after observing several patients with unstable neurologic deficits of mild-to-moderate degree progress to a severe fixed neurologic stroke adopted a successful approach of aggressive surgical management. They reported on 8 patients with stroke in evolution, each with a critical or unstable stenotic arterial lesion as defined by angiography, who underwent urgent revascularization. All 8 recovered completely without residual neurologic deficit. They concluded that patients with symptoms consistent with stroke in evolution differed from those with frank stroke in that infarction had not occurred and operation could prevent further brain damage. They recommended early operation, comparing their results to the dismal natural history of stroke in evolution.[39] They cautioned against operating on patients with profound stroke and also suggested that it is best not to attempt to reopen occluded vessels. This conclusion supported Millikan's[40] findings from 1972, which addressed the dismal prognosis for patients experiencing stroke in evolution when treated medically. Later, Mentzer et al[41] reported results similar to those of Goldstone and Moore, coming to the same conclusion that carotid endarterectomy is indicated in patients with fluctuating deficits or stroke in evolution, again noting that the natural history is for significant numbers to develop profound irreversible stroke. This group identified 43 patients with fluctuating neurologic deficits consistent with stroke in evolution. Of 26 patients treated nonoperatively, 5 improved, 17 sustained severe deficits and 4 died. Of 17 patients undergoing urgent operation, 12 had a complete neurologic recovery, 4 remained the same neurologically, and none worsened or died. In formulating recommendations the Ad Hoc Committee of the Society for Vascular Surgery and the North American Chapter of the International Society for Cardiovascular Surgery recognized Mentzer's favorable results as well as other anecdotal reports of dramatic improvement in patients undergoing emergent surgery and contrasted this to poorer results in patients managed medically. They recommended operation for stroke in evolution in carefully selected patients in centers recognized for excellence in the management of carotid disease.

UNFAVORABLE ANATOMY

Patients who are neurologically unstable and also harbor angiographic findings depicting anatomically compelling lesions for endarterectomy (free-floating thrombus, loose atheroma or preocclusive carotid string sign, etc.) constitute another subgroup in which early surgical intervention may avert the high risk of further neurologic deterioration (Fig. 8-1). Gertler et al[42] reviewed 29 such patients—2 (6.8%) died and 1 (3.4%) deteriorated neurologically following carotid endarterectomy. As the primary goal of carotid endarterectomy is stroke prophylaxis they concluded that removal of the potential embolic source and reperfusion of ischemic tissue carried lower risk than leaving these unstable lesions uncorrected. However, they also made note of the fact that these patients do carry a very high risk and emphasized careful dissection and avoidance of the carotid bulb prior to cross-clamping the artery.

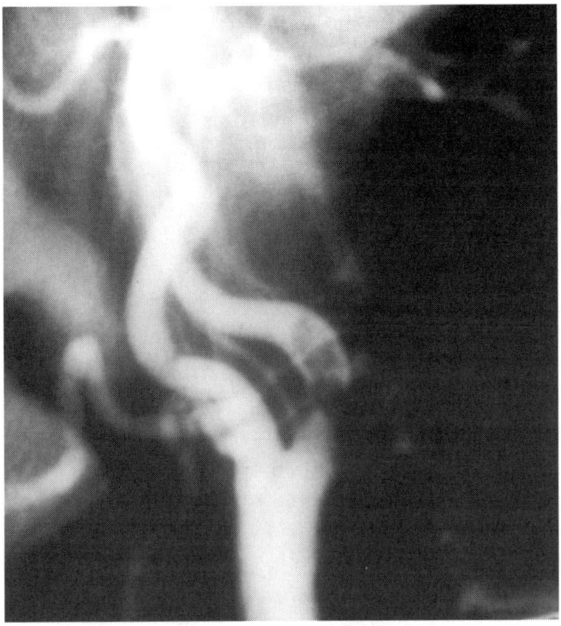

FIG. 8-1. Arteriography demonstrates free-floating thrombus occluding the carotid bifurcation with a patent distal internal carotid artery.

POST ENDARTERECTOMY STROKE

Both Najafi[17] and Kwaan[43] described effective reversal of neurologic deficits that developed during the immediate period following carotid endarterectomy. Following these reports and the reports of others it has become widely accepted that stroke from carotid occlusion following an apparently successful carotid endarterectomy is a clear indication for emergency re-exploration. There is little debate over potential benefits of urgent removal of thrombus to restore patency to the acutely occluded vessel in this setting. Most would agree that intervention needs to be immediate following the onset of symptoms without any delay to confirm radiographically the occlusion. This dogma is based on anecdotal reports and each postendarterectomy stroke patient needs an individualized treatment plan.

SMALL, FIXED DEFICITS

Whittemore et al[35] in 1984 suggested that the risk of subsequent occlusion of a stenotic carotid vessel occurring during the 4–6-week waiting period following stroke may outweigh the reported risk of neurologic morbidity from endarterectomy in patients with small, fixed deficits. Gasecki[36] came to similar conclusions following his review of the NASCET results, stating that "carotid endarterectomy can be undertaken safely in patients diagnosed with minor, non-disabling stroke, with or without evidence on CT scan." Piotrowski et al[44] found no difference in outcome when they compared two matched groups with moderate neurologic deficits. There was no difference in postoperative stroke and death rate observed between groups of patients operated on either within 6 weeks of a stroke or beyond the 6-week waiting period. Dosick et al[45] retrospectively reviewed the natural history of 19 patients following acute stroke and found 21% suffered a second cerebrovascular accident during the 4- to 6-week waiting period prior to endarterectomy. This review was followed by a prospective study that noted a 9.5% recurrent stroke rate within 6 weeks in a set of 74 patients with a clinical diagnosis of stroke and cortical infarcts on CT. This study went on to review 110 patients who underwent endarterectomy within 2 weeks of onset of a neurologic deficit lasting more than 24 hours and with no evidence of infarction by CT. A single patient suffered a postoperative stroke and no patients died. These results have led many vascular surgeons to believe that hemorrhagic infarct or extension of infarct following endarterectomy in patients with mild or resolved neurologic deficit and *normal* CT scan is unlikely, and the risk of early surgery in this subgroup should approach the risk seen in a patient operated on for transient ischemic attacks.

Little outcome data exists to support or condemn carotid endarterectomy in neurologically stable patients with moderate deficits and *abnormal* CT scan indicating a recent stroke. Numerous studies have shown that operation is relatively safe in patients with acute mild deficits regardless of the CT scan, but the numbers in these series are, unfortunately, small. Profound stroke with or without large areas of infarct on CT scan continues to be considered a contraindication to carotid endarterectomy.

Sannella[46] has recommended immediate contralateral carotid endarterectomy in patients with severe bilateral carotid disease and history of an acute, fixed neurologic deficit. Contralateral endarterectomy may improve ipsilateral perfusion via collaterals to a magnitude sufficient to maintain tissue viability within the "ischemic penumbra" without elevating pressure to a point that may result in hemorrhagic infarct. Sannella reported success in 13 patients with fixed neurologic deficits and CT scans proving stroke utilizing this novel approach. While numbers are small, the potential benefits of contralateral endarterectomy and the "dampening effect" of collateral circulation may warrant further investigation.

CONCLUSION AND RECOMMENDATIONS

Patients with critical carotid stenosis who suffer a stroke may subsequently worsen clinically either because of low flow or repeated emboli. Furthermore, the risk of significant second stroke is highest during the first few weeks and months following the initial event. Early operation, however, has an increased risk of stroke, as a relatively benign bland infarct can be converted into a hemorrhagic infarct.

Stroke patients with minimal deficits constitute a subgroup who should be considered for early operative intervention. The Ad Hoc Committee to the Joint Council of the Society for Vascular Surgery and the North American Chapter of the International Society for Cardiovascular Surgery have recommended a period of observation until the patients clinical course reaches a plateau. Patients with normal CT scans are candidates for early operation, as are those patients with small CT abnormalities. Early operation is usually not performed in patients with moderately sized infarcts seen on CT scan, especially if the abnormality enhances. Surgery, as always, needs to be performed by teams who have demonstrated acceptable results. The period of observation prior to operation may be from hours to a few days in patients with mild stroke.

Patients with waxing and waning symptoms and patients with stroke in evolution who have a related tight stenosis are candidates for emergency surgery. These patients should have a mild or at most a moderate deficit at the time of operation.

Stroke patients with profound neurologic deficits, particularly those with associated depressed level of consciousness carry a poor prognosis regardless of treatment and are not, in general, considered operative candidates. Since it is logistically difficult to diagnose carotid stenosis, rule out hemorrhage with a CT scan, commence operative intervention, and restore flow within 1–2 hours, carotid endarterectomy is currently contraindicated in these patients. Early operation increases the incidence of revascularization edema and hemorrhage; the risk of subsequent neurologic decline and mortality probably outweighs the risk of medical management. Severe stroke occurring secondary to carotid occlusion after operation or angiography are the exceptions to this dogmatic approach.

REFERENCES

1. Eascott HHG, Pickering GW, Rob CG. Reconstruction of the internal carotid artery in a patient with intermittant attacks of hemiplegia. Lancet 1954;2:994
2. North American Symptomatic Carotid Endarterectomy Trial (NASCET). Beneficial effect of carotid endarterectomy in symptomatic patients with high-grade carotid stenosis. N Eng J Med 1991;325:445–53
3. NASCET. Clinical alert: benefit of carotid endarterectomy for patients with high-grade stenosis of the internal carotid artery. National Institute of Neurological Disorders and Stroke. February 25, 1991
4. Hobson RW, Weiss DG, Fields WS, Goldstone J, Moore WS, Towne JB, Wright CB, and the Veterans Affairs Cooperative Study Group. Efficacy of carotid endarterectomy for asymptomatic carotid stenosis. N Eng J Med 1993;328:221–227
5. Breutman ME, Fields WS, Crawford ES, DeBakey ME. Cerebral hemorrhage in carotid artery surgery. Arch Neurol 1963;9:458–467
6. Fisher M, Adams RD. Observations on brain embolism with special reference to the mechanism of hemorrhagic infarction. J Neuropathol Exp Neurol 1951;10:92–94
7. Wylie EJ, Hein MF, Adams JE. Intracranial hemorrhage following surgical revascularization for treatment of acute stroke. J Neurosurg 1964;21:212–215
8. Rob GC. Operation for acute completed stroke due to thrombosis of the internal carotid artery. Surgery 1969;65:5:862–865
9. Thompson JE, Austin DJ, Patman RD. Endarterectomy of the totally occluded carotid artery for stroke. Arch Surg 1967;95:791–801
10. Thompson JE, Austin DJ, Patman RD. Carotid endarterectomy for cerebrovascular insufficiency. Ann Surg 1970;172:663
11. Giordano JM, Trout HM III, Kozloff L, Depalma RG. Timing of carotid endarterectomy after stroke. J Vasc Surg 1985;2:250–254
12. Blaisdell WF, Clauss RH, Galbraith JG, Imparato AM, Wylie EJ. Joint Study of Extracranial Arterial Occlusion. JAMA 1969;209:1809–1895

13. Fields WS. Selection of stroke patients for arterial reconstructive surgery. Am J Surg 1973;125:527–529
14. Ojemman RG, Crowell RM, Robertson GH, Fisher CM. Surgical treatment of extracranial carotid disease. Clin Neurosurg 1975;22:214–263
15. Rosenthal D, Borrero E, Clark MD, Lamis PA, Daniels WW. Carotid endarterectomy after reversible ischemic neurologic deficit or stroke; is it of value? J Vasc Surg 1988;8:527–534
16. Rob CG. Operation for acute completed stroke due to thrombosis of the internal carotid artery. Surgery 1969;65:862–865
17. Najafi H, Javid M, Dye WS, Hunter JA, Wideman FE, Julian OC. Emergency carotid thromboendarterectomy. Arch Surg 1971;103:610–14
18. Meyer FB, Sundt TM, Piepgras DG, Sandok BA, Forbes G. Emergency carotid endarterectomy for patients with acute carotid occlusion and profound neurologic deficits. Ann Surg 1986;203:82–89
19. Donaldson MC, Drezner AD. Surgery for acute carotid occlusion. Arch Surg 1983;118:1266–1268
20. Caplan LR, Skillman J, Ojemann R, Fields WS. Intracerebral hemorrhage after internal carotid endarterectomy: a hypertensive complication? Stroke 1978;9:457–60
21. Bernstien M, Flemming JFR, Beck JHN. Cerebral hyperperfusion after carotid endarterectomy: a cause of cerebral hemorrhage. Neurosurgery 1984;15:50–56
22. Solomon RA, Loftus CM, Quest DO, Correll JW. Incidence and etiology of intracerebral hemorrhage following carotid endarterectomy. J Neurosurg 1986;64:29–34
23. Pompselli FB, Lamparello PJ, Riles TS, Craighead CC, Giangola G, Imparato AM. Intracranial hemorrhage after carotid endarterectomy. J Vasc Surg 1988;7:248–255
24. Spetzler RF, Wilson CB, Weinstein P, et al. Normal perfusion pressure breakthrough theory. Clin Neurosurg 1978;25:651–672
25. Sundt TM Jr, Sharbrough FW, Peipgras DG, et al. Correlation of cerebral blood flow and electroencephalographic changes during carotid endarterectomy, with results of surgery and hemodynamics of cerebral ischemia. Mayo Clin Proc 1981;56:533–534
26. Harvey J, Rasmussen T. Occlusion of the middle cerebral artery. Arch Neurol Psychiatr 1951;66:20–29
27. Meyer, JS. Importance of ischemic drainage to small vessels in experimental cerebral infarcts. J Neuropath Exp Neurol 1958;17:571–585
28. Hachinski V, Norris JW. The reversibility of cerebral ischemia. In: Hachinski V, Norris JW. The acute stroke. Philadelphia: FA Davis, 1985:41–63
29. Lassen WA. The luxury-perfusion syndrome and its possible relation to acute metabolic acidosis localized within the brain. Lancet 1966;2:1113–1115
30. Ringelstein EB, Sievers C, Ecker S, Schneider PA, Otis SM. Noninvasive assessment of CO_2-induced cerebral vasomotor response in normal individuals and patients with internal carotid artery occlusions. Stroke 1988;19:963–969
31. Ringelstein EB, Van Eyck S, Mertens I. Evaluation of cerebral vasomotor reactivity by various vasodilating stimuli: comparison of CO_2 to acetazolamide. J Cereb Blood Flow Metab 1992;12:162–168
32. Wing SD, Norman D, Pollock JA, Newton TH. Contrast enhancement of cerebral infarcts in computed tomography. Radiology 1976;121:89–92
33. Ricotta JJ, Ouriel K, Green RM, DeWeese JA. Use of computerized cerebral tomography in the selection of patients for elective and urgent carotid endarterectomy. Ann Surg 1985;202:783–787
34. Little JR, Moufarrij NA, Furlan AJ. Early carotid endarterectomy after cerebral infarction. Neurosurgery 1989;24:334–338
35. Whitemore AD, Ruby ST, Couch MP, Mannick JA. Early carotid endarterectomy in patients with small fixed neurologic deficits. J Vasc Surg 1984;1:795–799
36. Gasecki AP, Ferguson GG, Eliasziw M, Clagett PG, Fox AJ, Hachinski V, Barnett MJ. Early endarterectomy for severe carotid artery stenosis after nondisabling stroke: results from the North American Symptomatic Carotid Endarterectomy Trial. J Vasc Surg 1994;20:288–295
37. Moore WS, Mohr JP, Najafi H, Robertson JT, Stoney RJ, Toole JF. Carotid endarterectomy: practice guidelines report of the Ad Hoc Committee to the Joint Council of the Society for Vascular Surgery and the North American Chapter of the International Society for Cardiovascular Surgery. J Vasc Surg 1992;15:469–479
38. Goldstone J, Moore WS. Emergency carotid artery surgery in neurologically unstable patients. Arch Surg 1976;11:1284
39. Millikan CH. Discussion. In: McDowell FH, Brennan RW (ed). Cerebral vascular diseases (Transactions of the Eighth Princeton Conference on Cerebral Vascular Disease). New York: Grune & Stratton, 1972:209–212

40. Millikan CH. Clinical management of cerebral ischemia. In: McDowell FH, Brennan RW (eds). Cerebral vascular disease, Eighth Conference. New York: Grune & Stratton, 1973;209
41. Mentzer RM, Finkelmeier RM, Crosby IK, Wellons MA. Emergency carotid endarterectomy for fluctuating neurological defects. Surgery 1981;89:60–66
42. Gertler JP, Blankensteijn JD, Brewster DC, Moncure AC, Cambria RP, LaMuraglia GM, Darling RC, Abbott WM. Carotid endarterectomy for unstable and compelling neurologic conditions: do results justify an aggressive approach? J Vasc Surg 1992;19:32–42
43. Kwaan JHM, Connolly JE, Sharefkin JB. Successful management of early stroke after carotid endarterectomy. Ann Surg 1979;190:676–678
44. Piotrowski JJ, Bernhard VM, Rubin JR, McIntyre KE, Malone JM, Parrent FM, Hunter GC. Timing of carotid endarterectomy after acute stroke. J Vasc Surg 1990;11:45–52
45. Dosick SM, Whalen RC, Gale SS, Brown WO. Carotid endarterectomy in the stroke patient: computed axial tomography to determine timing. J Vasc Surg 1985;2:214–219
46. Sannella NA. Bilateral severe carotid stenosis or occlusion and computed tomographic scan positive hemispheric stroke with neurologic deficit: immediate contralateral carotid endarterectomy. Ann Vasc Surg 1992;6:252–257

Management of Extracranial Cerebrovascular Disease, edited by Keith D. Calligaro et al.
Lippincott-Raven Publishers, Philadelphia © 1997.

9

Indications for Balloon Angioplasty and Stenting for Extracranial Artery Occlusive Disease

Robert D. G. Ferguson, John G. Ferguson

Carotid percutaneous transluminal angioplasty (PTA) is a relatively new form of cerebrovascular revascularization. This chapter focuses on high-pressure, non-elastomer balloon dilatation of vaso-occlusive arterial atherosclerotic lesions. There are two principle mechanisms by which arterial lesions reduce blood flow and cause cerebral ischemia or infarction:[1]

1. *in situ* atherothrombosis: arterial narrowing or occlusion caused by an atherosclerotic plaque (or myointimal proliferation), with or without associated thrombus, encroaching on the arterial lumen
2. artery-to-artery embolus: arterial narrowing or occlusion caused by plaque fragments or thrombi migrating from a more proximal source

Successful carotid PTA increases the crossectional area of the target artery[2] and initiates endoluminal remodeling. In theory, this can reduce the risk of recurrent ischemia by increasing flow reserve, improving perilesional rheology, and reconditioning endothelial function.

TRADITIONAL VERSUS ENDOVASCULAR CAROTID REVASCULARIZATION

Carotid surgery usually involves excision of a carotid bifurcation plaque (endarterectomy). The clinical effectiveness of carotid bifurcation endarterectomy was established by large randomized controlled trials (RCTs) in North America and Europe.[3,4,5,6] However, endarterectomy's risk-to-benefit ratio heavily depends on the procedural complication rate. Contemporary community-based audits[7,8,9] suggest that disability and death from carotid endarterectomy may be as high as 10%.[10,11,12] In addition to death and stroke, endarterectomy is associated with non-neurological procedural morbidity, including cranial nerve palsies, wound infection, septicemia, pulmonary embolism, congestive heart failure, and perioperative myocardial infarction.[3,5] Angioplasty of atherosclerotic carotid bifurcation lesions may minimize the complications of endarterectomy and surgical bypass in patients who have severely decreased vital capacity; a major surgical procedure within the previous 30 days; compensated congestive heart failure with moderate-to-severe systolic left-ventricular dysfunction; severe coronary artery disease and a strong indication for urgent coronary bypass surgery; myocardial infarction in the previous 6 months; recurrent symptomatic stenosis after carotid endarterectomy; target lesions or arteries that are technically unsuitable for reasons other than lesion location (*e.g.,* carotid revascularization after therapeutic neck irradiation); concurrent extracranial and intracranial carotid artery stenoses; and advanced age.[13]

In addition, carotid angioplasty or stenting appears to be feasible in patients with nonatherosclerotic target lesions due to fibromuscular hyperplasia, radiation damage, or intimal dissection with or without associated pseudoaneurysm.

Finally, PTA, in conjunction with thrombolytic agents, may permit earlier revascularization than surgical alternatives, in acute thrombotic or thromboembolic stroke due to extracranial carotid occlusion.

A definitive randomized controlled trial of carotid angioplasty's clinical effectiveness has, hitherto, been unfeasible. However, despite the technique's nascent state and the compromised baseline prognostic status of the patients studied to date, there is preliminary evidence supporting its *angiographic* effectiveness, with complication rates that are similar to those of community-based carotid.[14,15] Nevertheless, endarterectomy is the only carotid intervention for which there is Level I evidence of clinical effectiveness. Therefore, carotid bifurcation PTA should, with rare exceptions, be used only in protocols designed to assess the procedure's risks and benefits. Conversely, angioplasty may be proposed outside the aegis of a study protocol, when definitive evidence for the clinical effectiveness PTA alternatives, such as interarterial carotid lesion bypass, is lacking (*e.g.,* symptomatic, hemodynamically significant, prepetrous internal carotid or intrathoracic common carotid artery lesions, that are difficult to approach surgically, are typically amenable to PTA).

ADJUNCTS TO CAROTID ENDOVASCULAR REVASCULARIZATION

Adjunctive therapies, such as endoluminal stenting, may increase angioplasty's effectiveness while reducing procedural risks. Primary stenting has been advocated as an alternative to plain old balloon angioplasty (POBA). This stems from coronary RCTs that demonstrate better initial results and a lower rate of restenosis for stenting than POBA.[16,17] Secondary (rescue) stenting may be useful for angioplasty-induced dissection or spontaneous arterial occlusion due to plaque hemorrhage, with or without thrombosis; however, there are no published reports of definitive carotid stent studies, and the value of carotid stenting remains speculative. Moreover, the two stents that are approved by the Food and Drug Administration are susceptible to compression.

Stent deformability is an important issue in the carotid artery (Palmaz J. 2nd International Workshop on Interventional Radiology. Prague, June 15–17, 1995: personal communication); unlike epicardial coronary arteries, the carotid is susceptible to external compression. Indeed, empirical evidence (Roubin G. 6th Annual PTCA

Course. University of Alabama, Birmingham, September 1995: personal communication) suggests that stent crimping is real although its clinical consequences are uncertain. However, technology is advancing rapidly and the latest stent designs address the substantive deficiencies of extant devices.

SUMMARY

Angioplasty, with or without stenting, appears to be technically feasible in a broad spectrum of extracranial carotid pathologies. However, carotid angioplasty and stent-

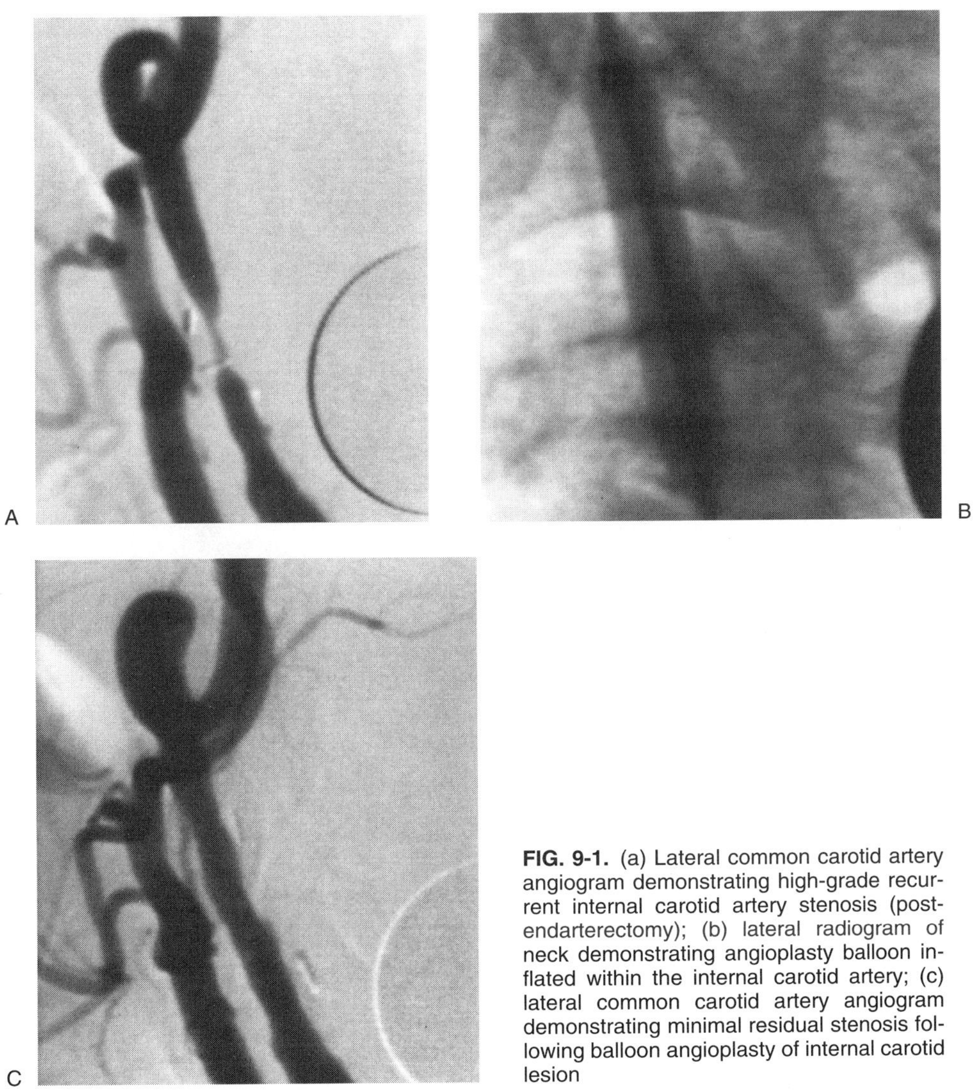

FIG. 9-1. (a) Lateral common carotid artery angiogram demonstrating high-grade recurrent internal carotid artery stenosis (post-endarterectomy); (b) lateral radiogram of neck demonstrating angioplasty balloon inflated within the internal carotid artery; (c) lateral common carotid artery angiogram demonstrating minimal residual stenosis following balloon angioplasty of internal carotid lesion

ing are in the early stages of clinical evaluation. There are no definitive reports concerning the long-term clinical and angiographic results of either procedure. Although preliminary short-term results are encouraging, the ultimate role of endovascular intervention for structural occlusive disease of the extracranial carotid is unclear; while there is no proof of angioplasty's *clinical* effectiveness, there is also no basis for asserting that it is technically ineffective or unsafe. We believe that the potential advantages of endovascular carotid revascularization warrant evaluation of its therapeutic role.

Until definitive studies comparing endovascular revascularization and endarterectomy are available, endovascular interventionists should refrain from treating carotid bifurcation lesions, that are amenable to endarterectomy, outside the framework of an IRB approved protocol that combines a standardized research protocol, a multidisciplinary neurointervention team, prospective multicenter data collection, and epidemiological as well as external oversight.

Large-scale RCTs are required to establish the relative merits of endovascular carotid intervention and endarterectomy in patients who are candidates for both procedures. However, randomized controlled studies are presently ill-advised given the state of the science in carotid PTA, the limited number of skilled PTA operators, and the rapid pace of technological development. PTA technology, techniques, and operator skills must stabilize before a definitive comparison of angioplasty and endarterectomy is feasible. The timing of large-scale RCTs is central to ensuring a fair test of angioplasty's therapeutic potential. Premature RCTs run a very real risk of underestimating the true value of endovascular carotid therapy.

A

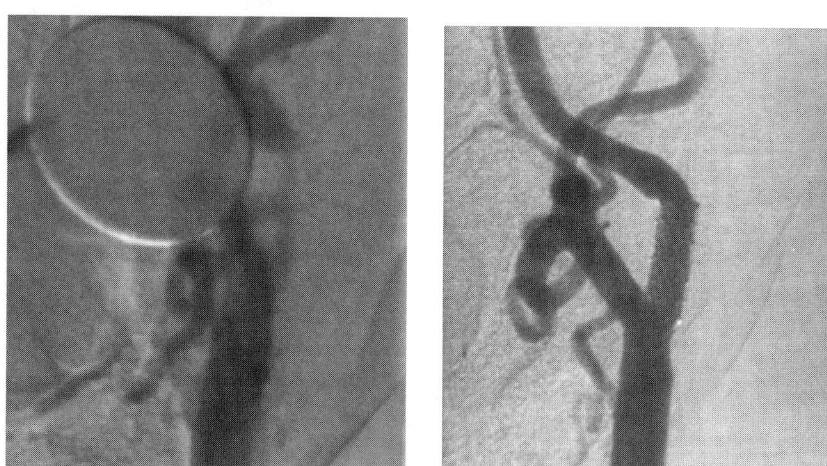

B

FIG. 9-2. (a) anteroposterior common carotid artery angiogram demonstrating high-grade ulcerated internal carotid artery stenosis; (b) anteroposterior common carotid artery angiogram demonstrating minimal residual stenosis following balloon angioplasty and stenting of internal carotid lesion

Figures 9-1 and 9-2 are examples of endovascular carotid intervention. Figure 9-1 shows angioplasty alone and Figure 9-2 shows angioplasty with adjunctive stenting.

REFERENCES

1. Classification of cerebrovascular diseases III. Stroke 1990;21(4):637–676
2. Landau C, Lange RA, Hillis LD. Percutaneous transluminal angioplasty. N Eng J Med 1994;330(14): 981–993
3. North American Symptomatic Carotid Endarterectomy Trial (NASCET). Beneficial effect of carotid endarterectomy in symptomatic patients with high-grade carotid stenosis. N Eng J Med 1991;325(7):445–453
4. European Carotid Surgery Trialists' Collaborative Group. MRC European Carotid Surgery Trial: interim results for symptomatic patients with severe (70%–99%) or mild (0–29%) carotid stenosis. Lancet 1991;337:1235–1243
5. Mayberg MR, Wilson SE, Yatsu F, et al. Carotid endarterectomy and prevention of cerebral ischemia in symptomatic carotid stenosis: Veterans Affairs Cooperative Study Program 309 Trialist Group. JAMA 1991;266:3289–3294
6. Investigators of the Asymptomatic Carotid Atherosclerosis Study (ACAS). Clinical Advisory on Carotid Endarterectomy for Patients with Asymptomatic Carotid Artery Stenosis. National Institute of Neurological Disorders and Stroke Clinical Alert, September 30, 1994
7. Brott T, Thalinger K. The practice of carotid endarterectomy in a large metropolitan area. Stroke 1984;15:950–955
8. Brott TG, Labutta RJ, Kempczinsky RF. Changing patterns in the practice of carotid endarterectomy in a large metropolitan area. JAMA 1986;255:2609–2612
9. Burns RJ, Willoughby JO. South Australian carotid endarterectomy study. Med J Austr 1991;154:650–653
10. Moore WS, Barnett HJM, Beebe HG, et al. AHA Scientific Statement. Special Report: Guidelines for Carotid Endarterectomy. A multidisciplinary Consensus Statement From the Ad Hoc Committee, American Heart Association. Circulation 1995;91(2):566–579
11. McCrory DC, Goldstein LB, Samsa GP, Oddone EZ, Landsman PB, Moore WS, Matchar DB. Predicting complications of carotid endarterectomy. Stroke 1993;24(9):1285–1291
12. Committee on Health Care Issues. Does carotid endarterectomy decrease stroke and death in patients with transient ischemic attacks? Ann Neurol 1987;22:72–76
13. Ferguson RDG, Ferguson JG. Carotid angioplasty: in search of a worthy alternative to carotid endarterectomy. Arch Neurol 1996: in press
14. Ferguson R, Ferguson J, Schwarten D, et al. Immediate angiographic results and in-hospital central nervous system complications of cerebral percutaneous transluminal angioplasty. Circulation (supplement) 1993;88(4):I–393
15. Goldstein LB, McCrory DC, Landsman PB, et al. Multicenter review of preoperative risk factors for carotid endarterectomy in patients with ipsilateral symptoms. Stroke 1994;25(6):1116–1121
16. Serruys PW, de Jaegere P, Kiemeneij F, et al. A comparison of balloon-expandable-stent implantation with balloon angioplasty in patients with coronary artery disease. Benestent Study Group. N Engl J Med 1994;331(8):489–95
17. Fischman DL, Leon MB, Baim DS, et al. A randomized comparison of coronary-stent placement and balloon angioplasty in the treatment of coronary artery disease. Stent Restenosis Study Investigators. N Engl J Med 1994;331(8):496–501

PART III

Surgical Technique of the Aortic Arch and the Extracranial Arteries

Management of Extracranial Cerebrovascular Disease, edited by Keith D. Calligaro et al.
Lippincott-Raven Publishers, Philadelphia © 1997.

10

Surgical Techniques for Symptomatic Aortic Arch Disease

Joseph S. Coselli, Luiz F. Poli de Figueiredo

The aortic arch is the segment of the aorta that extends from the leading edge of the origin of the right brachiocephalic trunk to the distal origin of the left subclavian artery. Symptomatic aortic arch disease reflects serious lesions and pathologies with the potential to lead to death in most cases.[1,2] Only surgical treatment of these lesions can modify the otherwise devastating consequences of aortic rupture or vital organ ischemia.

Interruption of cerebral blood flow and the special reconstructive techniques required to repair aortic arch disease are some of the special features that characterize this region as one of the most challenging for cardiac and vascular surgeons.

Following initial success with resection and graft replacement of the distal aortic arch in 1954[3] and the ascending aorta in 1956,[4] DeBakey reported the first successful complete aortic arch resection in 1957,[5] using an aortic homograft, cardiopulmonary bypass, and temporary antegrade brachiocephalic perfusion. The use of profound hypothermia and total circulatory arrest for brain protection in the treatment of adult aortic arch pathology was popularized by Griepp[6] in 1975, and the graft inclusion technique along with direct reattachment of arch vessels to openings in the graft by Crawford in 1981.[7] These have been considered the most important surgical advances contributing to the current acceptably low morbidity and mortality related to aortic arch replacement.[8,9]

ETIOLOGY AND PATHOLOGY

Although there are a number of different causes for aortic arch disease, the most frequent symptomatic lesions are aneurysmal dilatation or aortic dissections developed in weakened portions of the aortic wall. The forces generated by the pulsatile aortic pressure and high flow in the presence of localized or diffuse aortic wall alterations produce the conditions allowing for progressive aortic dilatation or dissection.

Syphilitic aortitis was the most common cause of arch aneurysms in the earlier studies.[10] In patients with contracted tertiary syphilis, approximately 10% have significant involvement of the cardiovascular system. Aneurysm is one of the least common manifestations of syphilic aortitis and is present in 5–10% of affected patients. Of these, 25% are fusiform and 75% are saccular. The condition leads to an inflammatory process affecting the aortic wall, resulting in medial destruction with granuloma formation and the development of saccular aneurysms. These aneurysms usually arise in the ascending or transverse segments of the aorta and are the most common presentation of syphilitic aortitis. Since the advent of effective antibiotic treatment for syphilis, these lesions have become distinctly uncommon.

The majority of aneurysmal lesions in the aortic arch are caused by medial degenerative disease or aortic dissection; the former leading to weakening and loss of elasticity of the aortic wall. As diffuse fusiform dilatation occurs, commonly there is extended involvement of the ascending aortic aneurysm, the aortic annulus and valve, descending thoracic, thoracoabdominal, and abdominal aorta. Diffuse atherosclerosis of the aortic intima is a frequently superimposed process, affecting mostly patients older than 60 years, many with associated chronic diseases. Less frequently, a localized weakening of the aortic wall secondary to atherosclerosis can result in a saccular aneurysm. This most frequently occurs along the lesser curvature of the distal transverse aortic arch.

Aortic dissection, after having progressed through the outer portion of the media, results in thinning of the outer wall of the false lumen and can lead to progressive dilatation and aneurysmal formation of the aortic arch. Usually the arch is affected by the extension of a dissection originated in the ascending aorta. A retrograde aortic arch dissection may also occur after a descending aortic tear. The aortic arch is the site of the intimal tear in only 15–25% of cases.[11,12]

Thoracic aneurysm is a prominent feature in Marfan syndrome, a hereditary connective tissue disorder characterized by cystic medial necrosis. Aortic dissection or aneurysm formation with rupture is the main cause of death in these patients. These aneurysms are frequently associated with marked dilatation of the sinuses of Valsalva and the aortic annulus, with annuloaortic ectasia causing loss of coaptation of aortic valve leaflets and with aortic insufficiency.[13]

A number of additional pathologic conditions are known to be responsible for weakening of the aortic wall leading to aneurysm formation. These include giant-cell[14] and Takayasu's aortitis,[15] infection (mycotic) of the aortic wall,[16] chest trauma, previous surgical procedure[17] or graft infection.[18]

Extensive occlusive aortic arch disease may be caused by arteritis or severe atherosclerosis; either of which is capable of affecting the ostium of the brachiocephalic vessels or of filling the lumen with laminated debris. Such a condition has the potential to increase the likelihood of cerebral embolism during manipulation for surgical procedures involving the ascending aorta, such as coronary artery revascularization or aortic valve replacement.[19,20] Cerebral or upper-extremity ischemia secondary to acute arterial thrombosis or atheroembolism also may occur. The presence of thick aortic arch plaques, larger than 4 mm, may contain thrombotic material superimposed and have been recently recognized as an independent potential source of cerebral emboli.[21]

CLINICAL MANIFESTATIONS

Asymptomatic aortic arch aneurysms are usually incidentally detected as superior mediastinal widening or mass on either a plain chest X-ray or computed tomography scan during evaluation for, frequently, an unrelated difficulty.

The most common symptom associated with aortic arch aneurysms is chest pain. The pain is sudden in onset, coincident with acute expansion of the aneurysm. The episode is usually anterior in location but is not infrequently referred to the back, shoulders, arms, neck, and jaw. The pain or discomfort, which may be chronic and of several months' duration, can signal imminent rupture with a sudden increase in intensity.

Various distinct symptoms may result from compression or erosion of adjacent structures. Erosion through the sternum and ribs forming a pulsatile palpable tumor was more commonly observed with syphilitic aortitis. Stretching and compression of the left vagus or recurrent laryngeal nerve may produce hoarseness from left vocal cord paresis or paralysis, sometimes the first symptom of an aortic arch aneurysm. Obstruction of the superior vena cava or innominate vein may produce venous stasis and distention of the veins in the neck, upper chest, and extremities. Compression of the trachea or mainstream bronchi can lead to partial or complete airway obstruction with respiratory distress, stridor, recurrent pulmonary infections, and lung collapse. Erosion of the airway may produce hemoptysis that can be massive and lethal. Similarly, severe dysphagia or massive hematemesis can occur from compression or erosion into the esophagus. Rupture may cause compression of the brachiocephalic vessels with loss of upper extremity pulses, carotid pulsation, or stroke (Fig. 10-1). More commonly, rupture of arch aneurysms cause sudden death from massive hemorrhage into the mediastinum, pericardium or pleural space. Rupture into large veins, pulmonary artery, or cardiac chambers can produce acute congestive heart failure accompanied by a continuous machinery type murmur.

Congestive heart failure can be the most common symptom of aortic arch aneurysm when it is an extension of an aortic root dilatation with aortic valve insufficiency. The decompensation is usually insidious, but overwhelming cardiac failure can be present.

Acute aortic dissection is usually manifested by excruciating substernal or intrascapular back pain, frequently described as tearing, and may mimic an acute myocardial infarction. A diversity in symptoms and unpredictable clinical findings can be expected and are the result of alterations in organ blood supply that may occur as the dissecting process progresses and the false lumen compresses or occludes the true lumen of the aorta or its major branches. Acute myocardial infarction, aortic valvular insufficiency, stroke, paraplegia, bowel ischemia, renal ischemia, upper and lower extremity ischemia can result individually or in any combination. Rupture generally occurs into the pericardium or into the pleural cavity, causing death from cardiac tamponade or exsanguination.[7,22]

Acute arterial thrombosis or atheroembolism may arise from ulcerative or occlu-

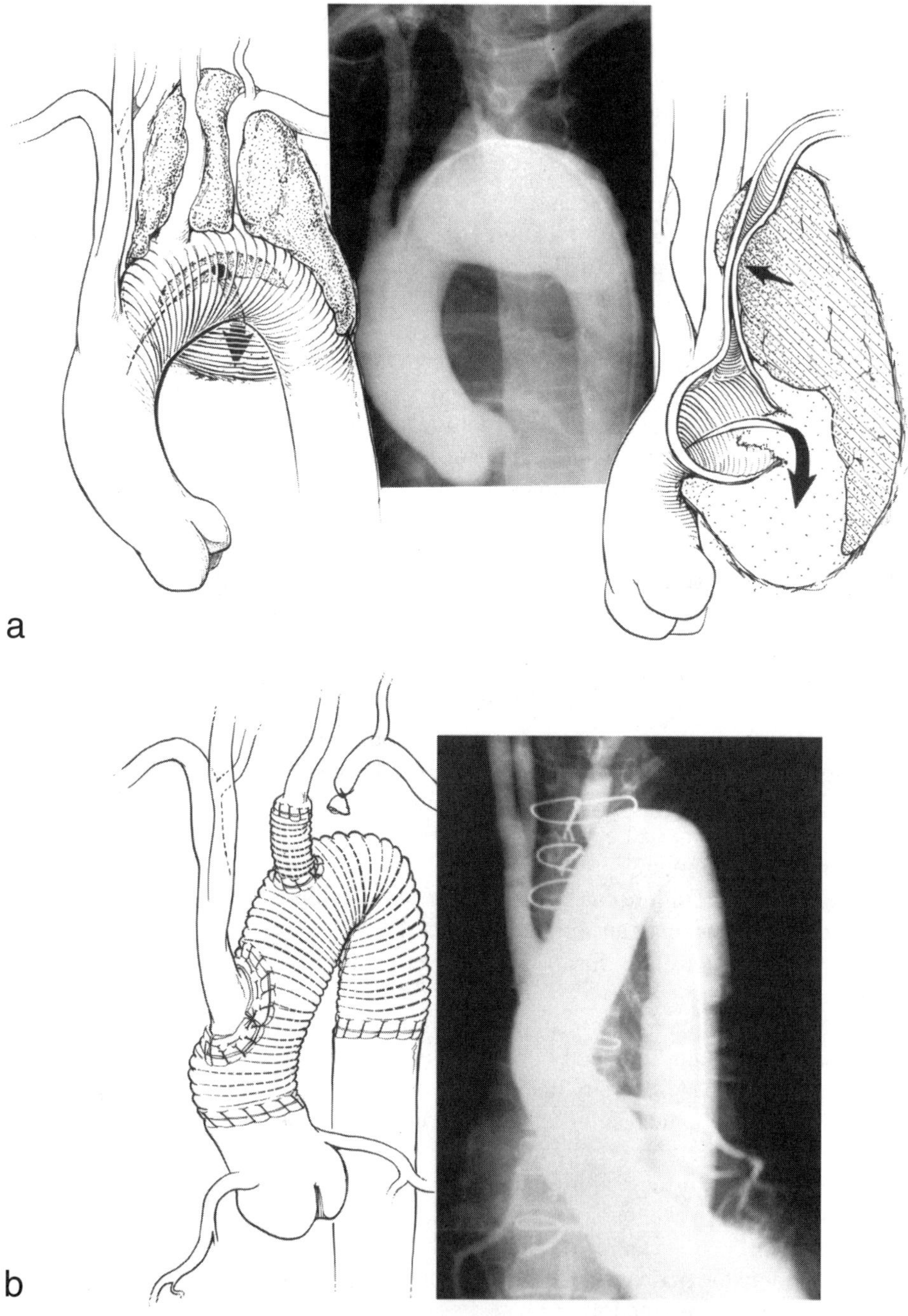

FIG. 10-1. (a) Ruptured transverse aortic arch aneurysm with compression of the left common carotid and left subclavian arteries, drawing and arteriogram; (b) postoperative drawing and arteriogram following resection and replacement of ruptured transverse aortic arch aneurysm.

sive aortic arch lesions, leading to transient or permanent stroke or upper extremity ischemia. Such lesions may involve the site of origin of the brachiocephalic arteries or the ascending or transverse arch intraluminal surface. Similar symptoms may arise as the result of acute aortic dissection or atheroemboli originating from the laminated thrombus that may be associated with fusiform aneurysmal enlargement.

DIAGNOSIS

Physical examination can be of limited value in establishing the nature and extension of aortic arch disease, but a detailed clinical evaluation is essential to determine the preoperative status of the cardiovascular system, including diminished and asymmetrical arterial pulsations, bruits, and murmurs. This is particularly important in cases of aortic dissection. Auscultation may identify associated aortic valvular insufficiency. Left vocal cord paresis or paralysis caused by left laryngeal nerve compression may be detected. Signs of neurological sequela from a prior cerebrovascular accident may also be present.

Plain chest x-rays can show enlargement of the superior mediastinal silhouette or a pronounced left-sided shadow. A prominent convex shadow to the right of the cardiac silhouette suggests enlargement of the ascending aorta. Displacement of the esophagus, trachea, or left main bronchus can be observed. A heavily calcified ascending aorta and arch can be usually detected on routine chest x-ray, anticipating problems for aortic cross-clamping during coronary artery bypass or ascending aorta and valve replacement.[19,20]

Aortography remains the gold standard for the evaluation of patients with, or suspected of having, aneurysm of the transverse aortic arch, providing the most information on a single examination. It allows visualization of the entire aorta and the status of the major arterial branches. Recent advances in angiographic technique and equipment allow for safer and faster studies, with less discomfort and radiation on newer imaging systems. Among the recent advances is digital angiography, a computerized method of acquiring angiographic images. The technique uses smaller amounts of intra-arterial contrast material, reduced levels of radiation, and captures images at a faster rate and can be electronically enhanced for improved contrast resolution. Aortography remains a superior technique for the precise evaluation of the origins of the brachiocephalic arteries and evaluation of their relationship to the true and false lumen in the presence of dissection. It can also locate the site of the intimal tear, essential in planning the proper surgical technique. Coronary angiography can be performed in patients over 50 years old or when coronary artery disease is suspected, identifying patients who would benefit from concomitant coronary artery bypass grafting. The presence of mural thrombus can mask the real size of aneurysms partially filled with intraluminal occupying thrombus; however, most anomalies and lesions in arch and associated branches may be clearly delineated.

Computed tomography (CT) scanning and magnetic resonance imaging (MRI) have proven sensitive in the evaluation of arch aneurysms and aortic dissection. They can determine the size, location, and extension of disease, the presence of mural thrombus, and diameter of the true and false lumen. Although these studies are valuable in evaluating the aortic lumen, characterization of atherosclerotic occlusive disease has yielded less than desirable results. These modalities have proven to be sensitive in studying the aortic wall and periaortic tissues (*i.e.,* rupture and postsurgical graft infection). Three-dimensional reconstructions have proven valuable in assessing branch vessels. Magnetic resonance angiography (MRA) images flowing blood and is used to assess vascular disease without the need for catheterization or injection of intravascular contrast agents. As a result of the necessary magnetic environment, MRI and MRA are of limited value in critically ill patients.

Transesophageal and transthoracic echocardiography are both useful, because they allow for a noninvasive method to distinguish between aortic dissections and ordinary chronic aneurysms. Either technique can identify the intimal flap between the true and false lumen and, frequently, the entry point into the false lumen. They are also used to evaluate the competence of the aortic valve and cardiac function. Recently, transesophageal echocardiography has been used to identify and characterize atherosclerotic aortic arch lesions in patients at risk for cerebral emboli and ischemic stroke.[21]

INDICATIONS FOR AORTIC ARCH REPLACEMENT

Elective repair of fusiform medial degenerative type aneurysms should be performed when the diameter is greater than 5 cm or, in the case of chronic dissection, when the combined diameter of the false and true lumen is 5 cm or greater. Patients with Marfan syndrome are treated somewhat more aggressively, as are patients with concomitant aortic valvular insufficiency or stenosis or coronary artery occlusive disease. Saccular aneurysms may present unpredictable progressive enlargement and should be treated electively when 3–4 cm in size. All postsurgical or posttraumatic false aneurysms should be treated before the development of symptoms. Postsurgical graft infection requires re-resection and replacement. Symptomatic branch vessel stenosis or intraluminal atherosclerosis justify surgical intervention.

Aortic arch replacement is indicated in all symptomatic patients with aortic arch aneurysms independent of the etiology. Emergency surgery is indicated whenever there is sudden expansion or persistent pain suggesting eminent rupture. Because of the extension of the aneurysm, concomitant repair of the ascending aortic aneurysm is usually required. Extension of aortic arch disease to the proximal descending aorta may also require simultaneous repair.

All patients with acute aortic dissection involving the ascending aorta should undergo immediate surgical repair, unless severe irreversible brain damage is present. If the aortic arch is not dilated and does not contain the origin of the intimal tear, the resection may be limited to the ascending portion of the aorta, leaving the aortic arch for long-term follow-up should progressive aortic arch dilatation occur. On the other hand, if the aortic arch does contain an intimal tear or if there is aneurysmal formation, emergency repair including replacement of the transverse arch is mandatory.

SURGICAL TREATMENT

The surgical repair of symptomatic disease involving the transverse aortic arch is in large part similar to that for asymptomatic pathology and is primarily by graft replacement, with the approach varying with the extent of disease.[9,23,24] Surgical reconstruction is carried out under total cardiopulmonary bypass, utilizing profound hypothermic circulatory arrest to protect primarily the brain and, secondarily, the body as a whole. Antegrade and reverse cardioplegia are employed for myocardial protection. Hypothermic circulatory arrest has the advantage of providing a bloodless operative field without the surgeon being encumbered with brachiocephalic clamps, cannulas, and tourniquets.

In the majority of patients, the exposure required is provided by an anterior midsternotomy incision. In patients in whom the very proximal aortic root is spared and who have significant descending or thoracoabdominal involvement, a left posterolateral thoracotomy or thoracoabdominal incision is utilized. In the latter circumstance, cardiopulmonary bypass is simply provided by femoro-femoral cannulation, and owing to the fact that the pericardium remains intact, left ventricular decompression is generally not required. In the former circumstance, required in the overwhelming majority of patients, bicaval cannulation or single atrial cannulation provides venous drainage, and pump return is established through femoral arterial cannulation. In patients with significant concomitant descending thoracic or thoracoabdominal aortic aneurysms with severe intimal atherosclerotic disease, an antegrade arterial perfusion cannula may be placed in the ascending aorta, even if aneurysmal. This is usually possible due to the fact that the ascending aorta is frequently spared of intimal disease in a relative fashion over the distal thoracic and abdominal aorta.

In either case, the patient is systemically cooled to achieve a temperature level providing an isoelectric electroencephalogram.[25] This generally requires 20–25 minutes of cooling. The brain temperature at the point of electrocerebral silence on a standard 10-lead montage is generally 18–20° C.[26] Acid-base balance is maintained using the alpha stat method of pH control. Hemodilution to a hemoglobin of 6–7 mg/dL is employed until rewarming at the completion of reconstruction is initiated, at which time hemoconcentration is begun. Extensive surgical dissection, looping, and clamping of the brachiocephalic vessels is not carried out. To avoid air embolism, the patient is maintained in an extreme Trendelenburg position during the reconstruction. The patient is returned to a horizontal position only after completion of arch replacement and reinstitution of cardiopulmonary bypass has filled the graft and aorta with blood and evacuated all air. The graft may then be clamped proximal to the anastomosis used to reattach the brachiocephalic vessels, reestablishing cerebral perfusion and allowing for rewarming of the patient for the remainder of the procedure, which is focused on proximal aortic reconstruction. Antegrade arterial reperfusion may be established by simple cannulation of the aortic graft at the arch level. Rewarming is continued to a rectal temperature of 37° C. The time period for circulatory arrest averages 25–30 minutes, but has varied from 15–75 minutes. Circulatory arrest beyond 40 minutes has been associated with an increased risk of cerebral ischemia and, beyond 60 minutes, with increased mortality. The period of rewarming generally requires 60–70 minutes.[8]

Most recently, in an effort to increase cerebral protection and provide safer prolonged periods of circulatory arrest, retrograde cerebral perfusion via the superior vena cava during arrest has been utilized. A Y-connection placed on the arterial line and another in the superior vena caval cannula line allow for oxygenated perfusion via only the superior vena caval cannula during the period of arrest.[27] A low-flow state using 300–500 mL/min with the proximal venous pressure monitored and kept at 20 mm Hg or less is carried out continuously. Persistent back bleeding from the brachiocephalic vessels, using this technique, reduces the risk of air embolism and embolic debris. Additionally, substrates from metabolism and oxygen may be provided to the brain in a retrograde fashion.[28]

Proximal aortic reconstruction is carried out during the rewarming period. During this portion of the procedure, the heart is protected by topical cooling and intermittent retrograde or antegrade cardioplegia. In most patients a simple end-to-end anastomosis is fashioned to the proximal aorta distal to the coronary artery origins. In patients in whom there is concomitant aortic valvular disease, an aortic valve replacement is carried out, and in those in whom coronary artery occlusive disease is present, coronary artery bypass grafting is established. In patients with annuloaortic ectasia and Marfan syndrome, composite valve graft replacement of the aortic root is employed. In the latter, reattachment of the coronary artery origins using buttons of aortic tissue directly to the graft is preferred. In the face of redo operation for patients requiring aortic root replacement in whom the coronary arteries are not accessible for proximal mobilization, a direct reattachment, a modification of the technique described by Cabrol, is utilized where a smaller, separate, transversely placed Dacron tube graft is used for coronary artery reattachment and reconstruction.[29]

In patients in whom the aneurysmal involvement is primarily the ascending aorta with a tapering effect of the aneurysm through the transverse aortic arch, a bevelled technique may be employed for transverse arch replacement (Fig. 10-2). In doing so, all of the lesser curvature of the transverse aortic arch is resected, leaving only the dorsum of the greater curvature containing the brachiocephalic vessels intact. In patients in whom there is generalized fusiform involvement of all of the transverse aortic arch, an end-to-end anastomosis is carried out to the proximal descending thoracic aorta under hypothermic circulatory arrest (Fig. 10-3). Following completion of this initial anastomosis, an opening is made in the graft, and the aorta surrounding the brachiocephalic vessels, generally as a group utilizing a single patch of aorta, is reattached to the opening in the graft, reconstructing the dome of the transverse aortic arch. The graft inclusion technique for aortic arch replacement has greatly simplified the procedure and decreased the intraoperative bleeding and time required for the reestablishment of cerebral perfusion. Modern grafts with the interstices sealed with either collagen or albumin have significantly reduced loss of blood through the interstices of the woven Dacron grafts employed in heparinized patients.

All patients with acute aortic dissection involving the ascending aorta or transverse aortic arch are treated as a surgical emergency.[30] It is less common for only the as-

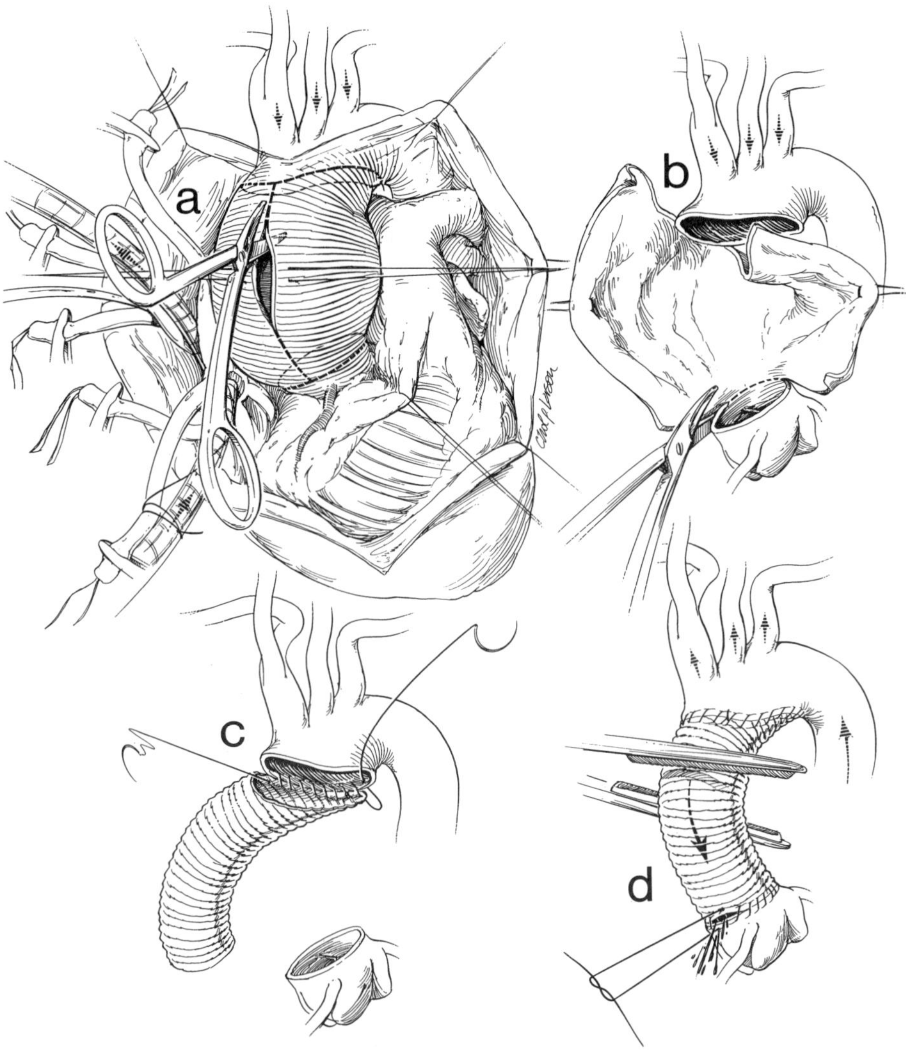

FIG. 10-2. (a–d) Illustration of operative technique for resection and replacement of ascending aortic and lesser curvature transverse aortic arch aneurysm using the bevel distal anastomosis approach.

cending aorta to be involved in the dissection process, DeBakey type II; most frequently the dissection extends through the transverse aortic arch and down the distal aorta. All patients surgically treated for proximal aortic dissection undergo resection and replacement of all of the ascending aorta (Fig. 10-4). Reconstruction is carried out with the routine use of deep hypothermic circulatory arrest. This allows for complete visualization of the entire transverse aortic arch and proximal descending tho-

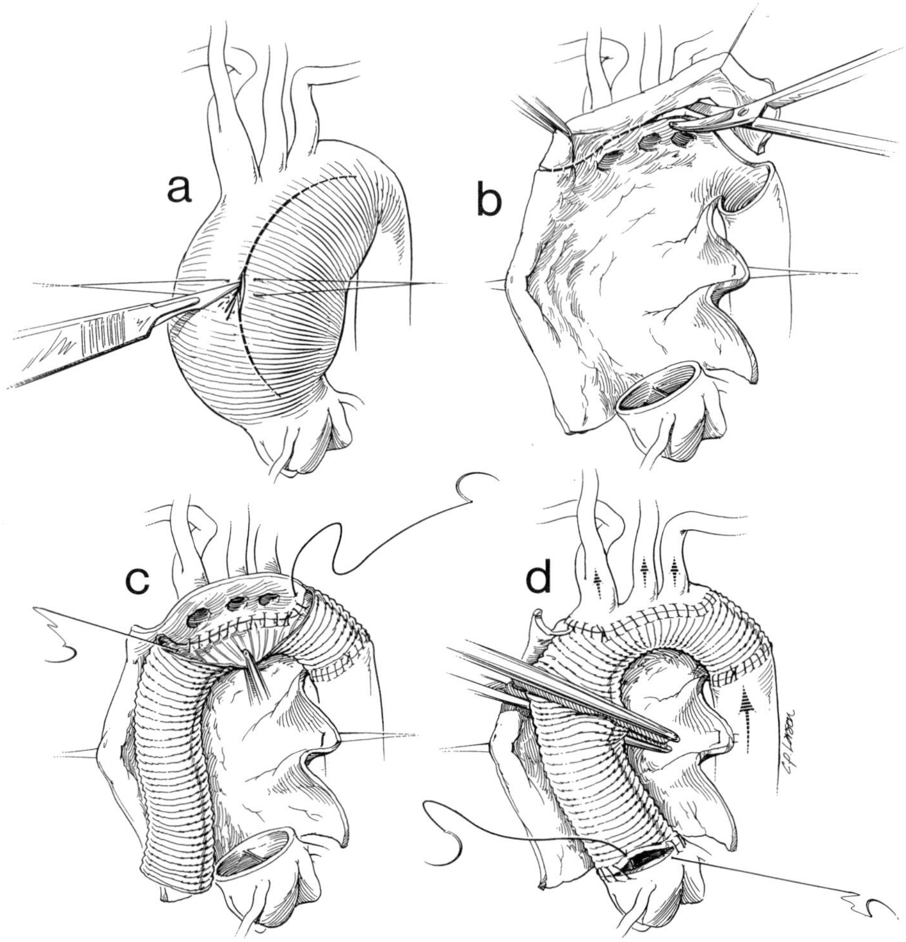

FIG. 10-3. (a–d) Illustration of operative technique for total transverse aortic arch replacement of a patient with fusiform aneurysm of ascending and transverse aortic arch showing reattachment of brachiocephalic vessels and supracoronary proximal anastomosis.

racic aorta through the lumen of the aorta. Additionally, the clamp is applied only to the aortic graft following distal anastomosis, avoiding injury to the friable intimal aorta since no clamp is applied directly to aortic tissues. The false lumen is obliterated, or closed, in the distal suture line, utilizing an open anastomosis that is reinforced with Teflon strips in patients with extremely thin and tenuous tissue. Reperfusion is established by cannulation of the aortic graft in order to avoid perfusion of the false lumen from retrograde flow during the rewarming period. Patients in whom the dissection originates in the transverse aortic arch or in whom tearing of the intimal layer involves the transverse aortic arch require a more extensive arch replacement with a distal anastomosis end-to-end to the descending thoracic aorta and reattachment of the brachiocephalic origins to an opening in the aortic graft.

In patients treated for chronic dissection, the techniques for aortic repair are similar to those described above with the exception that the wall between the true and the false lumen distally is excised (*i.e.,* fenestrated) as it proceeds through the proximal descending thoracic aorta in order that both the true and the false lumen may be perfused distally at the completion of the repair (Fig. 10-5). Further, prior to reconstruction of the transverse aortic arch, the wall between the true and the false lumen is completely excised, in effect creating a single lumen, following which standard techniques are employed. Should dissection extend up the innominate artery or left common carotid artery with aneurysmal involvement, these vessels are replaced with separate Dacron tube grafts.

The lesser curvature of the transverse aortic arch is not an infrequent location for the development of saccular atherosclerotic aneurysms. These are repaired with an approach using a median sternotomy. Again, deep hypothermic circulatory arrest is employed. In patients in whom the defect in the aortic wall encompasses 50% or less of the circumference, excision of the aneurysm and application of a Dacron patch is employed. With more extensive involvement a tube graft is inserted.

In patients treated for infection, including mycotic aneurysms or postoperative graft infection or false aneurysm involvement, standard techniques of replacement are utilized, employing wide debridement of involved mediastinal tissues and aortic wall. Reconstruction has been carried out in most cases with *in situ* reinsertion of prosthetic material, although homograft tissue is currently preferred.[18] Dead space in the anterior mediastinum is filled with muscle flaps from the chest wall or anterior abdominal wall, or omentum. This additionally provides viable tissue coverage of the aortic reconstruction and separation from the sternum.

Fistula formation may occur between an aneurysm involving the transverse aortic arch and the pulmonary artery, great veins, or cardiac chambers. These are treated by graft replacement, using the techniques described, and by closure of the fistula tract through the inner wall of the aortic aneurysm, employing either patch or direct primary closure.[31]

Calcific atherosclerotic intimal involvement of the ascending aorta and transverse aortic arch is potentially a source of emboli and acute and chronic cerebral ischemia. Additionally, these are associated with an increased morbidity and mortality for any cardiac surgical procedure requiring cross-clamping of the aorta. Profound hypothermia and circulatory arrest can be employed to allow direct visual inspection of the entire transverse aortic arch through a wide aortotomy.[20] This approach allows for the removal of ulcerated plaques and friable intimal debris prior to reconstruction of the transverse aortic arch for proximal aortic or cardiac surgery, reducing the risk of cerebral vascular accident. When friable intimal atherosclerosis extends up the innominate artery and left carotid artery, these vessels may require interposition tube graft replacement. In patients in whom severe stenosis of the origin of the innominate artery or left common carotid artery is present as an isolated phenomenon, individual graft replacement may be carried out without the use of cardiopulmonary bypass, em-

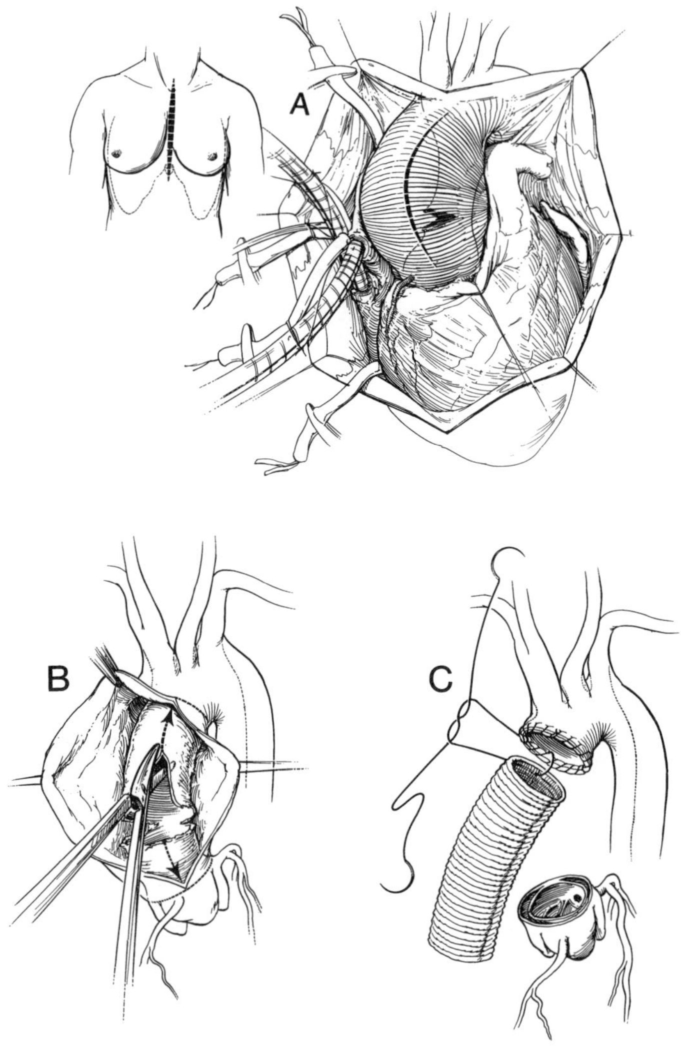

FIG. 10-4. (a–e) Illustration of operative technique for resection and graft replacement of entire ascending aorta for acute DeBakey type I aortic dissection employing hypothermic circulatory arrest and open distal anastomosis.

ploying a partial occluding clamp on the ascending aorta and distal grafting to the innominate or carotid arteries, varying with extent of involvement.

When aneurysmal disease involves the ascending aorta and transverse aortic arch and concomitantly involves the descending thoracic or thoracoabdominal aorta, a staged repair is employed. Provided that the distal aortic pathology is not symptomatic and is not disproportionately enlarged compared to the proximal aorta, the as-

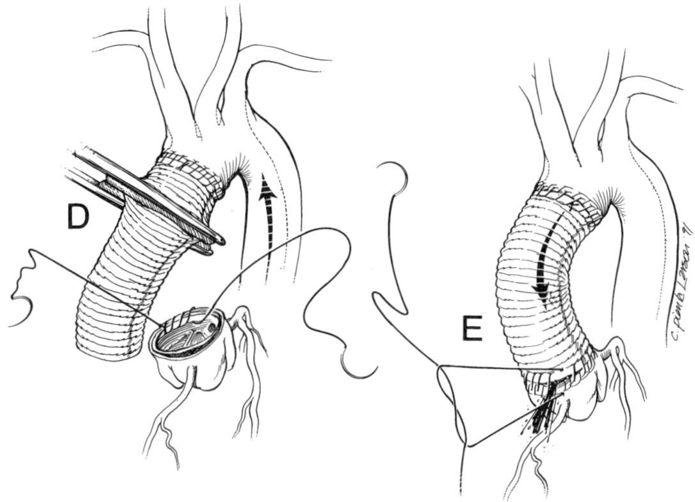

FIG. 10-4. (*continued.*)

cending aorta and transverse aortic arch are replaced as an initial procedure through a median sternotomy using the elephant trunk technique originally described by Borst[32] (Fig. 10-6). The arch repair is carried out in such a way as to allow for a portion of the Dacron graft to remain within the proximal descending thoracic aorta beyond the initial anastomosis positioned immediately distal to the left subclavian artery. Standard techniques are employed for brachiocephalic reattachment and proximal aortic reconstruction. The principle advantage of this technique is that minimal dissection is required in the region of the distal aortic arch during second-stage reconstruction, reducing the risk of injury to the recurrent laryngeal nerve, esophagus, and pulmonary artery (Fig. 10-7). Second-stage repair is generally carried out 4–6 weeks following the initial procedure.

RESULTS

The techniques employed for cerebral protection, namely deep hypothermia, circulatory arrest, and retrograde perfusion, have provided a reliable method to prevent brain damage during the replacement of the aortic arch. There is evidence suggesting that periods of 40 minutes of circulatory arrest during deep hypothermia rarely are associated with brain injury.[25] Increased occurrence of stroke was observed in a series of 656 patients[8] when the circulatory arrest time was longer than 40 minutes, and mortality rate was higher after 60 minutes.

Other factors can account for neurologic dysfunction in the postoperative period. There is a potential for brain embolization during the manipulation of the aortic arch, leading to focal neurologic deficits. Concomitant intracranial and extracranial arter-

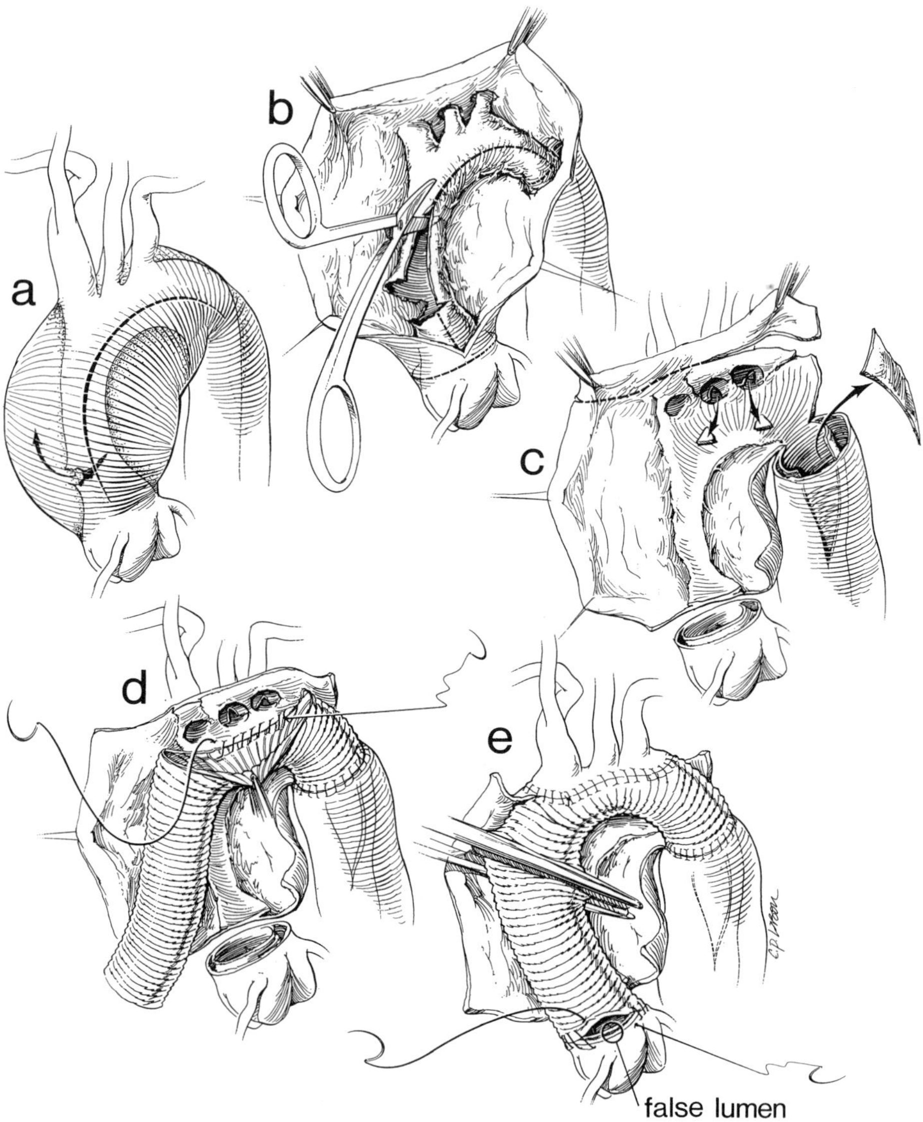

FIG. 10-5. (a–e) Illustration of operative technique for resection and replacement of ascending aortic and transverse aortic arch aneurysm in patient with chronic type I aortic dissection.

ial occlusive disease may be present in several patients, contributing to the development of cerebral hypoperfusion and reversible, nonfocal neurologic dysfunction. These events are usually manifested in the postoperative period by confusion, lethargy, or delirium. Increased age is an associated risk factor.

We recently reported our experience with 227 aortic arch replacements.[9] In this se-

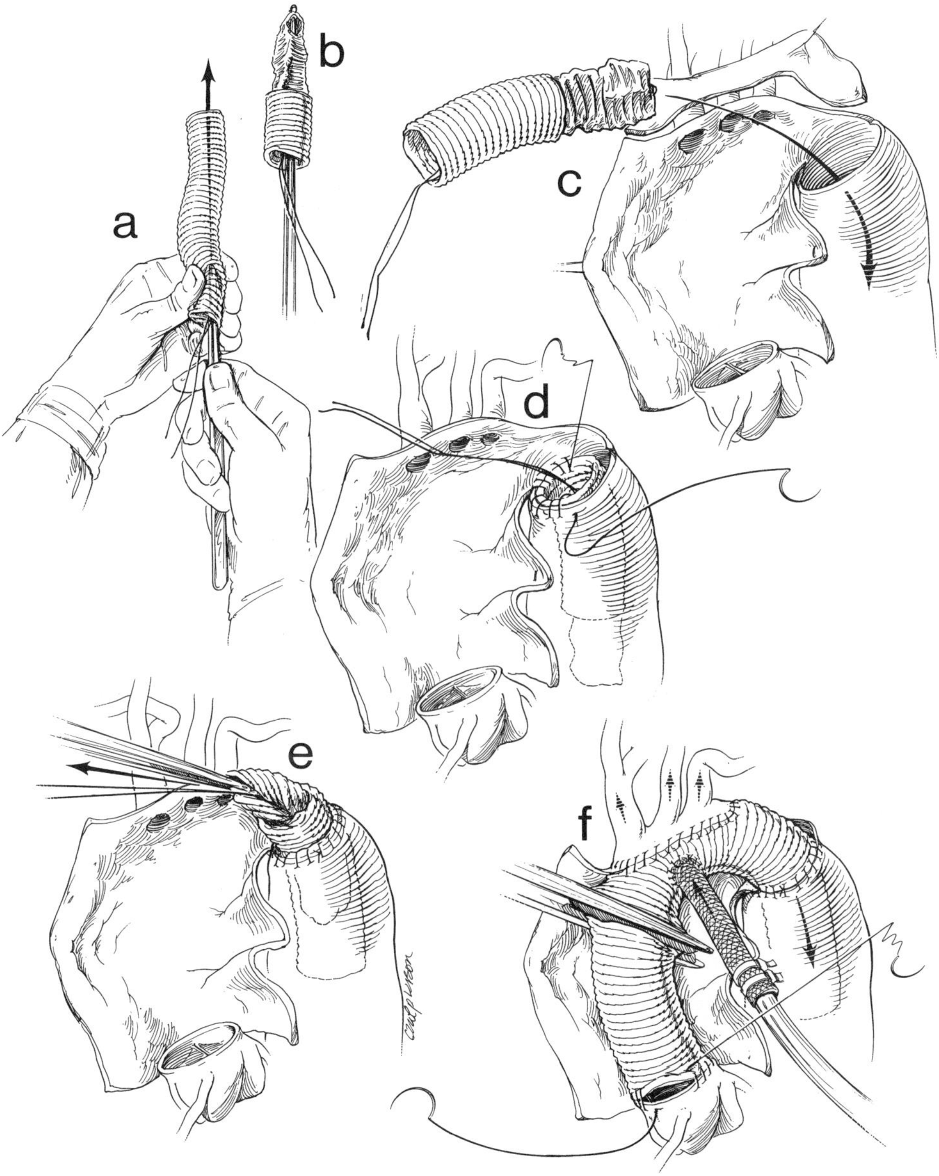

FIG. 10-6. (a–f) Illustration of operative technique for first stage of treatment of patient with mega aortic aneurysm showing the "elephant trunk" technique for replacement of the transverse aortic arch.

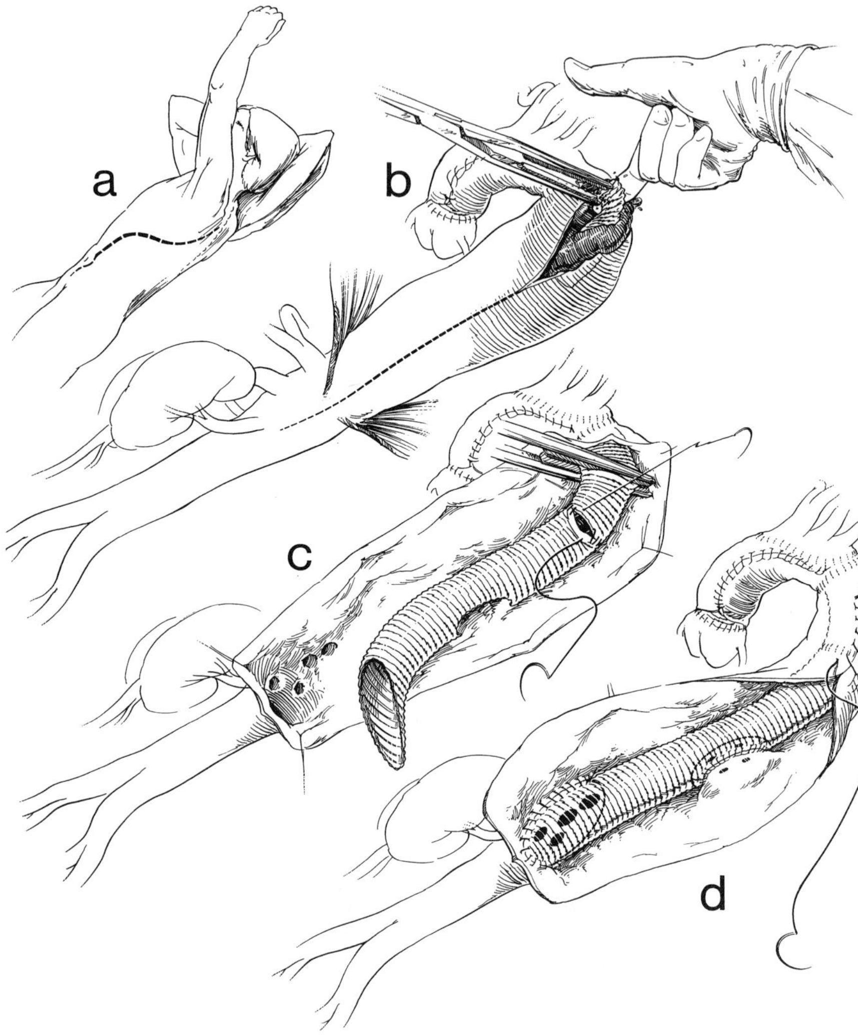

FIG. 10-7. (a–d) Illustration of operative approach for the second stage of treatment of patient with mega aorta with resection and replacement of thoracoabdominal aortic aneurysm following "elephant trunk" technique replacement of the transverse aortic arch.

ries, acute dissection was present in 21%, chronic dissection in 30%, and nondissecting aneurysms in 49%. In-hospital mortality was 6% and long-term mortality was 9%. The overall incidence of early stroke was 3.1%, while 3.5% developed early postoperative diffuse temporary encephalopathy.

The pathology affecting the transverse aortic arch remains diverse and technically challenging. Employing the surgical techniques described here, successful aortic arch replacement can be performed with acceptably low morbidity and mortality, consequently favorably altering the poor prognosis resulting from the natural history of this complex disease.

REFERENCES

1. Pressler V, McNamara JJ. Thoracic aortic aneurysm. Natural history and treatment. J Thorac Cardiovasc Surg 1980;79:489–498
2. Bickerstaff LK, Pairolero PC, Hollier LH, Melton LJ, Van Peenen HJ, Cherry KJ, Joyce JW, Lie JT. Thoracic aortic aneurysms: a population based study. Surgery 1982;92:1103–1108
3. DeBakey ME, Cooley DA. Successful resection of aneurysm of distal aortic arch and replacement by graft. JAMA 1954;155:1398–1403
4. Cooley DA, DeBakey ME. Resection of entire ascending aorta in fusiform aneurysm using cardiac bypass. JAMA 1956;162:1158–1159
5. DeBakey ME, Crawford ES, Cooley DA, Morris GC, Jr. Successful resection of fusiform aneurysm of aortic arch with replacement by homograft. Surg Gynecol Obstet 1957;105:657–664
6. Griepp RB, Stinson EB, Hollingsworth JF, Buehler D. Prosthetic replacement of the aortic arch. J Thorac Cardiovasc Surg 1975;70:1051–1063
7. Crawford ES, Saleh SA. Transverse aortic arch aneurysm: improved results of treatment employing new modifications of aortic reconstruction and hypothermic cerebral circulatory arrest. Ann Surg 1981;194:180–188
8. Svensson LG, Crawford ES, Hess KR, Coselli JS, Raskin S, Shenaq SA, Safi HJ. Deep hypothermia with circulatory arrest: determinants of stroke and early mortality in 656 patients. J Thorac Cardiovasc Surg 1993;106:19–31
9. Coselli JS, Büket S, Djukanovic B. Aortic arch operation: current treatment and results. Ann Thorac Surg 1995;59:19–27
10. Kampmeier RH. Saccular aneurysm of the thoracic aorta: a clinical study of 633 cases. Ann Intern Med 1938;12:624
11. Miller DC, Stinson EB, Oyer PE, Rossiter SJ, Reitz BA, Griepp RB, Shumway NE. Operative treatment of aortic dissections: experience with 125 patients over a sixteen year period. J Thorac Cardiovasc Surg 1979;78:365–382
12. Crawford ES, Kirklin JW, Naftel DC, Svensson LG, Coselli JS, Safi HJ. Surgery for acute ascending aortic dissection: should the arch be included? J Thorac Cardiovasc Surg 1992;104:46–59
13. Crawford ES, Coselli JS, Svensson LG, Safi HJ, Hess KR. Diffuse aneurysmal disease (chronic aortic dissection, Marfan, and mega aorta syndromes) and multiple aneurysms: treatment by subtotal and total aortic replacement emphasizing the elephant trunk operation. Ann Surg 1990;211:521–537
14. Lie JT. Aortic and extracranial large vessel giant cell arteritis: a review of 72 cases with histopathologic documentation. Semin Arth Rheum 1995;24:422–431
15. Robbs JV, Humann RR, Rajaruthnam P. Operative treatment of non-specific aortoarteritis (Takayasu's arteritis). J Vasc Surg 1986;3:605–616
16. Chan FY, Crawford ES, Coselli JS, Safi HJ, Williams TW. In-situ prosthetic graft replacement for mycotic aneurysm of the aorta. Ann Thorac Surg 1989;47:193–203
17. Crawford ES, Crawford JL, Safi HJ, Coselli JS. Redo operations for recurrent aneurysmal disease of the ascending aorta and transverse aortic arch. Ann Thorac Surg 1985;40:439–455
18. Coselli JS, Crawford ES, Williams TW Jr, Bradshaw MW, Wiemer DR, Harris RL, Safi HJ. Treatment of postoperative infection of ascending aorta and transverse aortic arch, including use of viable omentum and muscle flaps. Ann Thorac Surg 1990;50:868–881
19. Culliford AF, Colvin SB, Rohrer K, Baumann FG, Spencer FC. The atherosclerotic ascending aorta and transverse arch: a new technique to prevent cerebral injury during bypass: experience with 13 patients. Ann Thorac Surg 1986;41:27–35
20. Svensson LG, Sun J, Cruz HA, Shahian DM. Endarterectomy for calcified porcelain aorta associated with aortic valve stenosis. Ann Thorac Surg 1996;61:149–152
21. Amarenco P, Cohen A, Tzourio C, Bertrand B, Hommel M, Besson G, Chauvel C, Touboul PJ, Bousser MG. Atherosclerotic disease of the aortic arch and the risk of ischemic stroke. N Engl J Med 1994;331:1474–1479

22. DeBakey ME, McCollum CH, Crawford ES, Morris GC Jr, Howell J, Noon GP, Lawrie G. Dissection and dissecting aneurysms of the aorta: twenty-year follow-up of five hundred twenty-seven patients treated surgically. Surgery 1982;92:1118–1134
23. Coselli JS. Thoracic aortic aneurysms. In: Haimovici H. Vascular surgery (4th ed). East Norwalk, CT: Appleton & Lange, 1995;759–785
24. Coselli JS. Aneurysms of the transverse aortic arch. In: Baue AE. Sixth edition of Glenn's thoracic and cardiovascular surgery. East Norwalk, CT: Appleton & Lange, 1996;2239–2253
25. Coselli JS, Crawford ES, Beall AC Jr, Mizrahi EM, Hess KR, Patel VM. Determination of brain temperature for safe circulatory arrest during cardiovascular operation. Ann Thorac Surg 1988;45:638–642
26. Mizrahi EM, Patel VM, Crawford ES, Coselli JS, Hess KR. Hypothermic induced electrocerebral silence, prolonged circulatory arrest, and cerebral protection during cardiovascular surgery. Electroencephalogr Clin Neurophysiol 1989;72:81–85
27. Coselli JS. Retrograde cerebral perfusion via superior vena caval cannula for aortic arch aneurysm surgery. Ann Thorac Surg 1994;57:1668–1669
28. Pagano D, Boivin CM, Faroqui MH, Bonser RS. Retrograde perfusion through the superior vena cava perfuses the brain in human beings. J Thorac Cardiovasc Surg 1996;111(1):270–277
29. Cabrol C, Pavie A, Gandjbakheh I, et al. Complete replacement of the ascending aorta with reimplantation of coronary arteries: new surgical approach. J Thorac Cardiovasc Surg 1981;81:309–315
30. Crawford ES, Svensson LG, Coselli JS, Safi HJ, Hess MS. Aortic dissection and dissecting aortic aneurysms. Ann Surg 1988;208:254–273
31. Coselli JS, LeMaire SA, Van Cleve GD. Rupture of a dissecting thoracic aortic aneurysm into the pulmonary artery: successful surgical repair. J Cardiovasc Surg 1995;3:697–701
32. Borst HG, Walterbush G, Schaps D. Extensive aortic replacement using "elephant trunk" prosthesis. J Thorac Cardiovasc Surg 1983;31:37–40

Management of Extracranial Cerebrovascular Disease, edited by Keith D. Calligaro et al.
Lippincott-Raven Publishers, Philadelphia © 1997.

11

Regional Anesthesia for Carotid Endarterectomy

Thomas S. Riles, Mark S. Gold, Patrick J. Lamparello, Mark A. Adelman

In recent years anesthesiologists and surgeons have increasingly turned to regional and local anesthesia for surgical procedures. The most common reason for selecting regional over general anesthesia has been to decrease the cardiac and pulmonary risks. In vascular surgery this has become of particular importance as we extend the application of vascular reconstruction to patients who are older and present with more significant comorbidity. The interest in regional anesthesia has also been fueled by a desire to decrease the recovery and hospitalization time after an operation.

Although vascular surgeons commonly use regional anesthesia for lower extremity reconstruction, most have preferred general anesthesia for carotid surgery. The reluctance to use regional anesthesia for operations in the neck is due in part to lack of familiarity with the technique or discomfort working in the neck while the patient is awake. Others who have demonstrated excellent results performing carotid endarterectomy under general anesthesia simply have no particular reason to change a technique that has proven successful.[1–6]

Among the proponents of regional anesthesia for carotid surgery, the most commonly cited advantage is the ability to monitor accurately the patients' neurologic status during and immediately after the operation.[7–12] This points to the fact that the choice of anesthetic is closely related to the method by which the surgeon chooses to ensure cerebral protection during carotid clamping. From observations on the awake patient, it is known that 4% of the patients with a patent contralateral carotid artery and 25% of patients with an occluded contralateral carotid will develop neurologic symptoms with occlusion of the ipsilateral carotid.[13] With general anesthesia the surgeon is obliged to either identify those patients at risk for cerebral ischemia and provide cerebral protection by shunting them or, alternatively, to use a shunt in every patient. For those who prefer selective shunting, EEG monitoring or stump pressure measurements are the most common methods for selecting patients who need shunts. Although it is beyond the scope of this chapter to debate the issue of routine versus selective shunting, it is important to discuss the differences between various methods for selective shunting, since one of the methods is to monitor the neurologic status of the awake patient.

Stump pressure is reasonably reliable for selection, provided the threshold for shunting is <50 mm Hg.[14] At this threshold, however, approximately 40% of the patients will require a shunt. EEG is a more accurate method of determining the need for cerebral protection, but requires additional equipment and an experienced technician in the OR throughout the procedure. Centers that use EEG monitoring report ischemic changes necessitating a shunt in 15–42% of patients.[1,4–6,8] By comparison, surgeons who use regional anesthesia report alterations in neurologic status in 4–19% of patients.[8,11–13] One may conclude from this that EEG monitoring and stump pressure are overly sensitive and lead to more frequent shunting than may be necessary.[11]

In addition to the issue of monitoring during carotid clamping, we have found it advantageous to be aware of the patient's neurologic status immediately after restoration of blood flow and during the trip to the recovery room. Many of the neurologic problems become manifest at this time.[15] Observation of the nature of the deficit and the exact timing of its occurrence may give early insight into the cause and the best course of action.

Although often cited as an advantage,[10,11,16] there is very little data available to support the contention that regional anesthesia results in fewer cardiopulmonary complications for carotid endarterectomy. In one of the few papers to examine the issue, Allen and associates retrospectively compared 361 patients who had general anesthesia with 318 who had regional anesthesia, and found the incidence of cardiopulmonary complications to be half among those who had regional anesthesia (8.3% vs 4.6%, $p = 0.04$).[8] It is our belief that the advantages of regional anesthesia for patients at risk for cardiopulmonary complications are the same whether we are performing lower-extremity or carotid reconstruction. It is important to mention, however, that the use of regional anesthesia does not negate the need for close monitoring and aggressive treatment of the high-risk patient.

Some have argued that regional anesthesia for carotid surgery lowers the operative morbidity and mortality.[7,11,12] Whereas this may be true for a given surgeon or center, it is difficult to support this as a general statement. Excellent results have been reported in many centers using general anesthesia exclusively.[1–6] Other studies that have compared general and regional anesthesia have found no difference in stroke and death rates.[8,17,18] It is our view that although regional anesthesia improves the ability to monitor patients for cerebral ischemia and postoperative neurologic events, perioperative strokes are most often related either to technical errors at the time of the endarterectomy or reperfusion injuries, not the choice of anesthetic.

Whether regional anesthesia reduces the period of postoperative hypertension,[12] operating time,[8] or hospital stay[10,17,18] is unclear and will require further analysis.

TECHNIQUE

Essential to the administration of a cervical regional anesthetic is an understanding of the principal pain pathways from the area. The main pathways to the neck pass through nerve roots C2–C4. The distribution of these nerves covers the area from the base of the head down to the clavicle. Overlap of sensation may come from other dermatomes. T2 may innervate the lower neck. This is the next dermatome after C4, as C5–T1 forms the brachial plexus (Fig. 11-1). The third division of the trigeminal nerve provides sensation down to the edge of the mandible and in the region of the upper pole of the incision. Near the midline, there may also be overlap from the contralateral dermatomes. The carotid sheath has additional pain pathways through cranial nerves nine and ten.

There are several techniques to block all these pathways. We prefer to directly anesthetize nerve roots C2–C4 and then add additional superficial infiltration along the line of the incision and in the carotid sheath to block the secondary pathways.

The administration of a cervical block begins by carefully identifying and marking the anatomic structures necessary to find the cervical nerve roots and the superficial cervical plexus. The nerve roots emerge superior to the transverse process of each cervical vertebra. In the adult, the larynx overlies cervical vertebrae four through six and is useful to approximate the position of these structures. The notch of the thyroid cartilage marks the upper border of the larynx (C4), and the cricoid cartilage identifies the lower border (C6). Another C6 landmark is the point where the external jugular vein crosses the posterior border of the sternocleidomastoid muscle. With the patient's head turned to the contralateral side, a line can be drawn from the cricoid cartilage to the point where the external jugular vein crosses the muscle, marking the level of

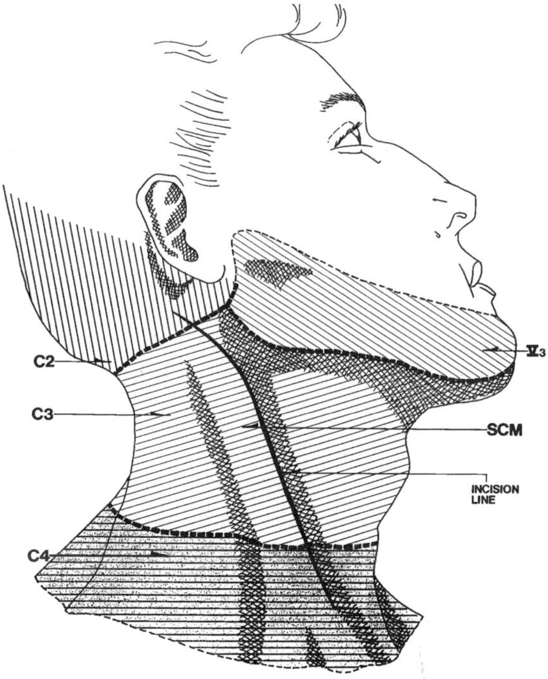

FIG. 11-1. The zones of innervation of nerve routes C2, C3, C4 and the lower branch of the trigeminal nerve (V3). The sternocleidomastoid muscle (SCM) is shown. (From Riles T, Gold M. Alternatives to general anesthesia for carotid endarterectomy. In: Moore W (ed.) Cerebral vascular surgery. Philadelphia: WB Saunders, 1995, with permission)

C6. A parallel line beginning at the notch of the thyroid cartilage identifies C4 (Fig. 11-2).

To determine the position of the C4 transverse process, the mastoid process is palpated and a mark is made 1 cm posteriorly. A line is drawn from this point perpendicular to the C4 line. Where the two lines intersect at right angles is the location of the C4 transverse process. The location of C2 and C3 is easily determined once the position of C4 is marked. Using the distance between the C4 and C6 line as a measure, the C2 process is that distance cephalad along the perpendicular line to the mastoid from the C4 point. The C3 process is halfway between C2 and C4 (see Fig. 11-2).

After marking the positions of the transverse process, the neck is prepped and draped. Using a 22-gauge 1.5-inch needle, the transverse processes are located by entering perpendicular to the skin. The depth varies with the body habitus of the patient. Once bone is located, the needle is pulled back slightly and directed cephalad. This is repeated until the needle is "walked off" the bone. The needle should not be inserted any more than 1–2 mm deeper than the bone, as deeper penetration can result in entering the subarachnoid space or the vertebral artery. After a negative aspiration, 5 cc of local anesthetic is injected slowly. This is repeated at the other two transverse processes. It is important to maintain communication with the patient continually, observing for a change in mental status that could occur with an intravascular or intrathecal injection.

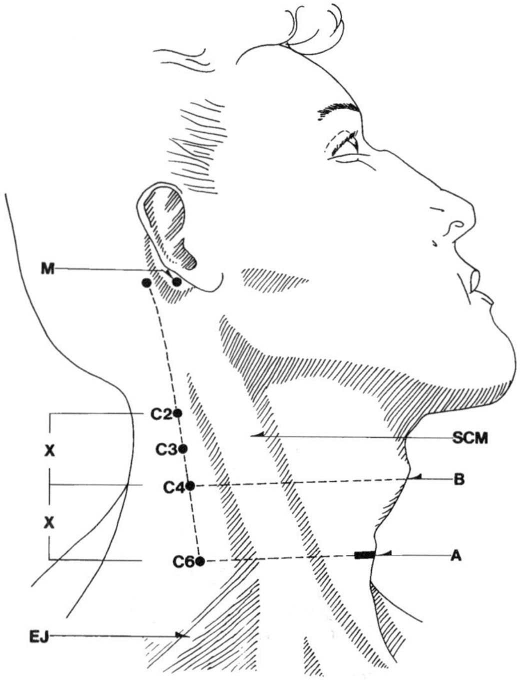

FIG. 11-2. Landmarks for locating and injecting the nerve routes C2 through C4. Landmarks include the cricoid cartilage (A), the thyroid cartilage (B), the sternocleidomastoid muscle (SCM), the mastoid bone (M), and the external jugular vein (EJ). C2 is located by measuring the same distance (x) cephalad from C4 as determined by the distance caudad to C6. C3 is half the distance between C2 and C4. (From Riles T, Gold M. Alternatives to general anesthesia for carotid endarterectomy. In: Moore W (ed.) Cerebral vascular surgery. Philadelphia: WB Saunders, 1995, with permission)

The superficial block is performed by injecting local anesthetic along the posterior border of the sternocleidomastoid muscle, particularly along the midpoint of the muscle, where the bulk of the superficial cervical plexus is located (Fig. 11-3). Anesthetic is also injected along the anterior border of the muscle and along the lower border of the mandible to ensure comfort along the line of the incision and to block any overlapping nerve pathways.

A variety of local anesthetics may be used for the cervical block. We have found that mepivacaine in a concentration of 1.5 percent gives an adequate block for approximately 4 hours. Approximately 30 cc of local anesthetic is necessary to block the neck. Since the neck is quite vascular, there may be a good deal of systemic absorption of anesthetic agent. To decrease the risk of anesthetic toxicity, absorption can be reduced by adding epinephrine in a concentration of 1:200,000. When local anesthetic is used at this volume and concentrations, the likelihood of reaching a toxic level is low for an average-sized adult. For smaller patients, either the volume or the concentration of the agent must be reduced.

Once the anesthetic is set, the patient's head is rotated to the contralateral side and secured. To keep the drapes off the patient's face and to allow access for the anesthesiologist, an Omni retractor is used to construct a frame over the upper head. A child's squeaker toy is placed in the hand of the patient contralateral to the side of the surgery. So as not to interfere with the movement of the hand, the arterial monitoring line is placed in the radial artery ipsilateral to the operation.

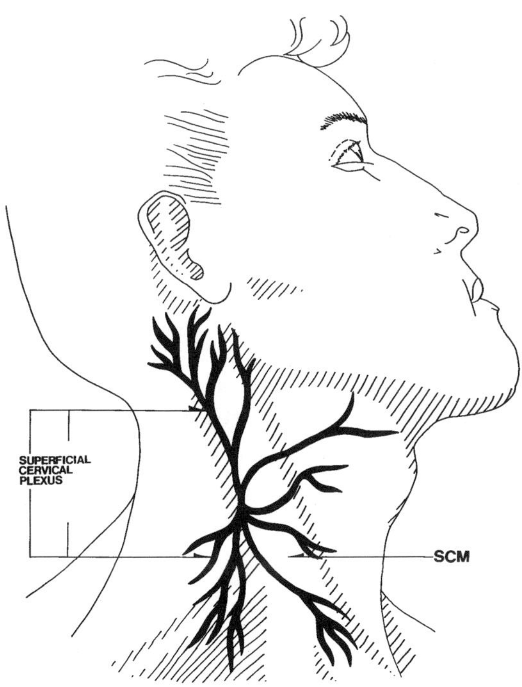

FIG. 11-3. The superficial cervical plexus radiating from its exit posterior to the sternocleidomastoid muscle (SCM). (From Riles T, Gold M. Alternatives to general anesthesia for carotid endarterectomy. In: Moore W (ed.) Cerebral vascular surgery. Philadelphia: WB Saunders, 1995, with permission.)

The neck is prepped and draped, and the procedure is performed in the conventional manner. If the patient shows any signs of discomfort, 0.5% lidocaine with epinephrine is infiltrated into the area with a 25-gauge needle. Additional anesthesia is often needed in the carotid sheath and occasionally for the fibers from the baroreceptors of the carotid bifurcation. Before making the arteriotomy, the surgeon test clamps the internal carotid artery. The patient is asked to count and squeak the toy in the contralateral hand for approximately 2 minutes. If there is no evidence of cerebral ischemia, the operation may proceed without a shunt. If the patient shows signs of monoparesis, aphasia, dysarthria, slowing of mentation, loss of consciousness, or confusion, the clamp is removed and preparations are made for shunting.

The vast majority of patients can tolerate the 1.5–2 hours of surgery with no more than the light sedation and periodic reassurances by the surgeon and anesthesiologist. Management of sedation is important during cervical block. The patient must be alert enough to respond to commands, thereby ensuring adequate cerebral blood flow. Some sedation may be needed, however, to allow the patient to tolerate the surgery. Small amounts of benzodiazepines, narcotics, propofol, or a combination of the three may be titrated to achieve the desired effect. Propofol has the advantage that it is extremely short acting, so if the patient becomes oversedated the effect will be short-lived.

Occasionally, especially in elderly patients, benzodiazepines cause disinhibition, resulting in restlessness and confusion. This can be differentiated from inadequate cerebral blood flow by reversing the benzodiazepine and flumazenil. Oversedation with narcotics can be reversed with small doses of naloxone. Caution must be exercised when using naloxone, because rapid administration may result in hypertension and congestive heart failure.

Occasionally, it is necessary to convert to general anesthesia with endotracheal intubation during the operation. Reasons for conversion may include patient discomfort, inability to cooperate, or claustrophobia. Other reasons include unusually difficult anatomy or prolonged operation. Under these circumstances, the surgeon may choose to complete the operation with the patient intubated and anesthetized. We have been able to convert to general anesthesia at any point in the operation without difficulty. This is done by first having the surgeon remove unnecessary instruments from the wound and place a sterile towel over the incision. The surgeon keeps his or her hand over the incision to prevent violation of the sterile field while the anesthesiologist folds back the drapes, removes the Omni retractor, and rotates the head to the midline. The patient is then anesthetized and intubated. Once the endotracheal tube is secured, the head is returned to the rotated position, the drapes are folded back to the head of the table, and the operation proceeds. We occasionally plan the operation in this manner to allow for test clamping of the carotid arteries before the patient is anesthetized in order to determine whether a shunt is necessary.

COMPLICATIONS

It is important that the anesthesiologist and surgeon be aware at all times of the possibility of several potentially serious complications of the cervical block anesthetic.

First, as with any local anesthetic, a potential exists for systemic toxic effects, with or without an intravascular injection. The manifestations of a local anesthetic toxicity may be neurologic (sedation, tinnitus, and seizures) or cardiac (conduction blockage, myocardial depression, arrhythmias, and cardiac arrest). The risk of central nervous system toxicity may be reduced by giving the patient intravenous benzodiazepine prior to performing the block. Although the risk is small, it is important that the individuals administering the block are knowledgeable about the management of local anesthetic toxicity.

Because of the close proximity of the vertebral arteries, extreme caution must be taken during the injection of the anesthetic agent. With the rich vasculature of the neck, an intravascular injection is a potential risk. It is important to make slow and careful injections with frequent aspirations and to maintain constant verbal communication with the patient, looking for signs of local anesthetic toxicity.

Another potentially serious complication is from an inadvertent intrathecal injection, resulting in a total spinal anesthetic. This may occur from injecting too deeply or from dissection of the anesthetic agent within the sheath of the nerve root back to the subarachnoid space. If this should occur, the patient may develop progressive paralysis of the extremities, become aphasic, and then lose consciousness, with loss of spontaneous responsiveness, within a matter of minutes. It is important to be alert to the possibility of this complication and to observe the patient carefully while blocking the neck. Prompt intubation and adequate ventilation will sustain the patient until the spinal anesthetic wears off. It is possible to continue the operation under general anesthesia if one is certain that the cause of the neurologic symptoms is the intrathecal injection.

An additional complication of cervical block is hematoma formation. This may occur if the needle enters a large blood vessel. Usually local compression alleviates the problem, but occasionally a hematoma will progress. If a hematoma occurs, one must be alert to the possibility of airway compromise.

SELECTION OF PATIENTS

In a recently reported series of 3,062 carotid endarterectomies, we used regional anesthesia in 90.1% of the cases. Comparing operations performed in recent years to those performed earlier, we have tended to use general anesthesia more often, but still prefer regional anesthesia in 82.8% of the cases (Fig. 11-4). We have no hesitation and, in fact, prefer regional anesthesia for secondary carotid surgery for recurrent stenosis.[19] Vascular surgeons and most anesthesiologists at our institution are familiar with both techniques and choose one or the other, based on what we feel will be best for a particular patient. Because we do not use EEG monitoring, the decision to use general anesthesia implies that we will routinely use a shunt unless other information assures us that the patient will have adequate collateral circulation with carotid clamping.

The decision to use general or regional anesthesia is often determined at the time of the initial consultation. If the patient has had a severe stroke or a neurologic con-

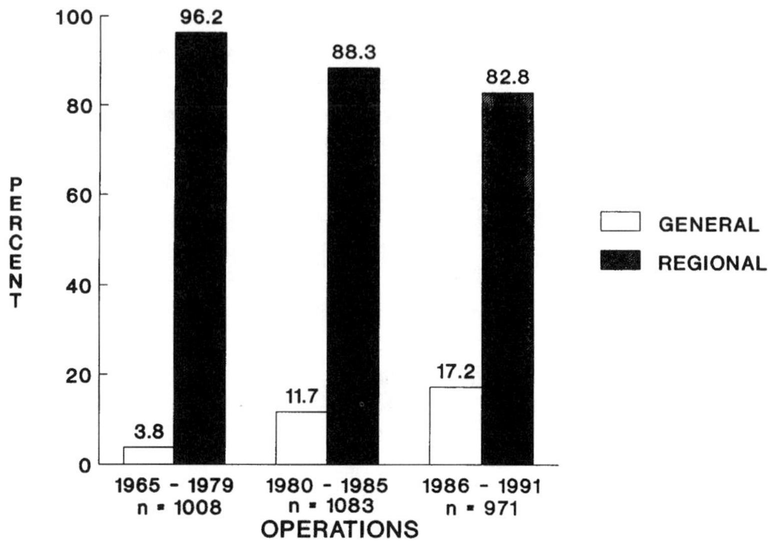

FIG. 11-4. The use of regional anesthesia for carotid endarterectomy at New York University, 1965–1991

dition that would make it difficult to cooperate during the operation, we would usually select a general anesthetic. Likewise, patients who are anxious or claustrophobic are felt to be poor candidates for regional anesthesia. Conversely, patients who have anatomy or plaque pathology that may make shunting difficult or patients with compromised cardiac or pulmonary function are urged to have a regional block. In the absence of these factors the patients are given the option of regional or general anesthesia. It is interesting to note that most patients, after asking a few questions about the technique and length of the surgery, choose to stay awake during the operation. Among the elderly in particular we find that there is more fear of the general anesthetic than the carotid repair.

The anesthetic choice is also discussed with the anesthesiologist and internist. Rarely, anatomic problems such as an unusually thick neck or difficult airway will influence the decision. If the patient becomes anxious or finds that being awake is uncomfortable while in the operating room, we have no hesitation in changing to general anesthesia. As mentioned earlier, conversion to general anesthesia is possible at any point during the operation.

SUMMARY

Regional anesthesia for carotid surgery is not for every patient and not for every surgeon. We feel that familiarity with the technique is very important. Although regional anesthesia does not ensure success, in some select cases it may make a difficult case relatively simple. In general, the more skills we can take into the operating room, the easier our task and the better the results for our patients. We find regional anesthesia a valuable technique for performing carotid surgery, a method that is easily learned and transported to other centers by our residents, and a choice that is appreciated by our patients.

REFERENCES

1. Whittemore AD, Kauffman JL, Kohler TR, Mannick JA. Routine electroencephalographic (EEG) monitoring during carotid endarterectomy. Ann Surg 1983;197:707–712
2. Hertzer NR, Beven EG, Greenstreet RC, et al. Internal carotid back pressure, intraoperative shunting, ulcerative atheromata, and the incidence of stroke during carotid endarterectomy. Surgery 1978;83: 306–312
3. Moore WS, Yee JM, Hall AD. Collateral cerebral blood pressure: an index of tolerance to temporary carotid occlusion. Arch Surg 1973;106:520–523
4. Towne JB, Bernhard UM. Neurologic deficit following carotid endarterectomy. Surg Gynecol Obstet 1982;154:849–852
5. Callow AD, Matsumoto G, Baker D, et al. Protection of the high-risk carotid endarterectomy patient by continuous electroencephalography. J Cardiovasc Surg 1978;19:55–64
6. Sundt TM, Jr, Sharbrough FW, Piepgras DG, Kearns TP, Messick JM, Jr, O'Fallon WM. Correlation of cerebral blood flow and electroencephalographic changes during carotid endarterectomy: with results of surgery and hemodynamics of cerebral ischemia. Mayo Clin Proc 1981;56:533–543
7. Connolly JE. Carotid endarterectomy in the awake patient. Am J Surg 1988;150:159–165
8. Allen BT, Anderson CB, Rubin BG, et al. The influence of anesthetic technique on perioperative complications after carotid endarterectomy. J Vasc Surg 1994;19:834–843
9. Benjamin ME, Silva MB, Jr, Watt C. Awake patient monitoring to determine the need for shunting during carotid endarterectomy. Surgery 1993;114:673–681
10. Collier PE. Carotid endarterectomy: a safe cost-efficient approach. J Vasc Surg 1992;16:926–933
11. Hafner CD, Evans WE. Carotid endarterectomy with local anesthesia: results and advantages. J Vasc Surg 1988;7:232–239
12. Corson JD, Chang BB, Leopold PW, et al. Perioperative hypertension in patients undergoing carotid endarterectomy: shorter duration under regional block anesthesia. Circulation 1986;741:II-4
13. Imparato AM, Ramirez A, Riles TK, Mintzer R. Cerebral protection in carotid surgery. Arch Surg 1982;117:1073–1077
14. Hobson RW, Wright DB, Sublett JW, Fedde CW, Rich NM. Carotid artery back pressure and endarterectomy under regional anesthesia. Arch Surg 1974;109:682–687
15. Riles TS, Imparato AM, Jacobowitz GR, et al. The cause of perioperative stroke after carotid endarterectomy. J Vasc Surg 1994;19:206–216
16. Peitzman AB, Webster MW, Loubeau JM, Grundy BL, Bahnson HT. Carotid endarterectomy under regional (conductive) anesthesia. Ann Surg 1982;196:59–64
17. Muskett A, McGreevy J, Miller M. Detailed comparison of regional and general anesthesia for carotid endarterectomy. Amer J Surg 1980;152:691–694
18. Gabelman CG, Gann DS, Ashworth CJ, Jr, Carney WI, Jr. One hundred consecutive carotid reconstructions: local versus general anesthesia. Amer J Surg 1983;145:477–482
19. Gagne PJ, Riles TS, Jacobowitz GR, et al. Long-term follow-up of patients undergoing reoperation for recurrent carotid artery disease. J Vasc Surg 1993;18:991

Management of Extracranial Cerebrovascular Disease, edited by Keith D. Calligaro et al.
Lippincott-Raven Publishers, Philadelphia © 1997.

12

Selective Shunting: Utility of EEG Monitoring and Carotid Stump Pressure

William H. Baker

The use of a temporary indwelling shunt during carotid endarterectomy is a controversial subject. This controversy has somewhat abated in recent years as the emphasis is currently on results, not methods. That is, a surgeon who has a stroke rate associated with operation that is 2% or less may use any technique he or she chooses. Those surgeons whose patients have higher stroke rates need to reexamine their technique. Thus, they may benefit from a discussion of EEG monitoring and stump pressures as they relate to selective shunting.

Some surgeons avoid this argument altogether by always using a shunt.[1] These surgeons readily acknowledge that 80–90% of their patients will not require the shunt. However, they would prefer to use the shunt rather than rely on any of the currently available methods used to test the safety of operation without shunt. In addition, they state that constant use of the shunt makes the surgeon adept in its use and the operation easier.

Other surgeons never use the shunt[2] and are in a distinct minority. Although occasional series have excellent results, when we attempted this approach those patients who had a low stump pressure and a contralateral internal carotid occlusion fared poorly sustaining an 11% stroke rate. More recently, carotid endarterectomy without a shunt has been performed utilizing EEG suppression with barbiturates. Further experience will be required before this technique becomes accepted.

Most surgeons prefer to perform carotid endarterectomy without the use of a temporary indwelling shunt. While the operation can be performed with the shunt in place, it makes the operation more difficult. Since 80–90% of the patients do not require the use of a shunt, surgeons have attempted to identify those patients utilizing a variety of means.

Some surgeons prefer to perform the operation under local anesthesia.[4] Cervical block is administered by either the anesthesiologist or the surgeon and is quite effective in anesthetizing the area. After the dissection has been completed the carotid artery is clamped. If the patient is asymptomatic after 3 minutes, the operation then proceeds in the usual manner. Should the patient experience a neurological deficit of any sort, a temporary indwelling shunt is inserted at that time. Excellent results have been reported using this technique.[5]

Most surgeons, however, prefer general anesthesia. There is greater patient comfort and the risk is slight. Thus, these surgeons must rely on some other method to select patients who may require a temporary indwelling shunt. Although sensory-somatic evoked potentials,[6] transcranial Doppler,[7] and cerebral blood flow[8] have been utilized in some centers, the electroencephalogram and carotid stump pressures have emerged as the most popular methods.

There exists an abundance of literature extolling the value of EEG to select patients who require a shunt.[8–12] Most of the older studies relied on 10–18-lead electroencephalograms. A technician was present in the operating room to record the EEG. In some series a neurologist was present to interpret the findings. There are a variety of abnormal ischemic patterns that are beyond the scope of this discussion. In general, if the tracings are unchanged, operation is performed without a shunt. Abnormal tracings include generalized slowing, lateralized slow wave activity or, in severe cases of ischemia, flattening of the hemispheric tracing. More recent papers tend to use compressed electroencephalographic or compressed spectral array analysis.[9] These techniques require fewer leads and with the use of fast Fourier analysis the computer converts the EEG to compressed spectral array form. Ischemic events are defined as a one-third or more amplitude attenuation for at least 30 seconds or unilateral decrease in the spectral edge frequency to less than 50% of its average value. The advantage of this latter technique is in its simplicity and interpretation.

The incidence of shunt placement based on EEG abnormalities is highly variable. Five hundred and eleven of 1,145 consecutive carotid endarterectomies reported by Sundt et al[8] utilized a temporary indwelling shunt. It should be noted that Sundt also relies upon the measurement of cerebral blood flow. Tempelhoff et al[9] shunted 14 of 97 patients (13.6%) utilizing the compressed spectral array analysis. Most other series report that 15–20% of their patients require a shunt. This incidence of shunt usage is slightly greater when compared to shunt usage during local (regional) anesthesia.

Whereas the EEG is a safe method to select patients for shunt usage, it is not a savior. Kresowik et al from the University of Iowa reported their experience of 458 patients.[13] The incidence of shunting was 15%. Nineteen strokes (4.1%) occurred in this patient cohort. Ten of the 19 strokes and 5 of 9 transient deficits were immediately apparent when the patient awoke from anesthesia. Of interest, 5 of the 10 patients with immediate stroke and all 5 of the patients with transient deficits had no ischemic EEG changes during the carotid endarterectomy. Thus, it is obvious that the EEG will not predict every patient who will suffer a neurologic deficit. It should be noted that this group utilized a 16-channel recorder for their study.

Carotid stump pressures were first introduced by Moore and Hall in 1969.[14] Two occluding vascular clamps are placed across both the external and the proximal common carotid artery. A needle placed into the common carotid distal to the clamp then measures the pressure reflected retrograde down the internal carotid artery (carotid stump pressure, back pressure). Operating at the San Francisco Veterans Administration Hospital they performed carotid endarterectomy under local anesthesia in 36 patients. Five patients (10%) were intolerant of carotid cross-clamping and lost consciousness. Their back pressures were 10, 19, 19, 20, and 22 mm Hg. All other patients who had a carotid artery back pressure greater than 25 mm Hg exhibited no neurologic changes. They concluded that a back pressure >25 mm Hg indicated carotid endarterectomy could be safely performed without a shunt.

Later, in the same city, Hayes et al from the University of California at San Francisco reported their experiences.[15] In this study patients who had a carotid artery stump pressure of 50 mm Hg or greater were spared neurologic complications. However, those patients with carotid artery stump pressures less than 50 did not fare as well. In the shunted group of 58 patients who had a low stump pressure, 3 had a temporary and 2 a permanent neurologic deficit. In the 15 patients with a low stump pressure in whom a shunt was not used, 1 temporary and 7 permanent deficits developed. Five of these latter 7 deficits were of a severe nature.

During my training I was impressed with the varying clinical application of the use of a temporary indwelling shunt. In those patients who had a low stump pressure but who, in addition, had a difficult end point, the shunt was extracted for seemingly long periods of time while attention was paid to this demanding technical problem. Yet, many of these patients did well. Thus, in 1970 we embarked on a plan of recording data in all patients, but shunting none.

Our preliminary results were published in 1977.[16] Our results at that time indicated that carotid endarterectomy could be performed safely without the use of a temporary indwelling shunt. There appeared to be no correlation between a low stump pressure and the development of an acute neurologic deficit following operation. Thus, our study continued until 1984.[3] By this time we had accumulated enough patients that it was obvious that a temporary indwelling shunt should be considered in a certain subset of patients. Those patients who had a carotid stump pressure of greater than 50 mm Hg all did well. Those patients who had a carotid artery stump pressure of less than 50 mm Hg and who, in addition, had a patent contralateral internal carotid artery also did well. Those patients who had both a contralateral occluded internal carotid artery and an ipsilateral stump pressure less than 50 mm Hg had a prohibitive stroke rate. There were 9 permanent deficits for a permanent stroke rate of 11%. Thus, we suggested in this paper that patients falling into this category be considered for a temporary indwelling shunt.

Littooy et al at the Hines Veterans Administration Hospital reported their experiences a few years later. In that series 2 of 7 patients who had a carotid artery stump pressure of less than 25 mm Hg had a devastating neurologic deficit following carotid endarterectomy.[19] Thus, the tenets enumerated by our 1984 study were further modified to include the use of a shunt in all patients with a carotid artery stump pressure of less than 25 mm Hg, regardless of the status of their contralateral internal carotid artery.

Other authors disagree with our numbers. Hobson and associates recorded carotid artery back pressures as high as 75 mm Hg[18] that were associated with neurologic deficits. Ricotta suggested that a level of 40 mm Hg was safe in patients without recent stroke.[19] Archie[20] and Beebe[21] have both noted that the stump pressure may vary during the operation. Archie[20] emphasizes that this variation is directly related to the variation in the systemic blood pressure. Archie also notes that a falsely elevated carotid stump pressure may be reported unless the surgeon takes the time and trouble to test occlude the distal internal carotid artery. In some instances there will be flow past an irregular plaque in the common carotid or external carotid artery, which subsequently elevates the pressure and gives the surgeon a false sense of security. In this clinic all patients have test occlusion with vascular pick-ups.

Hafner and Evans[5] compared carotid stump pressures and EEG tracings with the patient's neurologic status under local anesthesia. All patients who had a greater than 50 mm Hg carotid artery stump pressure did well and did not require a shunt. Two of 276 with an internal carotid artery stump pressure of 26–50 mm Hg required a shunt. Almost half of the 125 patients with a carotid artery stump pressure less than 25 mm Hg required a temporary indwelling shunt. The EEG had ischemic changes in 18 of 28 patients with a low stump pressure. All of these changes reverted with unclamping. None of these patients suffered a postoperative stroke. Four of 119 patients with stump pressures between 25 and 50 mm Hg had a stroke. Two of these patients exhibited EEG changes that resolved with shunt insertion, but two did not. Interestingly, two of 193 patients with stump pressures greater than 50 mm Hg suffered a postoperative stroke. In one of these patients there were no EEG changes. In the other patient EEG changes were unrelated to the operative occlusion, perhaps indicating an embolus. In 2 other patients EEG changes persisted, but neither of these patients suffered any neurologic complications. Thus, it can be seen that whereas in general there is a correlation between the EEG and the carotid artery stump pressure, this correlation is not necessarily comparable with the clinical situation. It was the conclusion of these authors that had the EEG or carotid stump pressure been used only, many patients would have been unnecessarily shunted. If, indeed, the presence of a shunt leads to an untoward clinical result as suggested by Green,[11] this finding is of great clinical significance.

The use of a temporary indwelling shunt does not ensure a good clinical result. Prioleau et al[22] reported that the incidence of stroke in four Charleston hospitals was 10.7%. When the cases were standardized, the incidence of stroke in 137 shunted cases was 9.5% and in 116 non-shunted cases was 0.9%. This data from a non-randomized series indicates only that the shunt will not salvage an otherwise poorly conceived and performed operation.

The use of a temporary indwelling shunt is a technique that every vascular surgeon needs to master. When to use the shunt is a matter of some controversy. The methods discussed in this chapter, namely EEG and carotid stump pressure, have been time tested by legions of surgeons. Both give good and reliable indications for the use of a shunt. Both techniques are recommended as excellent selectors.

I wish to emphasize that shunt usage is not the sine qua non of a successful operation. Technical perfection remains the hallmark of good patient care. During the initial dissection the bulb that contains offending atherosclerosis and clot cannot be manipulated. Clamps need to be applied in areas that are relatively free of atherosclerosis. The endarterectomy needs to be complete with special attention paid to the distal end point in the internal carotid artery. The closure should not compromise the vessel and the liberal use of patches is recommended. The shunt will not resurrect a bad operation. The shunt is used only to shepherd those relatively few patients who need it through operation without an ischemic neurologic event.

REFERENCES

1. Thompson JE, Talkington CM. Carotid endarterectomy. Ann Surg 1976;184:1–15
2. Ott DA, Cooley DA, Capa L, Coelho A. Carotid endarterectomy without temporary intraluminal shunt. Ann Surg 1980;191:708–714
3. Baker WH, Littooy FN, Hayes AC, Dorner DB, Stubbs D. Carotid endarterectomy without a shunt: the control series. J Vasc Surg 1984;1:50–56
4. Shaw DM, Darling RC, Chang BB, et al. Carotid endarterectomy in awake patients: its safety, acceptability, and outcome. J Vasc Surg 1994;19:1015–1020
5. Hafner CD, Evans WE. Carotid endarterectomy with local anesthesia: results and advantages. J Vasc Surg 1988;7:232–239
6. Schweiger H, Kamp H-D, Dinkel M. Somatosensory-evoked potentials during carotid surgery: experience in 400 operations. Surg 1991;109:602–609
7. Bergeron P, Benichou H, Rudondy P, Jausseran JM, Ferdani M, Courbier R. Stroke prevention during carotid surgery in high risk patients (value of transcranial Doppler and local anesthesia). J Cardiovasc Surg 1991;32:713–719
8. Sundt TM, Sharbrough FW, Piepgras DG, Kearns TP, Messick JM, Jr, O'Fallon WM. Correlation of cerebral blood flow and electroencephalographic changes during carotid endarterectomy. Mayo Clin Proc 1981;56:533–543
9. Tempelhoff R, Modica PA, Grubb RL, Jr, Rich KM, Holtmann B. Selective shunting during carotid endarterectomy based on two-channel computerized electroencephalographic/compressed spectral array analysis. Neurosurg 1989;24:339–344
10. Whittemore AD, Kauffman JL, Kohler TR, Mannick JA. Routine electroencephalographic (EEG) monitoring during carotid endarterectomy. Ann Surg 1983;197:707–713
11. Green RM, Messick WJ, Ricotta JJ, Charlton MH, Satran R, McBride MM, DeWeese JA. Benefits, shortcomings, and costs of EEG monitoring. Ann Surg 1985;201:785–792
12. Callow AD, Matsumoto G, Baker D, Cossman D, Watson W. Protection of the high risk carotid endarterectomy patient by continuous electroencephalography. J Cardiovas Surg 1978;19:55–64
13. Kresowik TF, Worsey MJ, Khoury MD, Krain LS, Shamma AR, Sharp WJ, Stern JA, Corson JD. Limitations of electroencephalographic monitoring in the detection of cerebral ischemia accompanying carotid endarterectomy. J Vasc Surg 1991;13:439–443
14. Moore WS, Hall AD. Carotid artery back pressure. Arch Surg 1969;99:702–710
15. Hayes RJ, Levinson SA, Wylie EJ. Intraoperative measurement of carotid back pressure as a guide to operative management for carotid endarterectomy. Surg 1972;72:953
16. Baker WH, Dorner DB, Barnes RW. Carotid endarterectomy: is an indwelling shunt necessary? Surg 1977;82:321–326
17. Littooy FN, Halstuk KS, Mamdani M, Calandra D, Hayes AC, Baker WH. Factors influencing morbidity of carotid endarterectomy without a shunt. Am Surg 1984;50:350–353
18. Hobson RW, Wright CB, Sublett JW, Fedde CW, Rich NM. Carotid artery back pressure and endarterectomy under regional anesthesia. Arch Surg 1974;109:682–687
19. Ricotta JJ, Charlton MH, DeWeese JA. Determining criteria for shunt placement during carotid endarterectomy. Ann Surg 1983;198:642–645
20. Archie JP. Technique and clinical results of carotid stump back-pressure to determine selective shunting during carotid endarterectomy. J Vasc Surg 1991;13:319–327
21. Beebe HG, Starr C, Slack D. Carotid artery stump pressure: its variability when measured serially. J Cardiovasc Surg 1989;30:419–423
22. Prioleau WH, Aiken AF, Hairston P. Carotid endarterectomy: neurologic complications as related to surgical techniques. Ann Surg 1977;185:678–683

Management of Extracranial Cerebrovascular Disease, edited by Keith D. Calligaro et al.
Lippincott-Raven Publishers, Philadelphia © 1997.

13

Clinical Applications of Transcranial Doppler in Patients with Cerebrovascular Disease

Anthony J. Comerota, Mira L. Katz

Transcranial Doppler (TCD) was introduced in 1982.[1] Since then, TCD ultrasonography has expanded the noninvasive diagnostic capability for patients with suspected cerebrovascular disease, permitting investigation of intracranial arteries that previously could be examined only by arteriography. TCD offers a hemodynamic evaluation, adding physiologic information to that provided by the anatomic evaluation of arteriography.

TCD applications have expanded rapidly and this technique is useful for a variety of clinical applications (Table 13-1). Based on the premise that knowledge of the intracranial circulation can assist clinicians in their assessment and treatment of patients with suspected occlusive cerebrovascular disease and to ensure that significant intracranial disease is not overlooked, TCD evaluation has been added to the noninvasive cerebrovascular examination in many vascular, radiology, and neurovascular laboratories.

This chapter reviews the applications of transcranial Doppler in patients with cerebrovascular disease, as well as a number of miscellaneous applications that may be of interest to physicians caring for these patients.

CEREBROVASCULAR APPLICATIONS

Diagnosis of Intracranial Disease

TCD offers the opportunity to detect intracranial artery stenosis,[2–9] occlusion,[10] aneurysms,[11–13] and AV malformations[13–16] in patients with suspected cerebrovascular disease. This is a new and potentially important addition to the noninvasive cerebrovascular examination. In order to assess accurately the intracranial vasculature, one must be aware of hemodynamic changes associated with intracranial (and extracranial) cerebrovascular disease and the importance of the natural history of the associated intracranial disease and its implications for treatment.

TABLE 13-1. *Clinical application of transcranial doppler in patients with cerebrovascular disease*

I. Cerebrovascular applications
  A. Diagnosis of intracranial disease
    1. stenosis
    2. aneurysm
    3. A-V malformation
  B. Evaluate collateral pathways
  C. Evaluate vertebrovascular insufficiency
  D. Evaluate subclavian steal
  E. Operative monitoring during carotid endarterectomy
    1. hypoperfusion
    2. emboli
  F. Cerebrovascular reserve
II. Miscellaneous applications
  A. Monitor vasospasm
  B. Predict stroke with sickle cell disease
  C. Evaluate migraine headache
  D. Evaluate brain death
  E. Epidemiologic studies

Stenosis

The characteristic alterations caused by an intracranial arterial stenosis include a focal increase in blood flow velocity, turbulence in the area of stenosis and a post-stenotic drop in velocity (Fig. 13-1). Stenoses can also produce bruits (low frequency enhancement around the baseline) or musical murmurs (band shaped enhancements symmetrical and parallel to the baseline).

Detectable intracranial stenoses are usually greater than 60% diameter reduction. Although absolute velocity criteria for intracranial stenoses are not reliable, a mean velocity of 80 cm/sec is a threshold for the anterior circulation that should cause concern. A mean velocity of 70 cm/sec is suspicious for a stenosis in the vertebrobasilar system. In general, any focal velocity increase of $\geq$25% should raise suspicion of an arterial narrowing.

Intracranial stenoses most commonly occur in the carotid siphon and in the middle cerebral artery (MCA), whereas the incidence of an isolated stenosis in the anterior or posterior cerebral arteries is low. The status of the cerebral tissue perfused has an important influence on intracranial velocity profiles. Lower velocities are found in patients with cerebral infarction due to decreased perfusion to the infarcted tissue. A patient without cerebral infarction preserves perfusion to the outflow bed and therefore will have appropriate velocity increases caused by an arterial stenosis.

TCD is somewhat limited in its ability to detect occlusion. These limitations are the result of inadequate transtemporal windows, anatomic variability, congenital aplasia, or severe hypoplasia of other intracranial arteries. If, however, an MCA Doppler signal is absent in the presence of a good transtemporal window, and high-quality Doppler signals obtained from other ipsilateral arteries, an MCA occlusion should be suspected. Additionally, an increase in the ipsilateral anterior cerebral artery velocity, due to perfusion through leptomeningeal collaterals, is corroborating evidence for MCA occlusion.

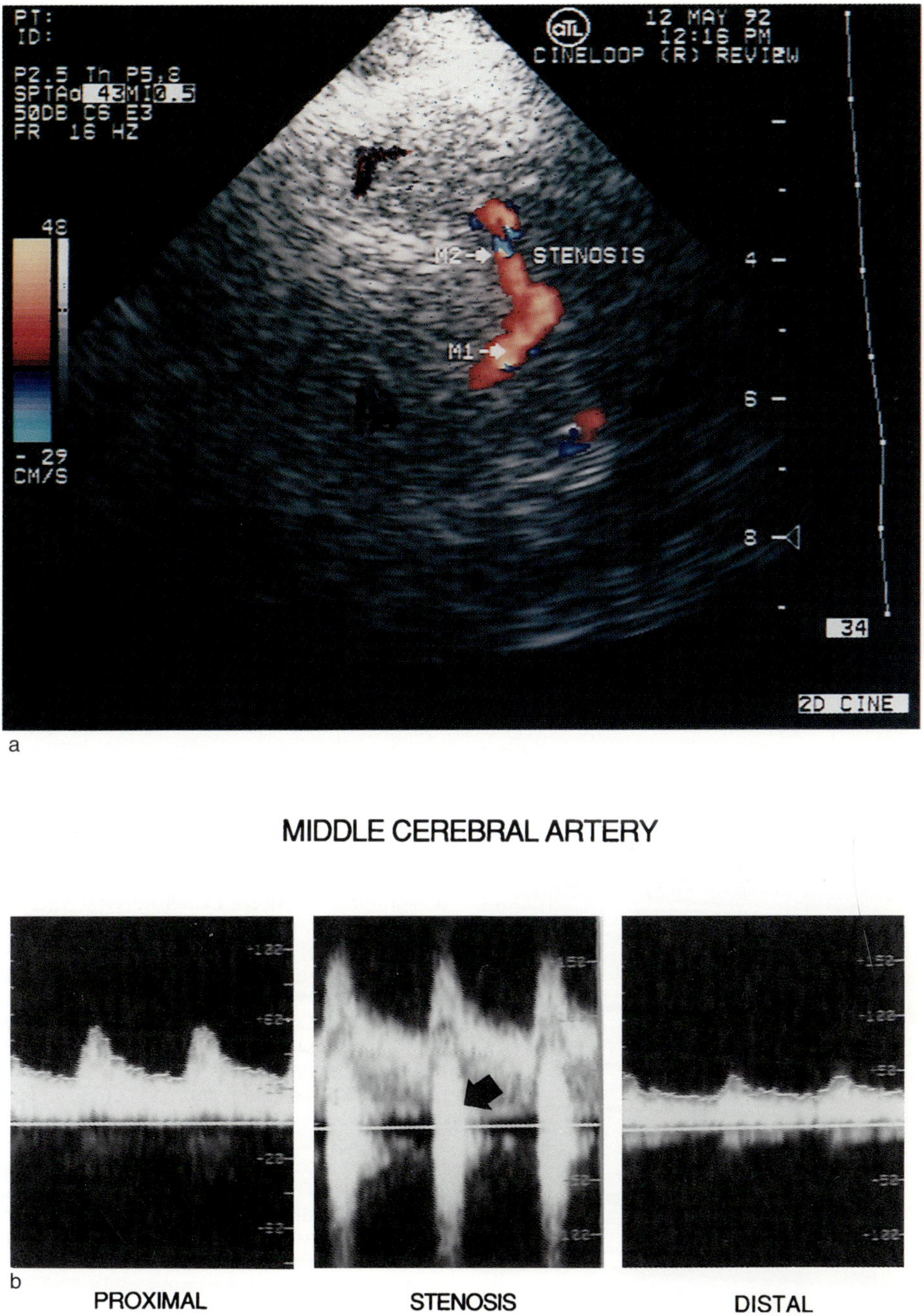

FIG. 13-1. An intracranial stenosis demonstrated by TCD. (a) Color changes demonstrate an increase in velocity in the M-2 segment of the middle cerebral artery; (b) Characteristic velocity changes associated with a stenosis demonstrate normal velocity signals proximal to the stenosis, increased velocity with an associated bruit (arrow) within the stenosis, and diminished velocity signals distally.

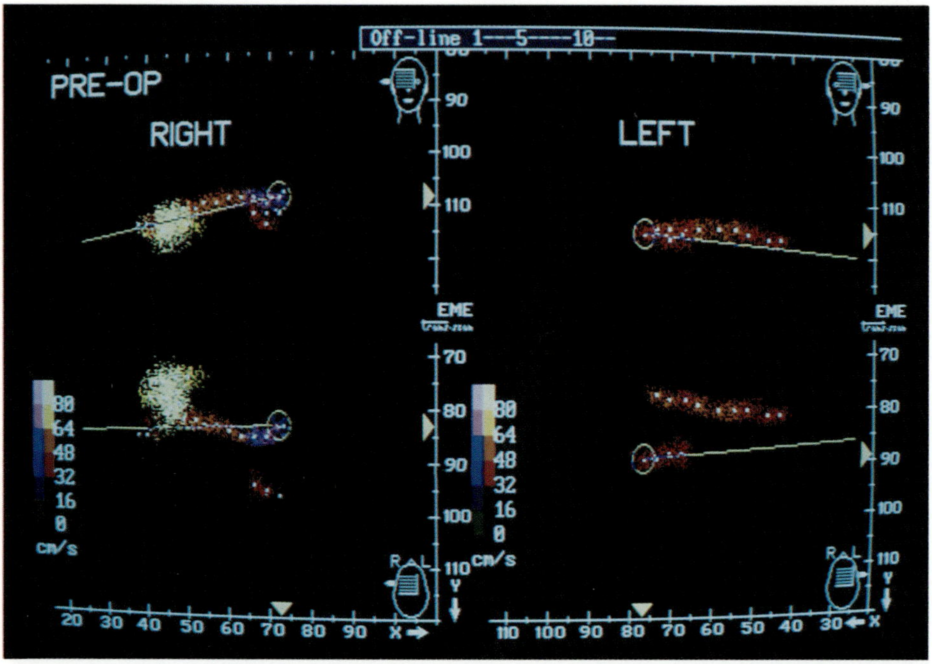

a

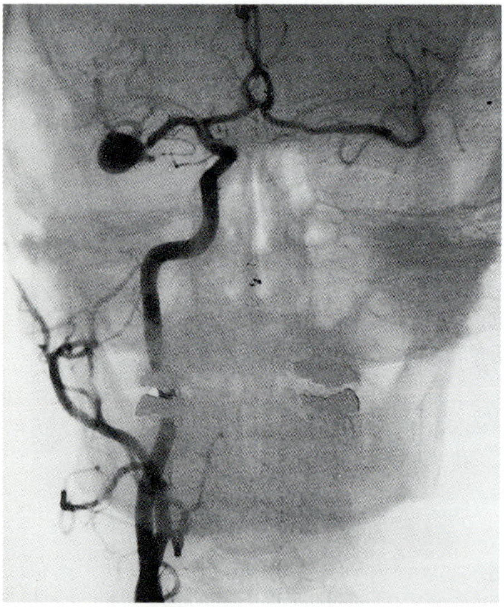

b

FIG. 13-2. This example demonstrates a TCD map of a patient with an intracranial aneurysm, which was found on a routine examination for a high-grade stenosis of left cervical internal carotid artery. (a) The anterioposterior and horizontal views of the right and left transtemporal map demonstrate a significantly increased velocity (>100 cm/sec) in the distal middle cerebral artery (MCA), which is recorded in yellow, indicating blood flow toward the transducer. Doppler signals from the distal MCA were turbulent and indicated the presence of an aneurysm. The right anterior cerebral artery (ACA) mapped in blue (flow away from the transducer) indicated increased velocity. On the left side, the ACA demonstrated reversed blood flow direction and is color-coded in red. These findings suggest cross-filling (right to left) via the anterior communicating artery; (b) The arteriogram confirmed the transcranial Doppler findings. A right middle cerebral artery aneurysm is demonstrated. Additionally, cross filling from the right to the left side via the anterior communicating artery confirmed the TCD findings.

The importance of an intracranial stenosis has been demonstrated in a number of reports. Carotid siphon stenosis has been associated with ipsilateral ischemic events following its diagnosis. Reports by Wechsler et al,[17] Craig et al[18] and Marzewski et al[19] demonstrated substantial morbidity associated with intracranial stenoses. On the other hand, Schuler et al[20] and, later, Borozan et al,[21] expanding on their earlier report, suggested that a carotid siphon stenosis was benign. Although this issue is not completely resolved, an understanding of the definition of "stenosis" in these reports is helpful. In the former reports most stenoses were >60% diameter reduction. This severity of disease influences flow characteristics and is generally considered to be "hemodynamically significant." In the latter reports, however, patients who had a 20% or more diameter reduction lesion were included. It is likely that such minimal disease is not associated with appreciable morbidity and certainly does not cause hemodynamic abnormalities.

A severe extracranial carotid stenosis may well warrant correction even in association with intracranial disease. However, the prognosis for additional neurologic events after successful carotid endarterectomy may be influenced by intracranial lesions, particularly if the lesion is a high-grade stenosis. As more patients are being offered carotid endarterectomy without preoperative arteriography, the opportunity to evaluate the intracranial circulation anatomically is erased in these patients. Therefore, if one is to evaluate properly the etiology of neurologic events remote from carotid endarterectomy in this patient group, TCD may be useful.

Aneurysms

In general, the ability of TCD to detect a patent intracranial aneurysm depends on its location and its size (Fig. 13-2). Sensitivities have been reported from 0–85%.[12,13] In the most optimistic report, Baumgartener and colleagues[12] identified 85% (23 of 27) of nonthrombosed aneurysms having a diameter of 6–25 mm. Four nonthrombosed aneurysms with a mean diameter of 5 mm were not detected and, of course, 3 thrombosed aneurysms were also missed. One would not expect TCD to detect thrombosed intracranial aneurysms since there is no blood flowing in the aneurysm sac. Martin and colleagues[13] were unable to detect any of 11 angiographically identified intracranial aneurysms in 5 patients; however, each of those aneurysms was ≤5 mm.

If transcranial color Doppler imaging is used, differentiation of a dilated vessel from color artifact can be difficult, since the high color gain settings required during transcranial imaging cause color spill-over into the adjacent tissue. Additionally, vessel tortuosity or branching may be misdiagnosed as an aneurysm.

Arteriovenous Malformations

An arteriovenous malformation (AVM) is a developmental anomaly in which blood flows directly from the arterial circulation to the venous circulation without intervening capillaries. In an AVM the resistance is low compared to the normal cerebrovascular resistance. Arteries that supply the AVM are designated "feeders" to distinguish them from the arteries that supply the surrounding neural tissue. Since they carry a large volume of blood, feeders are usually larger in diameter and characterized by an increased velocity, reduced pulsatility, and reduced responsiveness to CO_2.[14–16] The venous drainage comprises enlarged veins that carry pulsatile arterialized blood. The danger of an AVM is that the tissue normally supplied by the involved arterial circulation may become ischemic if the shunt is severe.

TCD can demonstrate the hemodynamics of an AVM as well as its anatomic location. A standard TCD examination is performed in these patients with special attention given to the intracranial arterial velocities, pulsatility indices and direction of flow. The increased velocities often approach those associated with vasospasm following subarachnoid hemorrhage; however, the pulsatility index tends to be lower because vascular resistance is low.

The sensitivity of detecting intracranial AVMs depends on their size, location, and the number and length of the main feeders. Lindegaard et al[14] reported that TCD detected 93% (26 of 28) of the AVMs evaluated in their series. The 2 AVMs that were not detected were both less than 2 cm.

Petty et al[15] studied 15 patients with AVMs that had 19 feeding arteries, and evaluated the outcome of therapy, comparing the final hemodynamics of those treated with embolization (10 feeding arteries) compared to surgical resection (9 feeding arteries). The initial diagnosis and treatment outcomes were confirmed angiographically in all patients. Post-treatment TCD examinations were performed on average 8 days following intervention. Both surgery and embolization resulted in similar changes in hemodynamics, demonstrating a decrease in velocity and an increase in the pulsatility indices. Although there were greater hemodynamic changes in the surgically treated group, this trend did not reach statistical significance. This study demonstrates that TCD can reliably evaluate the hemodynamic outcome of treatment of AVMs.

Collateral Pathways

Transcranial Doppler identifies the intracranial arterial collateral patterns in patients with extracranial arterial stenosis.[6,22,23] An artery providing collateral circulation usually demonstrates increased flow velocity, characterized by diffuse velocity increases throughout the length of the artery, unlike the focal increase in velocity found with an arterial stenosis.

The three main collateral pathways identified by TCD are:

1. The anterior communicating artery (ACoA), providing a collateral from hemisphere to hemisphere
2. The ophthalmic artery (OA), providing a collateral from the extracranial external carotid artery (ECA) to the intracranial internal carotid artery (ICA) through the orbit

3. The posterior communicating artery (PCoA), providing a collateral from the posterior to the anterior circulation (or vice-versa)

In our experience, the most commonly found collateral pattern in patients with significant extracranial carotid disease is through the anterior communicating artery (ACoA)[24] (Fig. 13-2). The characteristics of this collateral pathway include:

An increase in the velocity of the contralateral anterior cerebral artery
Turbulent Doppler signal and increased midline velocity (secondary to increased velocity through the ACoA)
Reversal of blood flow in the ipsilateral ACA

The external carotid or ophthalmic artery collateral pathway via the orbit is confirmed by demonstrating flow reversal in the ophthalmic artery, which carries the blood from the ECA to the intracranial ICA. Collateral perfusion from the posterior circulation via the posterior communicating artery to the anterior circulation is the third pattern and is found most often in patients with significant bilateral extracranial carotid disease. In patients with severe vertebral artery disease, this flow pattern may be reversed, thereby providing blood to the posterior circulation from the anterior.

There has been a good correlation of TCD with arteriography for the identification of collateral pathways. Lindegaard et al[22] demonstrated a 94% (29 of 31) sensitivity for the anterior communicating artery pathway and 87% (26 of 30) for the posterior communicating artery. Likewise, Grolimund et al[6] found a 94% (16 of 17) sensitivity for the ACoA and 88% (7 of 8) for the PCoA, with an 89% (8 of 9) sensitivity for the ACA collateral pathway via the orbit. However, a recent study that included six medical centers reported a sensitivity of only 62% (18 of 29) for the ACoA but 100% (7 of 7) for the OA collateral pathway.[23]

Potential errors in these correlative studies occur because arteriography does not always demonstrate true physiologic conditions. Differences between the TCD and arteriography may be due to the pressure of contrast injection during the arteriogram and, therefore, TCD may provide a more accurate indication of functional collateral blood flow than arteriography. Additionally, the posterior collateral is often difficult to visualize even when present and represents a source of technical error during transcranial Doppler examinations.

Vertebrobasilar Insufficiency

The symptoms of vertebrobasilar insufficiency are often nondescript, and patients with suspected vertebrobasilar disease are frequently difficult to evaluate. Although arteriography remains the definitive diagnostic evaluation, many patients are not fully evaluated because of its associated morbidity.[25]

Transcranial Doppler has been used to assess the intracranial hemodynamics and particularly the vertebrobasilar system in these patients. The techniques of assessing the posterior circulation have been established.[26] Intracranial stenoses are identified by focal elevations in mean blood flow velocity, which are often associated with a distal loss of signal pulsatility. Although the absence of a signal suggests arterial occlusion, arterial hypoplasia or anatomic variability are also possibilities. Marked loss of pulsatility unassociated with focal intracranial stenosis often indicates severe proximal vertebral artery disease.

Kinsella et al[27] evaluated the impact of transcranial Doppler on the management of 107 consecutively referred patients with suspected vertebrobasilar insufficiency. These authors interviewed referring physicians before and after the results of the TCD examination were reported. Interestingly, management changed in 42% of the patients after the TCD results were given and there was a 58% reduction in the use of angiography ($p = 0.04$) and a 128% increase in the use of aspirin ($p = 0.005$).

Color-coded imaging of the vertebral basilar system improves diagnostic capabilities. Several investigators have shown that imaging of the vertebrobasilar system in addition to the Doppler findings enable accurate identification of the intracranial vertebrobasilar arteries and improves the reliability of the TCD evaluation.[28,29]

It appears that TCD examination of patients with suspected vertebrobasilar insufficiency can have a significant impact on patient management. We believe this is especially true when the index of suspicion of vertebrobasilar disease is relatively low and there is a desire to avoid angiography.

Subclavian Steal Syndrome

The subclavian steal syndrome is characterized by symptoms of brain stem ischemia associated with a stenosis or occlusion of the left subclavian, the innominant or the right subclavian arteries proximal to the origin of the vertebral artery. A stenosis causes the pressure in the affected upper extremity to be lower than normal, producing a pressure gradient that causes flow reversal in the ipsilateral vertebral artery, becoming especially prominent during exercise of the involved arm. When this occurs, the vertebral artery acts as the major collateral to the upper extremity, thereby "stealing" blood from the basilar artery and brain stem as a result of retrograde blood flow. If the volume of blood flow is large enough and the brain stem becomes ischemic, the patient may experience neurologic symptoms.

When subclavian steal is suspected, a standard TCD examination is performed with particular attention focused on blood flow direction and velocities of the vertebral arteries and the basilar artery. Since blood flow is normally away from the transducer in the vertebrobasilar system, flow toward the transducer indicates flow reversal of the vertebral or basilar artery, which is evidence of a steal. Most commonly, flow reversal is found only in a single vertebral artery, suggesting a vertebral-to-vertebral steal, without flow reversal in the basilar artery.[30–33]

In many patients flow reversal at rest is absent, or one might observe alternating flow, with reversal occurring during end diastole. This may represent a latent steal, and maneuvers designed to reduce outflow resistance of the upper extremity should be performed. Such maneuvers include either exercise of the involved arm or post-occlusive reactive hyperemia while blood flow in the vertebral artery is monitored.

Our preference is postocclusive reactive hyperemia. This maneuver frequently uncovers a latent steal and demonstrates flow reversal in the affected vertebral artery (Fig. 13-3). The role of basilar artery blood flow in suspected subclavian steal has been evaluated by TCD. In most patients, resting basilar artery blood flow is not reduced, but may become abnormal if the contralateral vertebral artery (or subclavian) is also diseased. Reports have demonstrated that basilar artery blood flow is resistant to velocity changes during flow reversal in the vertebral arteries, and that actual flow reversal in the basilar artery is rare.[30,31]

Ringelstein[30] demonstrated flow reversal in the vertebral arteries in 91 patients; however, alternating or flow reversal in the basilar artery was demonstrated in only 1 of 48 patients with latent steal. Alternating flow or reversal of flow in the basilar artery was documented in 12 of the remaining 43 patients, with permanently reversed flow in the affected vertebral artery. Interestingly, each of these 12 patients had disease of the contralateral subclavian or feeding vertebral artery. This careful study demonstrates that reversal of blood flow in the basilar artery is not a common finding in patients with suspected or documented subclavian steal.

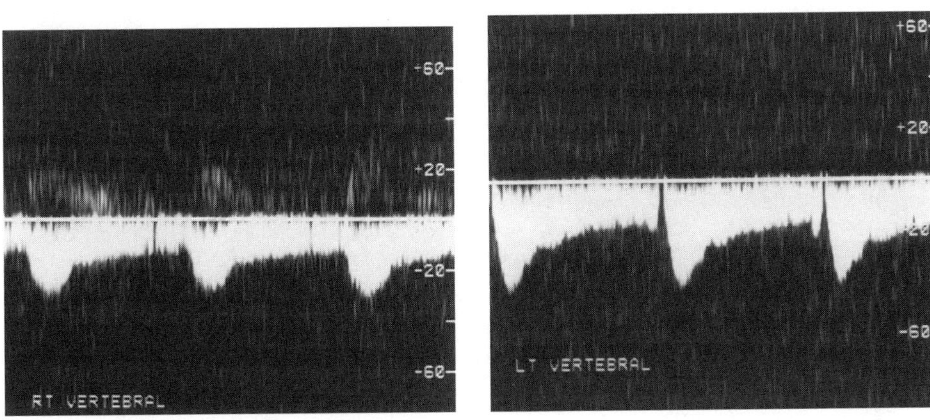

a b

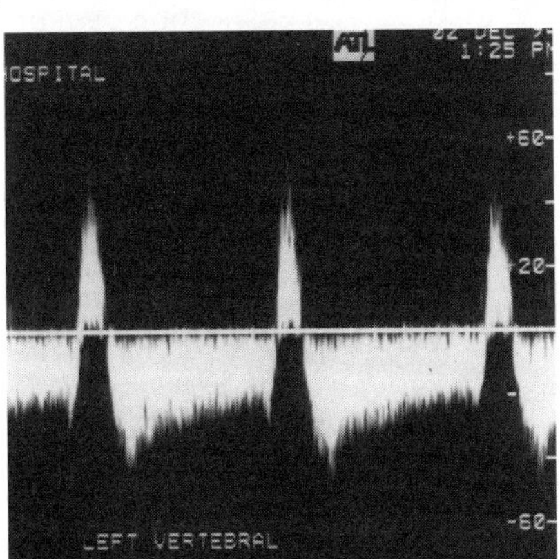

c

FIG. 13-3. Example of a patient with a 50% stenosis of the left subclavian artery, demonstrating characteristic blood flow changes at the end of the cardiac cycle in the left vertebral artery. (a) Normal velocity profile of the distal right vertebral; (b) Velocity profile of the left vertebral artery, demonstrating that blood flow diminished to zero at end diastole; (c) Following postocclusive reactive hyperemia there is flow reversal in the left vertebral artery at end diastole.

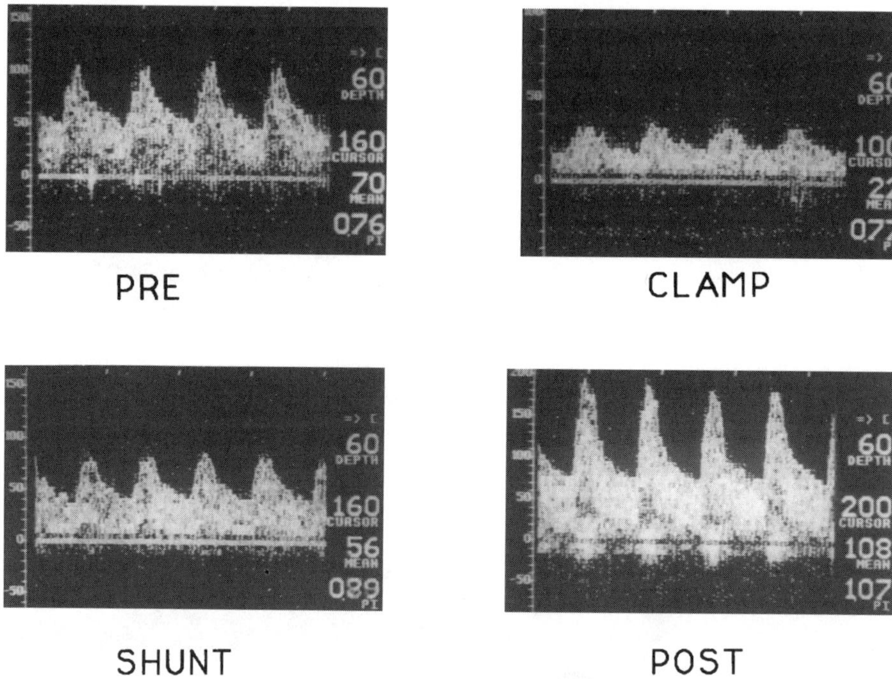

FIG. 13-4. Monitoring of middle cerebral artery velocity profiles during carotid endarterectomy. This patient's preclamp mean MCA velocity was 70 cm/sec, which decreased to 22 cm/sec during carotid clamping. This was associated with a concurrent slowing in the patient's EEG. After placing a carotid shunt, the MCA velocity increased to 56 cm/sec and the EEG reverted to normal. In the immediate postoperative period, the mean velocity increased to 108 cm/sec, demonstrating the characteristic hyperemia that can occur after a high-grade carotid stenosis has been corrected.

Monitoring During Carotid Endarterectomy

TCD monitoring during carotid endarterectomy offers real-time detection of alterations of intracranial arterial blood flow velocity in the ipsilateral cortex (Fig. 13-4). It has the advantage of continuous monitoring and as such may offer advantages over intermittent methods of monitoring such as Xenon studies or somatosensory evoked potential (SEP) information. TCD monitors the capacity of the intracranial collateral system to maintain middle cerebral artery blood flow during carotid clamping, indicating the need for carotid shunting. Observations during monitoring of MCA perfusion during carotid endarterectomy have led to TCD's use for detection of embolic phenomenon during the operative procedure.

Hypoperfusion

It is intuitive that a patient with good collateral circulation will preserve cerebral perfusion (middle cerebral artery velocity profile) during carotid clamping compared to the patient with poor intracranial collateral circulation. In general, middle cerebral artery velocities greater than 20 cm/sec or reductions in middle cerebral artery velocity of less than 65% compared to preclamp values are consistent with good collateral blood flow. Velocity reduction of 65% or more in the middle cerebral artery is required to demonstrate abnormalities in the somatosensory evoked potential. However, some patients may have no recordable middle cerebral artery profile yet maintain normal somatosensory-evoked potentials.[34] This information suggests that most neurologic deficits following carotid endarterectomy are the result of thromboembolic complications rather than hypoperfusion.

Some patients, however, are put at risk of ischemic neurologic dysfunction during carotid clamping, and the debate as to which patient requires shunting continues. The initial role for TCD monitoring for carotid endarterectomy was to identify those patients with a significant drop in middle cerebral artery perfusion, indicating the need for carotid shunting. Investigators who performed TCD and simultaneous EEG recordings have demonstrated that abnormalities in EEG occurred only when middle cerebral artery velocity diminished by >50% on carotid clamping.[35,36] Interestingly, they found that EEG changes always appeared within 2 minutes after documenting a significant decrease in MCA flow velocity. As expected, flow velocity changes were observed prior to the onset of neurologic deficits in patients operated under regional anesthesia. While it is true that patients with EEG slowing, marked decrease in regional cerebral blood flow, and abnormal somatosensory evoked potentials had significantly diminished middle cerebral artery velocity changes, the converse is not true—many patients with significant drops in MCA velocity did not have the corresponding EEG, regional cerebral blood flow, or SEP changes.[37–39] Therefore, it appears that the aforementioned MCA velocity changes with clamping would be sensitive but not specific for patients requiring shunting during carotid clamping.

TCD allows surveillance of the functioning of the shunt used during carotid endarterectomy. Decreased shunt flows are immediately reflected by a drop in MCA velocity and, therefore, shunt position and function can be immediately corrected should abnormalities occur.

Emboli

In addition to monitoring hemodynamic changes of the middle cerebral artery during carotid endarterectomy, the occurrence of intraoperative embolic signals have been observed. These high-frequency signals are detected during dissection, after the arteriotomy is performed and shunts are inserted, and after release of the carotid clamps. The emboli detected during the initial phase of the operation (*i.e.,* before the artery is open) must be the result of formed emboli, such as atheroma, particles of fractured thrombi or platelet aggregates.[38] Air emboli can occur following the arteriotomy (*i.e.,* during shunt insertion or after release of the vascular clamps). Interestingly, it has been observed that most new objectively documented cerebral infarcts occurred when more than ten embolic signals were observed during the initial dissection phases of the operation.[41] Additionally, Gaunt and colleagues[42] monitored 91 patients undergoing carotid endarterectomy. Twenty-three patients had particulate emboli during the carotid dissection, which correlated with a significant deterioration in postoperative cognitive function in 11 of these 23 patients.

Air emboli, however, appear to have a different natural history. Spencer and colleagues[40] demonstrated air bubble emboli in 62% of 56 patients following the release of carotid clamps. Cerebrovascular symptoms were present postoperatively in only 1 of those patients who had embolic signals. It appears that air bubble emboli do not necessarily produce postoperative symptoms; however, patients with persistent formed-element emboli are at higher risk for postoperative neurologic dysfunction or cerebral infarction.

In carefully studied patients, TCD may offer clinically relevant information about middle cerebral artery hemodynamics and embolic phenomenon during the course of carotid endarterectomy. This type of information may affect the technique of carotid endarterectomy and may potentially modify the course of the operation in order to reduce the occurrence of these embolic signals. However, if TCD monitoring is to become routine, it will depend on improving the ease of the monitoring and the confidence of interpreting the velocity patterns.

Cerebrovascular Reserve

Cerebral blood flow is maintained over a wide range of perfusion pressures by vasoconstriction and by vasodilation of the intracranial arterioles. TCD offers a noninvasive means to evaluate whether the extracranial carotid system can supply additional perfusion during periods of vasodilation. Patients who have exhausted their cerebrovascular reserve cannot increase perfusion in response to further vasodilatory stimuli, and these patients are thought to be at risk of ischemic brain injury if perfusion is diminished.

CO_2 can be used to enhance cerebral blood flow in both hemispheres. The CO_2 levels can be increased by having patients inhale up to a 5% concentration of CO_2, or merely by breath holding. The CO_2 affects the distal cerebral arteries but does not cause diameter increases of the large basal arteries.[43] Since changes in velocity do not reflect diameter variation of the proximal middle cerebral artery, TCD monitoring of that segment is a reliable indicator of cerebrovascular reserve.

Ringelstein and colleagues[44] evaluated the vasomotor reserve in 40 healthy volunteers and 40 patients with cerebrovascular disease. In the volunteers hypercapnia increased mean MCA velocity by 55.2% and hypocapnia was associated with a 35.3% decrease in MCA velocity. The 40 patients with unilateral ICA occlusion had significantly lower vasomotor reactivity on the occluded side, showing a 45.2% increase in velocity compared to a 67.7% increase on the nonoccluded side ($p < 0.0001$). Interestingly, the vasomotor reactivity was significantly lower in patients with symptomatic ICA occlusion compared to those with asymptomatic occlusions (37.6% versus 62.9%, $p < 0.006$).

Marcus and Harrison[45] evaluated breath-holding methods to inhalation of defined concentrations of CO_2. Each method correlated significantly with the degree of stenosis in 23 patients with extracranial carotid occlusive disease. They concluded that the breath-holding technique is a convenient screening method to assess CO_2 reactivity and can be applied much more easily because it does not require administration of CO_2.

Kleiser and Widder[46] measured CO_2 reactivity in 85 patients with ICA occlusion to evaluate the risk of stroke. Patients were categorized according to their CO_2 reactivity and were prospectively followed for a mean of 38 months. In the group thought to have sufficient CO_2 reactivity, 8% developed a TIA or prolonged reversible deficit; however, none had a stroke. In patients with a diminished or exhausted cerebrovascular reserve, 32% developed an ipsilateral event (stroke in 8 and TIA in 4, $p < 0.01$).

Webster et al[47] recently demonstrated the important prognostic value of diminished cerebrovascular reserve as monitored by Xenon perfusion studies. TCD is less cumbersome and has the potential of greater application in these high-risk patients.

MISCELLANEOUS APPLICATIONS

Vasospasm

Cerebral vasospasm is a serious complication following subarachnoid hemorrhage (SAH) and is a significant cause of morbidity and mortality. Early diagnosis and treatment can reduce the devastating consequences of this complication. Severe vasospasm produces an increase in blood flow velocity associated with a pressure drop distal to the spastic segment. Patients can compensate for these changes and maintain cerebral blood flow through their collateral circulation and by cerebral autoregulation. With increased intracranial pressure or exhaustion of cerebrovascular reserve, cerebral blood flow can be reduced to critical levels resulting in ischemia or infarction.

Prior to TCD, arteriography was the only method to diagnose vasospasm. The arteriographic diagnosis of vasospasm is subjective, variable in timing, difficult to measure, and has been associated with significant interobserver variability.[48] Arteriography can be risky in these patients and therefore is limited as a monitoring technique. The arterial narrowing produced by the spasm causes an increase in blood flow velocity that can be quantified by TCD.[49–54] The evaluation of vasospasm over time and its response to treatment also can be monitored by TCD. Since the increase in velocity detected by TCD often precedes the onset of neurologic deterioration, TCD can be used to determine the correct timing for surgical intervention or the need to continue or intensify pharmacologic intervention.[52]

Middle cerebral artery mean velocities of 100–120 cm/sec correlate with mild vasospasm when compared with arteriography. Moderate vasospasm is defined by velocities in the 120–200 cm/sec range, and severe vasospasm is characterized by velocities exceeding 200 cm/sec. Mean velocities >200 cm/sec indicate that the patient is at risk of reduced cerebral blood flow. Additionally, a rapid increase (>25 cm/sec/day) in velocity in the first few days after an intracranial hemorrhage is associated with a poor prognosis.[50] Musical murmurs have also been observed in patients being monitored for vasospasm, although their clinical relevance is uncertain.[55]

Predicting Stroke in Sickle Cell Disease

TCD is now being used to evaluate patients with sickle cell disease. Hemoglobin S tends to form intracellular polymers that distort red blood cells, and sickle cell disease is characterized by chronic hemolytic anemia. Cerebral infarction in these patients is associated with an occlusive vasculopathy involving the terminal internal carotid, the middle cerebral, and the anterior cerebral arteries. Prevention of stroke may be feasible with transfusion therapy if patients at risk can be identified.

Adams and colleagues[56] performed TCD examinations in 190 patients (age at entry was 3–18 years) with sickle cell disease. A TCD was considered abnormal if velocities exceeded 170 cm/sec. The TCD was normal in 167 patients and abnormal in 23. The clinical and hematologic parameters were similar between the two groups. Seven patients had a stroke, and in 6 of these patients the TCD was abnormal. These results indicate that TCD may be a useful method to assess the risk of stroke and perhaps alter management plans in patients with sickle cell disease.

Migraine Headache

The evaluation of patients with vascular headaches is a relatively new application for TCD.[57–63] A routine examination should be performed during the headache-free period and compared to the findings in the patient during the headache attack. Serial examinations are required for proper evaluation of these patients, therefore careful recording of the best window and location of the intracranial vessels is required.

Findings observed during migraine headaches include increased velocities, asymmetry of corresponding intracranial arteries, intracranial arterial bruits, or musical murmurs.

Thie and colleagues[59] performed TCD examinations on 109 consecutive patients with migraines and on 40 healthy volunteers. They found an increase in mean blood flow velocity of the intracranial arteries, and more intracranial bruits during the attack, with greater changes in the posterior cerebral artery velocity response to eye closing in migraineurs during the headache-free period compared with controls.

When 18 patients were evaluated during a headache attack, distinct differences were observed in patients with common migraines (without prodromes) compared to patients with classic migraine headaches (with transient visual or other sensory or motor prodromes).[60] Patients with common migraines had decreased intracranial velocities, increased pulsatility, and intracranial bruits that often disappeared compared to patients with classic migraines, who demonstrated an increase in velocities, a decrease in pulsatility, and in whom intracranial bruits became more prominent or newly developed.[59] The TCD findings were diffuse and did not correlate with the side of the headache or the neurologic aura. Such objective hemodynamic information may assist in the differential diagnosis of headaches of unknown etiology. These findings may be used to explain the pathophysiology of migraines and the changes in cerebral blood flow velocity during the attacks. This TCD information may become an important clinical tool in the evaluation and treatment of these patients.

Brain Death

Although clinical criteria for brain death have been established,[64] most hospitals require additional studies to confirm the diagnosis. TCD is noninvasive, portable, inexpensive, quick, and easily repeated.

Cerebral perfusion pressure (CPP) is the difference between the systemic arterial pressure (SAP) and the intracranial pressure (ICP). Cerebral circulatory arrest occurs when the intracranial pressure equals or exceeds the systemic arterial pressure.

During normal conditions the ICP is less than the SAP, and end-diastolic flow velocities are approximately 50% of the peak systolic velocity. Increased ICP increases peripheral resistance, thereby causing a decrease in the diastolic flow velocity, and the systolic peaks of the spectral wave forms assume a spiked appearance (increased pulsatility). As the ICP increases and approaches the diastolic SAP, the end-diastolic perfusion is reduced. When ICP is equal to the diastolic SAP, diastolic flow velocity disappears and only systolic peaks are detectable. If the ICP continues to increase (further drop in cerebral perfusion pressure) a diastolic flow component of the spectral wave form velocity reappears in the reversed direction. This characteristic TCD wave form is often referred to as the "to-and-fro" waveform. This signal reflects the oscillating movement of the blood column in the larger intracranial arteries, which are reflected from the arterioles, indicating no perfusion of the brain parenchyma. When the CPP approaches zero, three different TCD wave forms have been described; the oscillatory signal (to and fro), short systolic spike signals, or the absence of a signal that was previously present. Variations of these TCD patterns exist and progression from one stage to the next does not necessarily imply irreversible progression to brain death.

Investigators have emphasized TCD as a method to confirm the clinical diagnosis; however, it is not used alone to establish brain death.[65–69] These reports indicate that signals should be obtained from several intracranial arteries through different windows, because individual patients may have variable amounts of associated intracranial disease. The study by Powers et al suggested that representative TCD signals alone were inadequate and that Doppler signals with a net flow velocity $<$10 cm/sec in the MCA was a sensitive determinant of brain death.[68]

REFERENCES

1. Aaslid R, Markwalder TM, Nornes H. Noninvasive transcranial Doppler ultrasound recording of flow velocity in basal cerebral arteries. J Neurosurg 1982;57:769–774
2. Spencer MP, Whisler D. Transorbital Doppler diagnosis of intracranial arterial stenosis. Stroke 1986;17(5):916–921

3. Lindegaard KF, Bakke SJ, Aaslid R, Nornes H. Doppler diagnosis of intracranial artery occlusive disorders. J Neurol Neurosurg Psychiatry 1986;49:510–518
4. Niedekorn K, Neumayer K. Transcranial Doppler sonography: a new approach in the noninvasive diagnosis of intracranial brain artery disease. Eur Neurol 1987;26:65–68
5. Hennerici M, Rautenberg W, Schwartz A. Transcranial Doppler ultrasound for the assessment of intracranial arterial flow velocity. Part 2. Evaluation of intracranial arterial disease. Surg Neurol 1987;27:523–532
6. Grolimund P, Seiler RW, Aaslid R, et al. Evaluation of cerebrovascular disease by combined extracranial and transcranial Doppler sonography: Experience in 1,039 patients. Stroke 1987;18: 1018–1024
7. deBray JM, Joseph PA, Jeanvoine H, et al. Transcranial Doppler evaluation of middle cerebral artery stenosis. J Ultrasound Med 1988;7:611–616
8. Ley-Pozo J, Ringelstein EB. Noninvasive detection of occlusive disease of the carotid siphon and middle cerebral artery. Ann Neurol 1990;28:640–647
9. Rorick MB, Nichols FT, Adams RJ. Transcranial Doppler correlation with angiography in detection of intracranial stenosis. Stroke 1994;25:1931–1934
10. Kaps M, Damian MS, Teschendorf V, Dorndorf W. Transcranial Doppler ultrasound findings in middle cerebral artery occlusion. Stroke 1990;21:532–537
11. Harders A. Intra-aneurysmal flow pattern. In: Neurosurgical applications of transcranial Doppler sonography. New York: Springer Verlag, 1986
12. Baumgartner RW, Mattle HP, Kothbauer K, Schroth G. Transcranial color-coded duplex sonography in cerebral aneurysms. Stroke 1994;25:2429–2434
13. Martin PJ, Gaunt ME, Naylor AR, et al. Intracranial aneurysms and arteriovenous malformations: transcranial color-coded sonography as a diagnostic aid. Ultrasound Med Biol 1994;20:689–698
14. Lindegaard KF, Grolimund P, Aaslid R, Nornes H. Evaluation of cerebral AVM's using transcranial Doppler ultrasound. J Neurosurg 1986;65:335–344
15. Petty GW, Massaro AR, Tatemichi TK, et al. Transcranial Doppler ultrasonographic changes after treatment for arteriovenous malformations. Stroke 1990;21:260–266
16. Manchola IF, DeSalles AAF, Foo TK, et al. Arteriovenous malformation hemodynamics: a transcranial Doppler study. Neurosurg 1993;33:556–562
17. Wechsler LR, Kistler JP, Davis KR, Daminski MJ. The prognosis of carotid siphon stenosis. Stroke 1986;17:714–718
18. Craig DR, Meguro K, Watridge C, et al. Intracranial internal carotid artery stenosis. Stroke 1982;13: 825–828
19. Marzewski DJ, Furlan AJ, St Louis P, et al. Intracranial internal carotid artery stenosis: Long-term prognosis. Stroke 1982;13:821–824
20. Schuler JJ, Flanigan DP, Lim LT, et al. The effect of carotid siphon stenosis on stroke rate, death and relief of symptoms following elective carotid endarterectomy. Surgery 1982;92:1058–1067
21. Borozan PG, Schuler JJ, LaRosa MP, et al. The natural history of carotid siphon stenosis. J Vasc Surg 1984;1:744–749
22. Lindegaard KF, Bakke SJ, Grolimund P, et al. Assessment of intracranial hemodynamics in carotid artery disease by transcranial Doppler ultrasound. J Neurosurg 1985;63:890–898
23. Babikian V, Sloan MA, Tegler CH, et al. Transcranial Doppler validation pilot study. J Neuroimaging 1993;3:242–249
24. Comerota AJ, Katz ML, Hosking JD, et al. Is transcranial Doppler a worthwhile addition to screening tests for cerebrovascular disease? J Vasc Surg 1995;21:90–97
25. Earnest F, Forbes G, Sandok BA, et al. Complications of cerebral angiography: prospective assessment of risk. AJR 1984;142:247–253
26. Aaslid R. Transcranial Doppler examination techniques. In: Aaslid R (ed.) Transcranial Doppler sonography. New York: Springer Verlag, 1986:39–60
27. Kinsella LJ, Feldman E, Brooks JM. The clinical utility of transcranial Doppler ultrasound in suspected vertebrobasilar ischemia. J Neuroimaging 1993;3:115–122
28. Kaps M, Seidel G, Bauer T, Behrmann B. Imaging of the intracranial vertebrobasilar system using color-coded ultrasound. Stroke 1992;23:1577–1582
29. Becker G, Linder A, Bogdahn U. Imaging of the vertebrobasilar system by transcranial color-coded real-time sonography. J Ultrasound Med 1993;12:395–401
30. Ringelstein EB. A practical guide to transcranial Doppler sonography. In: Weinberber J (ed.). Noninvasive imaging of cerebral disease;1989:75–121

31. Bornstein NM, Krajewski A, Norris JW. Basilar artery blood flow in subclavian steal. Can J Neurol Sci 1988;15:417–419
32. Hennerici M, Klemm C, Rautenberg W. The subclavian steal syndrome: a common vascular disorder with rare neurologic deficits. Neurol 1987;37 (Suppl 1):316–317
33. Klingeolhofer J, Conrad B, Benecke R, Frank B. Transcranial Doppler ultrasonography of carotid-basilar collateral circulation in subclavian steal. Stroke 1988;19:1036–1043
34. Padayachee TS, Gosling RG, Bishop CC, et al. Monitoring middle cerebral artery blood velocity during carotid endarterectomy. Br J Surg 1986;73:98–100
35. Nedey C, Barjoud H, Chateland P, et al. The role of intraoperative transcranial Doppler monitoring in carotid artery surgery. Ann Vasc Surg 1995;9(3):247–251
36. Boysen G. Cerebral hemodynamics in carotid surgery. Acta Neurol Scand 1973 (suppl):149–152
37. Otis SM, Rongelstein EB. Transcranial Doppler sonography. In: Bernstein EF (ed.). Recent advances in noninvasive diagnostic techniques in vascular disease. St. Louis: CV Mosby, 1989.
38. Thiel A, Russ W, Zeiler D, et al. Transcranial Doppler sonography and somatosensory evoked potential monitoring in carotid surgery. Eur J Vasc Surg 1990;4:597–602
39. Jansen C, Vriens EM, Eikelboom BC, et al. Carotid endarterectomy with transcranial Doppler and electroencephalographic monitoring: a prospective study in 130 operations. Stroke 1993;24: 665–669
40. Spencer MP, Thomas GI, Nicholls SC, Sauvage LR. Detection of middle cerebral artery emboli during carotid endarterectomy using transcranial Doppler ultrasonography. Stroke 1990;21:415–423
41. Jansen C, Ramos LMP, van Heesewijk JPM, et al. Impact of microembolism and hemodynamic changes in the brain during carotid endarterectomy. Stroke 1994;25:992–997
42. Gaunt ME, Martin PJ, Smith JL, et al. Clinical relevance of intraoperative embolization detected by transcranial Doppler sonography during carotid endarterectomy: a prospective study of 100 patients. Br J Surg 1994;81:1435–1439
43. Huber P, Handa J. Effect of contrast material, hypercapnia, hyperventilation, hypertonic glucose and papaverine on the diameter of the cerebral arteries. Investig Radiol 1967;17–32
44. Ringelstein EB, Sievers C, Ecker S, et al. Noninvasive assessment of CO_2-induced cerebral vasomotor response in normal individuals and patients with internal carotid artery occlusions. Stroke 1988;19: 963–969
45. Markus HS, Harrison MJG. Estimation of cerebrovascular reactivity using transcranial Doppler, including the use of breath-holding as the vasodilatory stimulus. Stroke 1992;23:668–673
46. Kleiser B, Widder B. Course of carotid artery occlusions with impaired cerebrovascular reactivity. Stroke 1992;23:171–174
47. Webster MW, Makaroun MS, Steed DL, et al. Compromised cerebral blood flow reactivity is a predictor of stroke in patients with symptomatic carotid occlusive disease. J Vasc Surg 1995;21:338–345
48. Eskesin V, et al. Observer variability in assessment of angiographic vasospasm after aneurysmal subarachnoid hemorrhage. Acta Neurochir 1987;87:54–57
49. Aaslid R, Huber P, Nornes H. Evaluation of cerebrovascular vasospasm with transcranial Doppler ultrasound. J Neurosurg 1984;60:37–41
50. Aaslid R, Huber P, Nornes H. A transcranial Doppler method in the evaluation of cerebrovascular vasospasm. Neuroradiology 1986;28:11–16
51. Seiler RW, Grolimund P, Aaslid R, et al. Cerebral vasospasm evaluated by transcranial ultrasound correlated with clinical grade and CT-visualized subarachnoid hemorrhage. J Neurosurg 1986;64: 594–600
52. Harders AG, Gilsbach JM. Time course of blood velocity changes related to vasospasm in the circle of Willis measured by transcranial Doppler ultrasound. J Neurosurg 1987;66:718–728
53. Sekkar LN, Wechsler LR, Yonas H, et al. Value of transcranial Doppler examination in the diagnosis of cerebral vasospasm after subarachnoid hemorrhage. Neurosurg 1988;22:813–821
54. Sloan MA, Haley EC, Kassell NF, et al. Sensitivity and specificity of transcranial Doppler ultrasonography in the diagnosis of vasospasm following subarachnoid hemorrhage. Neurology 1989;39: 1514–1518
55. Aaslid R, Nornes H. Musical murmurs in human cerebral arteries after subarachnoid hemorrhage. J Neurosurg 1984;60:32–36
56. Adams R, McKie V, Nochosl F, et al. The use of transcranial ultrasonography to predict stroke in sickle cell disease. N Engl J Med 1992;326:605–610
57. Gawael MJ, Krajewski A. Intracranial hemodynamics in cluster headaches. Headache 1988;28: 484–487

58. Thie A, Spitzer K, Lachenmayer L, Kunze K. Prolonged vasospasm in migraine detected by noninvasive transcranial Doppler ultrasound. Headache 1988;28:183–186
59. Thie A, Fuhlendorf A, Spitzer K, Kunze K. Transcranial Doppler evaluation of common and classic migraine. Part I. Ultrasonic features during the headache-free period. Headache 1990;30:201–208
60. Thie A, Fuhlendorf A, Spitzer K, Kunze K. Transcranial Doppler evaluation of common and classic migraine. Part II. Ultrasonic features during attacks. Headache 1990;30:209–215
61. Zanette EM, Agnoli A, Roberti C, et al. Transcranial Doppler in spontaneous attacks of migraine. Stroke 1992;23:680–685
62. Silvestrini M, Cupini LM, Troisi E, et al. Estimation of cerebrovascular reactivity in migraine without aura. Stroke 1995;26:81–83
63. Totaro R, De Matteis G, Marini C, Prencipe M. Cerebral blood flow in migraine with aura: a transcranial Doppler sonography study. Headache 1992;32:446–451
64. President's Commission. Guidelines for the determination of death. JAMA 1981;246:2184–2186
65. Ropper AH, Kehne SM, Wechsler L. Transcranial Doppler in brain death. Neurology 1987;37: 1733–1735
66. Kirkham FJ, Levin SD, Padayachee TS, et al. Transcranial pulsed Doppler ultrasound findings in brainstem death. J Neurol, Neurosurg, and Psychiatry 1987;50:1504–1513
67. Hassler W, Steinmetz H, Gawlowski J. Transcranial Doppler ultrasonography in raised intracranial pressure and in intracranial circulatory arrest. N Neurosurg 1988;68:745–751
68. Powers AD, Graeber MC, Smith RR. Transcranial Doppler ultrasonography in the determination of brain death. Neurosurgery 1989;24:884–889
69. Petty GW, Mohr JP, Pedley TA, et al. The role of transcranial Doppler in confirming brain death: sensitivity, specificity and suggestions for performance and interpretation. Neurology 1990;40:300–303

Management of Extracranial Cerebrovascular Disease, edited by Keith D. Calligaro et al.
Lippincott-Raven Publishers, Philadelphia © 1997.

14

Carotid Artery Patch

Gary Giangola

Patch reconstruction of the carotid artery after endarterectomy is a well-accepted method of closure. This technique is just one part of the operation. It is probably no less or more important than many other steps in the procedure, all of which contribute to the final result. As Imparato has emphasized, patch angioplasty alone will not improve results and indeed may worsen them if too wide a vessel is created.[1] Some surgeons prefer the technique as a routine and others use it selectively. The end points for a particular surgeon to examine in judging this technique are perioperative stroke, recurrent stenosis, and complications from use of the additional surgery. An attempt is herein made to examine the technique, the benefits, the various patch materials, and problems with patch angioplasty of the endarterectomized carotid artery.

TECHNIQUE

When saphenous vein is to be the patch material, I routinely expose it in the groin under local anesthesia (0.5% lidocaine) to begin the operation, prior to the cervical incision. The vein is exposed at the origin, visualizing the fossa ovalis, to ensure that the saphenous, and not an anterior branch, is the vein exposed and to increase the chance that the remaining vein will maintain patency. The vein is not excised at this time of the operation. The wound is packed with a moist sponge and tension is released on the wound retractor.

During carotid endarterectomy one must be certain that the arteriotomy extends well distal and proximal from the respective intimal end points. I prefer a deep endarterectomy plane that removes all evidence of smooth muscle cells. The patch is begun distally and both the medial and lateral sides are sewn. The proximal portion of the vein patch can be held up to visualize the suture line from within at this most critical portion of the reconstruction. After the distal patch is placed to just proximal to the distal intimal edge, the proximal portion of the patch is sutured down. One must take care not to invaginate the proximal patch into the common carotid lumen. The lateral wall is completed first to allow the uncompleted segment to be partially filled with heparinized saline while the final portion of the reconstruction is performed. Liberal use of heparinized saline in the artery while the endarectomy and closure are performed prevents small thrombi from accumulating. Back bleeding from the internal, followed by the external, carotid vessels is performed. Finally, the common carotid is released and clamped to flush any thrombotic material, and the remaining segment is then copiously irrigated with heparinized saline. Flow is restored first to the external, followed by the internal carotid vessel. If regional anesthesia is used it is important to assess the neurologic status at this point to allow the surgeon to determine the exact cause of neurologic symptoms, should they occur. The groin wound is closed with interrupted absorbable sutures for the fascia. I prefer to place a central intravenous line through the proximal saphenous vein so that postoperative blood pressure changes can be quickly and reliably treated.

Whether vein or fabric is used for the patch, care must be taken to avoid a widening to the point of creating an aneurysm. Usually 3–4 mm width of patch is sufficient.

RECURRENT STENOSIS

In spite of the fact that carotid endarterectomy has become a well-accepted and commonly performed procedure since its introduction in the early 1950s, there remains disagreement as how to best close the vessel. Most surgeons would agree that patch angioplasty is required in at least selected cases. One reason given to support patch closure is a reduced rate of recurrent stenosis. Recurrence rates after carotid endarterectomy have been reported to be from 0 to 29%, with women having consistently higher rates.[2–8] The reasons for higher recurrence rates in women are not known but may have to do with the smaller average size of the vessel. Early recurrent stenoses can result from technical errors, which may not be significant enough to cause early thrombosis (Fig. 14-1). Bandyk et al showed an increased rate of recurrent stenosis and occlusion if flow disturbances were present after endarterectomy.[18] Occasionally, the junction between a wide patch and the normal distal internal carotid will be interpreted as a relative stenosis on Duplex ultrasonography (Fig. 14-2).

Late recurrent stenoses are usually attributed to atherosclerosis. These should be defined as those lesions that were not present after surgery and develop after one year. Hemodynamics at the bifurcation, smoking, and other risk factors for atherosclerosis are implicated as the causes of these lesions.[9,25] Hemodynamic factors that lead to

- Retained thick intima
- Incomplete endarterectomy - retained media smooth muscle cells
- Distal edge of abruptly tapering patch
- Buckling of back wall
- Vascular clamp injury

FIG. 14-1. Early recurrent stenosis

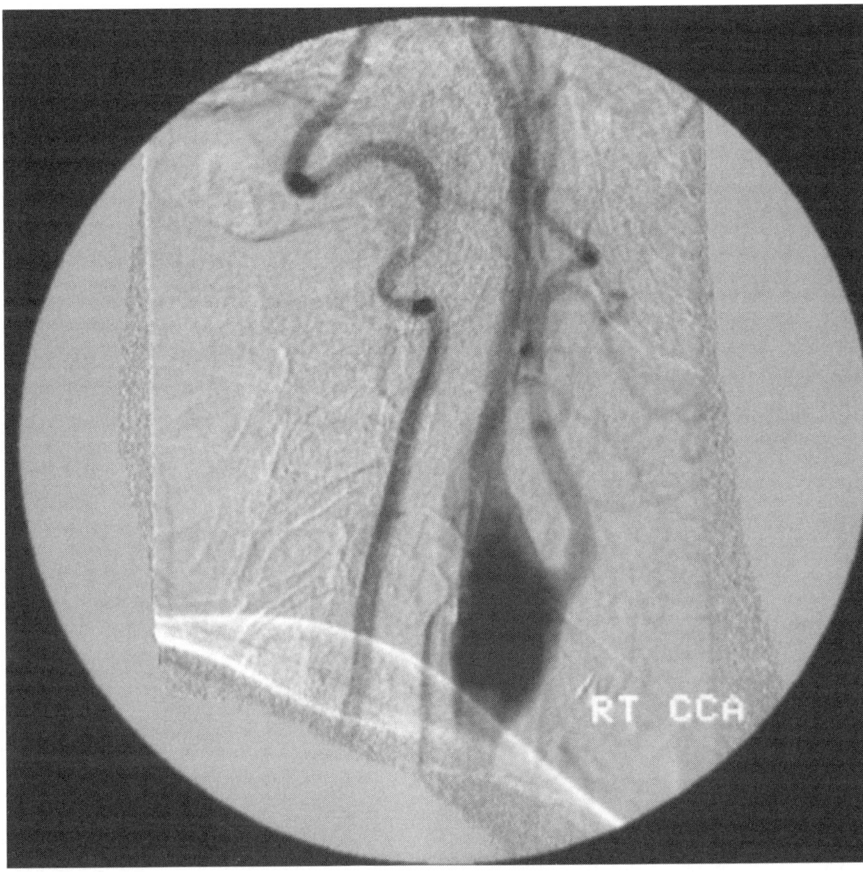

FIG. 14-2. Angiogram. No stenosis identified; carotid endarterectomy; wide patch; 1 year after surgery. Duplex 50–79% stenosis.

recurrent stenoses and atherosclerotic plaques are complex. Imparato has stressed that the vessel is patched to alter these factors and not to widen the vessel.[10] He has stated that "the effective use of patch grafting requires that it be utilized in conjunction with maneuvers to deal with several mechanisms that can result in operative site stenosis or occlusion."[1] This must be considered in interpreting series that report on any one particular technique.

Many authors have shown the benefits of patch angioplasty after carotid endarterectomy. Archie presented 200 consecutive patients, half with vein patch and the other half closed primarily. Of the first 108 operations, all but 8 had primary closure, and of the last 95 all had patch angioplasty except for 3. Restenosis or thrombosis occurred in 9% of the non-patched group as opposed to 0% in the patched arteries.[10] Hertzer more recently examined this issue in a prospective study performed at the Cleveland Clinic in 1989. Recurrent stenosis was least with vein patch angioplasty.

Patch versus primary closure was compared in a large group that consisted of over 900 carotid endarectomies from 1983 to 1985 at the Cleveland Clinic. The equally sized cohorts both had respectively good data. Hertzer's conclusions were that even good results could be made better by the use of a venous patch. Early stroke rates were 3.1% in the non-patched, compared to 0.7% in the patched. Early thrombosis was reduced from 3.1 to 0.5% by patching. Recurrent stenosis was also improved from 31 to 9.0% in 3 years[11] (Fig. 14-3). Eikelboom et al also demonstrated the benefit of carotid patching in a controlled, almost completely randomized group of 129 carotid endarterectomies. They compared vein patch with primary closure, with 1-year follow-up that included duplex scanning and DSA exams early and again at 1 year. Recurrent stenoses were seen in 21% of primary closures, compared to 3.5% of those patched (Fig. 14-4). The results were even more striking in women who had recurrent stenoses of 55% when primarily closed, compared to 0% with primary closure.[12] Others have also shown the benefit of vein patching.[4] Based on this data many surgeons routinely or selectively patch. Indications given for selective patching include "small arteries," recurrent stenoses, and women.[3,5,7]

There are reports revealing mixed results with patching. Clagett et al reported a higher incidence of restenosis with patching than without.[12] Just 1 woman, however, was included in this group of 136 patients. The study design was randomized and prospective but 30 patients were excluded for "obligatory" patch. This same group, in a later paper, showed no significant difference in restenosis between patched and unpatched arteries.[16] Other authors who have questioned the benefit of patch angioplasty have data that show equal results with or without the technique. Katz et al did not find a statistical difference between polytetraflouroethylene (PTFE) patched vessels and primary closure, due to the small group sizes. However, 2 of 49 vessels developed recurrent stenoses with primary closure as opposed to 0 of 51 with patch closure.[15] Curley et al showed no differences in recurrent stenosis between vein patch, bifurcation advancement, and primary closure.[17] Each group consisted of only approximately 20 patients and follow-up was at just 1 year. The overall incidence of recurrent stenosis was 13.8%.

	Follow-up	Number	Restenosis
Hertzer 1987			
Primary	3 yrs.	483 pts.	31%
Patch	3 yrs.	434 pts.	9%
Archie 1986			
Primary	30 mos.	100 pts.	9 %
Patch	30 mos.	100 pts.	0 %

FIG. 14-3. Patch versus primary closure

	Follow-up	Number	Stenosis
Katz 1987			
Primary	12 mos.	47 pts.	19%
Patch	12 mos.	42 pts.	2%
Eikelboom'88			
Primary	12 mos.	62 pts.	21%
Patch	12 mos.	67 pts.	4%

FIG. 14-4. Vein patch versus primary closure

The true incidence of carotid restenosis is difficult to ascertain completely. One must distinguish between recurrent and persistent stenoses. In addition, patch reconstruction of the artery, especially if the patch is wide, can be interpreted as a relative stenosis on duplex ultrasonography (see Fig. 14-2). Bandyk underscores the importance of distinguishing between recurrent stenosis and residual disease. Completion studies that revealed a normal reconstruction had a 0% incidence of restenosis at 2 years as opposed to a 21% incidence if a defect was identified at the time of surgery.[18] The overall incidence of recurrent stenosis, however, appears to be approximately 5–15% at 3 years after surgery. Symptomatic stenosis is approximately 1–5% during this same time period.

PERIOPERATIVE COMPLICATIONS

Patch closure may also decrease the incidence of thrombotic complication around the time of surgery (Fig. 14-5). Archie,[11] Hertzer,[13] and Ouriel[3] have shown significantly less complications with patch reconstruction of the vessel. In addition, those

	Number	TIA/CVA
Archie 1986		
Primary	100 pts.	4 %
Patch	100 pts.	0 %
Hertzer 1987		
Primary	483 pts.	3.1%
Patch	434 pts.	0.7%
Ouriel 1987		
Primary	49 pts.	10.2%
Patch	53 pts.	0 %

FIG. 14-5. Carotid surgery—early results. Primary closure versus patch

	Number	TIA/CVA Thrombosis
Rosenthal '90	1000 pts.	
Primary	250 pts.	4.5%
PTFE	250 pts.	4.5%
Dacron	250 pts.	4.0%
Vein	250 pts.	0.8%
Myers 1994	163 pts.	
Primary	64 pts.	3.0%
Vein	61 pts.	1.6%
Obl.Vein	38 pts.	5.3%

FIG. 14-6. Carotid surgery—early results. Primary closure versus patch

authors whose data generally do not favor patch closure, have improved results when vein patch closure is performed routinely (Fig. 14-6).[16,30]

The reasons to patch the carotid artery at the time of endarterectomy are to prevent recurrent stenosis and to decrease the complication rate of surgery. Fietsam et al studied primary versus narrow and wide patch reconstructions of the canine carotid artery with intra-arterial pressure, electromagnetic, and pulsed Doppler ultrasound flow meter measurement analyses.[31] The primarily closed vessels showed moderate increases in both systolic and diastolic velocities as well as significant pressure gradients across the closure. In addition, he showed an approximately 15% diameter stenosis in the primarily closed vessels (native vessel 4 mm average diameter). Hirschl et al found remarkably turbulent flow, whether or not the vessel was patched, but these changes were more significant for those that were. Patch sizes were not mentioned.[32]

Author	Incidence % (pts.)	Vein Origin	Day of Rupture
O'Hara 1992	0.5% (3/1691)	Ankle	2.3 days
Riles 1990	0.13% (3/2275)	Ankle	2-5 days
Eikelboom'88	1.5% (1/67)	Ankle	2 days
Tawes 1991	0.7% (13/1760)	Ankle 12 Groin 1	1-21 days

FIG. 14-7. Vein patch rupture

Archie has demonstrated the importance of size of the donor vein and its relationship to rupture pressure as well as the significance of the size of the patch reconstruction.[28] Based on his experimental studies the recommendation given was to choose saphenous vein from the groin rather than the smaller-sized ankle vein. In addition he stressed the importance of keeping the patch repair narrow.

Carotid patch material other than saphenous vein is commonly used.[14] Dacron has been used for many years without reported increased complications.[19] Biosynthetic patches have also been utilized in the carotid position.[20] Recently, PTFE has found increased use as a carotid patch.[21] Aside from some reported increased needle-hole bleeding, results appear as favorable as with other patch material.[22–24]

The use of saphenous vein from the ankle has been reported to result in patch rupture (Fig. 14-7).[26–29] Of 20 vein patch ruptures reported, all except 1 have been ankle vein. Only one undocumented ruptured vein was harvested from the groin as determined by a mail questionnaire conducted by the Western Vascular Society.[27] Archie has offered that the smaller diameter veins are at greater risk of rupture.[28] It seems prudent that ankle vein should not be used as patch material on the carotid artery.

REFERENCES

1. Imparato AM. The role of patch angioplasty after carotid endarterectomy. J Vasc Surg 1988;7:715–716
2. Thomas M, Otis SM, Rush M, et al. Recurrent carotid artery stenosis following endarterectomy. Ann Surg 1984;200:74
3. Ouriel K, Green RM. Clinical and technical factors influencing recurrent carotid stenosis and occlusion after carotid endarterectomy. J Vasc Surg 1987;5:702
4. Sanders EACM, Hoeneveld H, Eikelboom BC, et al. Residual lesions and early recurrent stenosis after carotid endarterectomy. J Vasc Surg 1987;5:731
5. Bernstein EF, Torem S, Dilley RB. Does carotid restenosis predict an increased risk of late symptoms, stroke, or death? Am Surg 1990;212:629
6. Atnip RG, Wengrovitz M, Gifford RRM, et al. A rational approach to recurrent carotid stenosis. J Vasc Surg 1990;11:511
7. Eikelboom BC, Ackerstaff RG, Hoeneveld H, et al. Benefits of carotid patching: a randomized study. J Vasc Surg 1988;7:240–247
8. Ten Holter JBM, Ackerstaff RGA, Schwartzenberg GWST, et al. The impact of vein patch angioplasty on long-term surgical outcome after carotid endarterectomy. J Cardiovasc Surg 1990;31:58
9. Clagett GP, Rich NM, McDonald PT, et al. Etiologic factors for recurrent carotid artery stenosis. Surgery 1983;93:313–318
10. Imparato AM, Weinstein GS. Clinicopathologic correlation in postendarterectomy recurrent stenosis. J Vasc Surg 1986;3:657–662
11. Archie JP. Prevention of early restenosis and thrombosis-occlusion after carotid endarterectomy by saphenous vein patch angioplasty. Stroke 1986;17:901–905
12. Clagett GP, Patterson CB, Fisher DF, et al. Vein patch versus primary closure for carotid endarterectomy. J Vasc Surg 1989;9:213–223
13. Hertzer NR, Beven EG, O'Hara PJ, et al. A prospective study of vein patch angioplasty during carotid endarterectomy. Ann Surg 1987;206:628–635
14. Katz D, Snyder SO, Gandhi RHMD, et al. Long-term follow-up for recurrent stenosis: a prospective randomized study of expanded polytetrafluoroethylene patch angioplasty versus primary closure after carotid endarterectomy. J Vasc Surg 1994;19:198–205
15. Katz MM, Jones GT, Degenhardt RD. The use of patch angioplasty to alter the incidence of carotid restenosis following thromboendarterectomy. J Cardiovasc Surg 1987;28:2–8
16. Meyers SI, Valentine RJ, Chervu A. Saphenous vein patch versus primary closure for carotid endarterectomy: long-term assessment of a randomized prospective study. J Vasc Surg 1994;19:15–22

17. Curley S, Edwards WS, Jacob TP. Recurrent carotid stenosis after autologous tissue patching. J Vasc Surg 1987;4:350–354
18. Bandyk DF, Kaebnick HW, Adams MB. Turbulence occurring after carotid bifurcation endarterectomy: a harbinger of residual and recurrent stenosis. J Vasc Surg 1988;7:261–274
19. Shultz GA, Zammit M, Sauvage LR. Carotid artery patch angioplasty: a ten year experience. J Vasc Surg 1987;3:475–478
20. Pratesi C, Pulli R, Michelagnoli S, et al. Biosynthetic patch in carotid angioplasty. J Vasc Surg 1992;26:1–7
21. Carney WI, Lilli MP. Intraoperative evaluation of PTFE, Dacron and autogenous vein as carotid patch materials. Ann Vasc Surg 1987;1:583–586
22. Lord RS, Raj TB, Stary DL, et al. Comparison of saphenous vein patch, PTFE, and direct arteriotomy closure after carotid endarterectomy. Part 1. J Vasc Surg 1989;9:521–529
23. McCready RA, Siderys H, Pittman JN, et al. Delayed postoperative bleeding from PTFE carotid artery patches. J Vasc Surg 1992;4:661–663
24. LeGrand DR, Linehan RL. The suitability of expanded PTFE for carotid patch angioplasty. Ann Vasc Surg 1990;3:209–212
25. Baker JD. Recurrent stenosis of the carotid artery: incidence, diagnosis, prognosis, and management. In: Moore W (ed.). Surgery for cerebrovascular disease. Philadelphia: W. B. Saunders Company, 1987:703–713
26. Riles TS, Lamparello PJ, Giangola G, et al. Rupture of the vein patch: a rare complication of carotid endarterectomy. Surgery 1990;107:10–12
27. Tawes RL, Treiman RL. Vein patch rupture after carotid endarterectomy: a survey of the western vascular society members. Ann Vasc Surg 1991;1:71–73
28. Archie JP, Green JJ. Saphenous vein rupture pressure, rupture stress and carotid endarterectomy vein patch reconstruction. Surgery 1990;4:389–396
29. O'Hara PJ, Hertzer NR, Krajewski LP, et al. Saphenous vein patch rupture after carotid endarterectomy. J Vasc Surg 1992;15:504–509
30. Rosenthal D, Archie JP, Garcia-Rinaldi R, et al. Carotid patch angioplasty: immediate and long-term results. J Vasc Surg 1990;12:326–333
31. Fietsam R, Ranval T, Cohn S, et al. Hemodynamic effects of primary closure versus patch angioplasty of the carotid artery. Ann Vasc Surg 1992;6:443–449
32. Hirschl M, Bernt RA, Hirschl MM. Carotid endarterectomy of the internal carotid artery with and without patch angioplasty: comparison of hemodynamical and morphological parameters. Int Angiol 1989;6:10–15

Management of Extracranial Cerebrovascular Disease, edited by Keith D. Calligaro et al.
Lippincott-Raven Publishers, Philadelphia © 1997.

15

Vertebral Basilar Insufficiency: A 25-Year Experience with Proximal Subclavian and Vertebral Artery Lesions

William H. Edwards, Sr.

Major arteriosclerotic lesions at the origin of the brachiocephalic arteries rarely cause irreversible neurologic changes, but symptoms and disability do occur. The proximal subclavian artery (SA) should be discussed within the context of vertebral basilar ischemia (VBI) because diseases of the proximal SA may result in hind-brain ischemia in addition to symptoms in the arm and hand. Operative intervention for stenosis of the SA may correct VBI symptoms. The same may apply to lesions of the innominate artery, but much less frequently.

Vertebral basilar transient ischemic (VBTI) attacks or basilar artery hypoperfusion may result from diminished vertebral artery flow or embolic events. Symptoms include vertigo, ataxia, dizziness, syncope, transient motor sensory changes—sometimes bilateral, visual disturbances, and "drop attacks." The excellent collateral circulation to the arm usually minimizes symptoms of the arm and hand, unless microemboli occur. Surgical correction of stenotic or ulcerated lesions will usually relieve symptoms but the best operative approach will depend on the site of the obstruction or the multiplicity of arteries involved. Our plan for the surgical management of these arterial lesions has evolved over the past 25 years, giving us a good perspective of treatment options.

The history of surgery of the vertebral basilar system has been well-reviewed by Carney.[1] For centuries there was little point in being concerned about the vertebral artery (VA) because the surgical limitations made operation hazardous. The VA remained a reclusive vessel with the features of a hedgehog hiding behind the cervical foramina, difficult to get close to and always ready to attack.[2] Willis[3] describes very clearly the vascular anatomy of the brain, including the VB and anterior spinal arteries. In 1853, Maisonneueve ligated the first part of the VA for trauma. In 1883 Rudolph Matas also ligated the VA but his patient died 17 days postoperatively of septic cerebral emboli.

In 1864, Smythe[4] created surgical history by ligating an aneurysm of the first part of the VA in a 32-year-old man who had had previous ligation of SA artery and developed perfuse secondary bleeding. It should be noted that before the patient died he suffered what Smythe then recognized as subclavian steal syndrome.

The first successful surgical correction for proximal brachiocephalic occlusive disease was performed by Cate and Scott in 1957.[5] They performed a thromboendarterectomy on the VA and left SA in a patient with disabling VBI. This was reported at the meeting of the Society for Vascular Surgery (SVS) in June of 1958 but was not published until January of 1959 in Surgery. In June of 1958 (3 days prior to the SVS meeting), Crawford and DeBakey performed their first elective vertebral endarterectomy. The Houston case appeared in the JAMA in October of 1958.[6]

DIAGNOSTIC STUDIES

In evaluating some 9,000 patients with cerebral symptoms, an operation was performed in 688 (8%) for significant stenosis of the proximal vertebral, subclavian, or innominate arteries. Clinical manifestations ranged from dizziness and ataxia to paresthesias and visual disturbances (Fig. 15-1). For the past decade, our operative procedure has been to perform an anastomosis between the end of the subclavian or VA, distal to the occlusive disease, and the adjacent carotid artery transposition.

Arch aortography is the diagnostic roentgenographic technique used most frequently to visualize subclavian and vertebral lesions (Fig. 15-2). Although we use this method on occasion, we prefer percutaneous retrograde brachial and carotid angiography for high-quality films with detailed visualization of both extracranial and intracranial arterial distribution.

In the early years of evaluating patients with cerebral disease, the origins of the vertebral and subclavian arteries were not routinely visualized. Surgical intervention

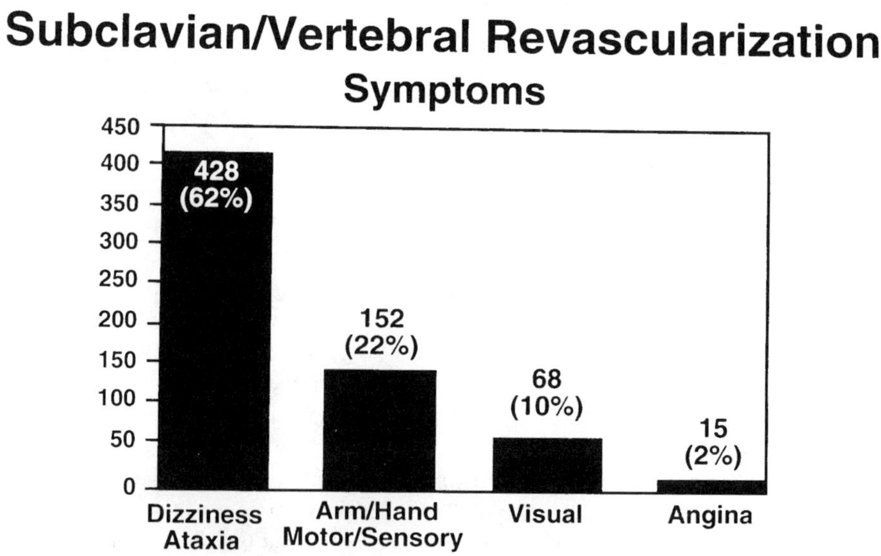

FIG. 15-1. Symptoms in patients with brachiocephalic stenosis

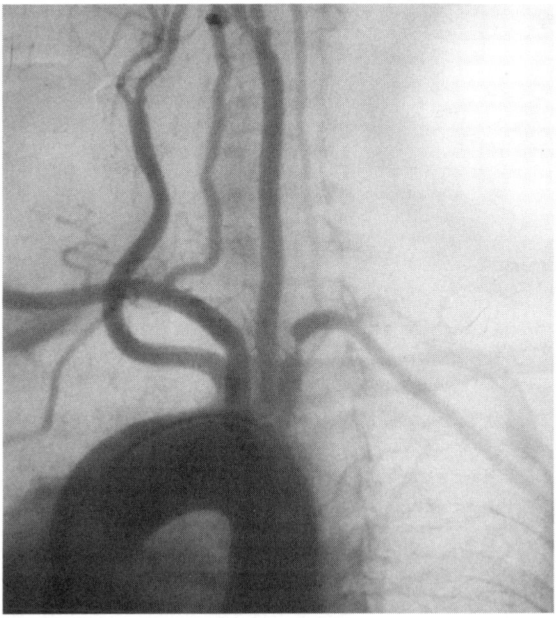

FIG. 15-2. Arch aortogram with proximal left subclavian stenosis

was more formidable and most symptoms were thought to be relieved by corrective carotid surgery when disease was present. The continued occurrence of nonhemispheric symptoms, coupled with better techniques of diagnosis and improved surgical techniques, prompted the complete evaluation of total cerebral flow in all patients evaluated for cerebral symptoms.

ANATOMY

The right subclavian, a branch of the innominate artery, is shorter than the left and less susceptible to atherosclerotic disease or traumatic disruption. The left is a common site for atherosclerotic disease, as well as the site of decelerating injuries. In its intrathoracic segments, the SA travels with the vagus and phrenic nerves, which cross anteriorly. The phrenic nerve lies laterally while the vagus is more medial in the neck. As it enters the neck the artery comes in posterior proximity to the thoracic duct, which emerges from the posterior mediastinum to curve outward and drain into the jugular–subclavian–venous confluence.

The first segment of the SA ends at the take-off of the VA, which generally arises just proximal to the internal mammary artery. It generally arises in a somewhat posterior position from the SA. In up to 5% of the population, the VA on the left side may originate from the aorta.

The first segment of the vertebral extends from its origin to the level of C-6, where it enters the cervical spine (Fig. 15-3). The length of the VA available for surgical cor-

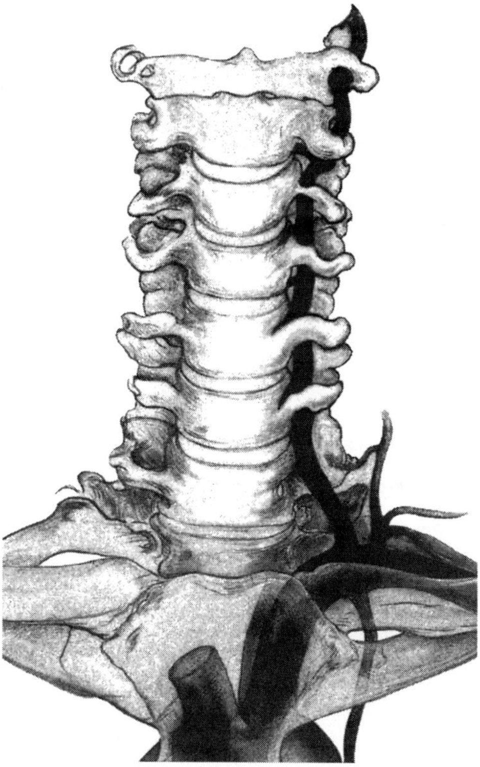

FIG. 15-3. Vertebral artery in its cephalad course. (Modified from Pernqopf E, Atlas of topographical and applied human anatomy. Baltimore, MD: Urban and Schwarzenberg, 1980:245)

rection depends on the level that the SA extends into the neck before it passes under the scalenus anticus muscle. If the subclavian arches high out of the thoracic outlet, there will then be a short segment of vertebral available.

OPERATIVE APPROACH

The three basic operations of endarterectomy, bypass grafting, and direct arterial anastomosis (transposition) are all suitable for stenotic lesions of the brachiocephalic or VA. The exposure of the origins of the innominate, subclavian, and left carotid are limiting factors in performing an endarterectomy.

An extrathoracic approach is most commonly used in the exposure of the base of the right subclavian and common carotid, but adequate control of the innominate cannot be obtained with this technique. A blind endarterectomy of the proximal innominate is possible, but is fraught with hazards and is not recommended.

A sternal splitting incision gives excellent exposure for the arch of the aorta and the innominate artery. With this approach, the endarterectomy can be performed with partial aortic occlusion. A similar approach and technique can be used for the proxi-

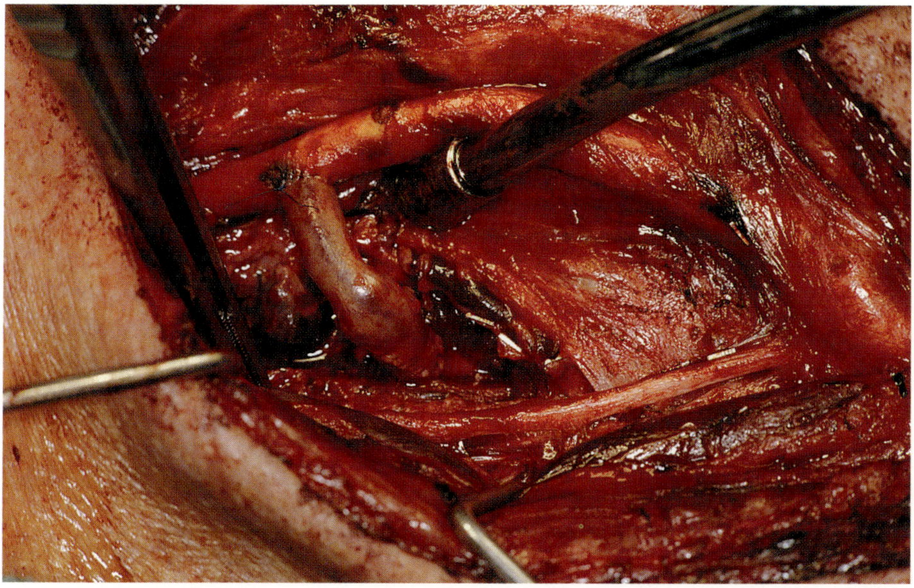

FIG. 15-4. Carotid–vertebral bypass with autogenous tissue

mal left carotid artery. The ease and safety of splitting the sternum and the stability achieved on closure makes this an excellent surgical approach.

ENDARTERECTOMY

Endarterectomy of the VA requires control of the proximal and distal SA. Distally, this may require division of the scalenus anticus muscle, as well as the internal mammary artery and thyrocervical trunk. Identification and preservation of the phrenic nerve are necessary. On the left side, any exposure of the VA needs careful division of the thoracic duct to prevent lymph drainage. Care is taken to avoid injury to the vagus and recurrent laryngeal nerve.

Removal of the diseased intima in the proximal VA continues to be the operation utilized by many surgeons when operating for VA stenosis. Either a transsubclavian incision with dissection and extraction of the intima or a combined subclavian and vertebral incision with more direct visualization of the distal intima can be used. Control of the distal intima at the point of termination of the endarterectomy is required. A patch graft is useful in this type of operation to prevent narrowing in what may well be a small vessel. Although possible, shunting is fraught with technical problems and probably is not necessary. Heparinization can be safely achieved with 5000 units intravenously. Reversal at the termination of the endarterectomy is accomplished with 50 mg of protamine sulfate.

With the technical problems involved in an endarterectomy of the VA or brachiocephalic vessels, we feel that bypass grafting and direct anastomosis offer safer, better long-term results and can be obtained with an extrathoracic approach.

BYPASS GRAFTING

As advances have been achieved in arterial reconstructive surgery, bypass grafts have, for the most part, supplanted endarterectomy.

The first bypass grafts for proximal innominate and subclavian stenosis were aortic to distal SA. This involved an intrathoracic and extrathoracic incision and the associated difficulties of tunneling a graft through the thoracic outlet. Realization that the distal subclavian or the axillary, as well as the ipsilateral, carotid could be used as the donor artery for bypass was a major step in simplification of the treatment of proximal brachiocephalic occlusive disease.

For an extrathoracic bypass to be successful, one of the three brachiocephalic arteries should not be involved with significant stenosis. In our experience, this is usually the left carotid followed by the innominate. The proximal subclavian on the left is the most frequently involved.

For a left subclavian stenosis, a left carotid to left subclavian bypass will restore flow relieving symptoms. Either synthetic or autogenous tissue may be used, but most surgeons prefer autogenous tissue. Currently, polytetrafluoroethylene (PTFE) is a good second choice. Bypassing in this manner is ineffective if proximal left vertebral stenosis is present along with subclavian disease. For isolated lesions of the VA, a bypass also may be used (Fig. 15-4 following page 154). Autogenous saphenous vein functions well.

Similarly, for lesions of the right subclavian, the right common carotid can be utilized for bypass.

A patent SA may be used to originate a bypass graft in the area of the scalenus anticus or, more distally, its axillary segment. There are proponents of both subclavian–subclavian or axilloaxillary bypasses. The axilloaxillary is probably the easier and safer to perform and, when completed, leaves a graft with little angulation.

DIRECT ANASTOMOSIS

Some years ago, we discontinued the use of endarterectomy for lesions of the vertebral or proximal brachiocephalic arteries. Since then we have used direct arterial anastomosis alone or in combination with a bypass graft. Our early experience was a side-to-side subclavian-to-common carotid anastomosis (Fig. 15-5). We subsequently extended the operation to include side-to-side vertebral-to-common carotid artery. As our operative experience continued, we found that an end of subclavian- or vertebral-to-carotid artery was a better anastomosis with no tension and was also easier to perform. The direct anastomosis, however, cannot be used with innominate stenosis.

The use of the common carotid artery to restore flow to the subclavian or VA has been criticized because of the potential for siphoning blood from the distal carotid flow. Experimental studies, as well as our clinical experience, indicate this concern

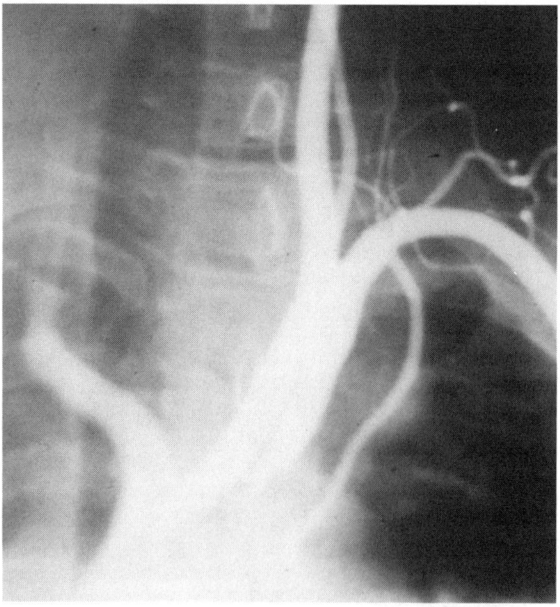

FIG. 15-5. Postoperative side-to-side subclavian-to-carotid transposition

to be unfounded. We are careful, however, that there is no internal carotid artery stenosis, as well as being certain that the inflow from the arch is adequate. In our experience, the proximal left common carotid is the least frequently involved of all the extracranial cerebral vessels.

The incision is placed just above the clavicle, extending from the suprasternal notch laterally for 7 to 8 cm. The platysma and sternocleidomastoid muscles are divided (Fig. 15-6). This exposes the common carotid artery and the internal jugular vein with the vagus nerve between and deep to the jugular vein. At this point, cephalad and caudad dissection along the course of the jugular vein and carotid artery facilitates the deeper dissection that will follow, as well as preparing a portion of the carotid artery for anastomosis. We generally loop the vagus nerve with a Vesseloop to remind us of its location. Care is taken not to stretch the nerve. The jugular vein and vagus nerve are retracted laterally and the common carotid medially. The exposure from this point on is beneath the deep cervical fascia and does not require exposure of the scalenus anticus muscle or phrenic nerve. Visualization of these structures alerts the surgeon that the dissection is too far lateral. On the right side, the recurrent laryngeal nerve

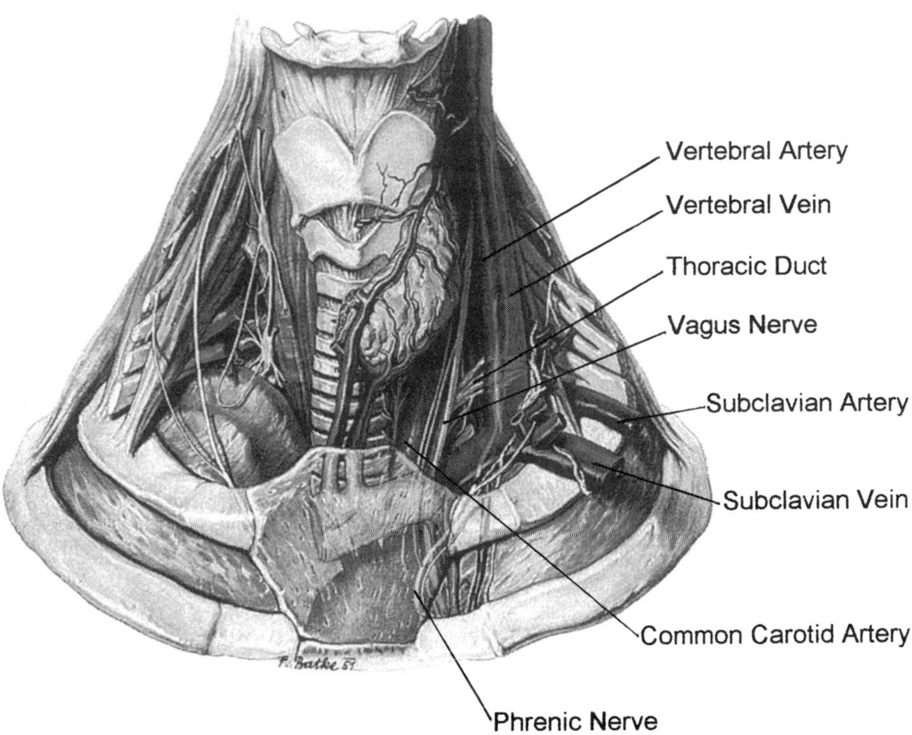

FIG. 15-6. Exposure of first portion of left vertebral artery. (Modified from Pernqopf E, Atlas of topographical and applied human anatomy. Baltimore, MD: Urban and Schwarzenberg, 1980:240)

looping over the subclavian may at times need identification. The ansa subclavia is usually visualized. On the left side, the thoracic duct is identified, ligated, and divided. If the subclavian is the involved vessel, then a portion of the subclavian proximal to the vertebral must be free for the anastomosis. Care is taken not to injure the recurrent laryngeal nerve. It is generally not necessary to disturb the internal mammary or thyrocervical trunk. Preservation of the internal mammary may be important in patients with the potential for coronary artery disease. If the vertebral is the involved vessel, it is unnecessary to expose the subclavian artery. The VA is the first branch of the subclavian artery, arises from its posteriosuperior aspect, and has no branches at this level. This is important in identification. The thyrocervical trunk arises from the anterior aspect of the subclavian, branches almost immediately, and can be mistaken for the vertebral. In an occasional patient, the vertebral may arise from the aortic arch but will follow the same course in the neck to enter the bony canal. The vertebral is cleared of tissue from its origin to its disappearance behind the longus coli muscle. It is sometimes necessary to divide some of the sympathetic fibers, crossing the vertebral to obtain a sufficient length of the VA.

The patient is informed of the possibility of a Horner's syndrome. This will depend on the need to divide sympathetic fibers in exposing the VA. It should not occur in exposure of the SA. It has not been a long term problem in any patient.

The common carotid artery, having previously been dissected, is ready for use in the anastomosis. The involved vertebral or subclavian is transected and the stump appropriately occluded. The cut vessel is tailored by incising its medial wall in the case of the vertebral and usually just trimming in the case of the subclavian. The carotid is occluded and opened at the chosen site. We have found that a Goosen punch works well to create an adequate opening in the carotid artery. We use an internal shunt only when a combined internal carotid endarterectomy is performed in conjunction with direct anastomosis. The anastomosis is accomplished with 6-0 monofilament nylon on a special small curved needle designed to facilitate the anastomosis in the small vessels. No tension exists on the completed anastomosis. Loop magnification is extremely helpful. Following completion of the anastomosis, the wound is closed in layers without drainage.

Total operative time is about 1 hour and 15 minutes, and patients are usually ready to leave the hospital on the first or second day after operation.

Both bypass grafting and a direct arterial anastomosis can be employed as long as there is one brachiocephalic artery not involved with stenosis.

DISCUSSION

Traditionally, the brain has been divided anatomically into the cerebral hemispheres and the hind brain (*i.e.,* the contents of the posterior fossa). The occipital and temporal lobes, however, are commonly supplied by the vertebral basilar system and the anatomical terms do not reflect this important clinical and physiologic division. The terms "fore brain" and "hind brain" have been redefined for clinical usefulness:

	Subclavian	Vertebral
Asymptomatic	188 (97%)	172 (61%)
Symptomatic		
Improved	5 (3%)	185 (27%)
Not improved	0	55 (8%)

FIG. 15-7. Results of 90% follow-up extending to 24 years

fore brain includes the brain supplied by the anterior middle cerebral arteries and the hind brain includes the brain supplied by the posterior cerebral artery and the contents of the posterior fossa. An anomalous Circle of Willis with a hypoplastic communicating artery makes the patient more vulnerable to strokes.[7]

Transient brain ischemia may be due to systemic factors such as reduced cardiac output or postural hypotension. Arterial obstruction proximal to the Circle of Willis may produce ischemia in the direct vascular bed of the artery or in a more remote site. Thus, hind brain ischemia can result from carotid occlusion (*i.e.,* perfusion of the parietal lobe may be normal and that of the posterior fossa decreased even though high flow exists within the vertebral basilar system). Obstruction proximal to the Circle of Willis is preferably treated by carotid or VA reconstruction to enhance collateral capacity of the Circle of Willis. Generally, large vessels carry more blood for a longer period of time than small vessels.

Clinically, Williams and Wilson[8] describe the full scope of hind-brain symptoms and point out that half of patients have visual problems while two thirds have vertigo, ataxia, or dizziness. They recognized that symptoms were primarily related to reduced flow and not to infarcts because the symptoms are generally reversible. Symptoms, however, can be misleading.

A general consideration is that patients who would benefit from surgical correction of highly stenotic or ulcerative lesions should be considered for VA reconstruction.

For the past 25 years, we have performed direct arterial anastomoses when dealing with stenotic lesions of the proximal subclavian or VA. A total experience with direct anastomosis now numbers 697 procedures. The operative morbidity and mortality is low and the results we feel justify operative intervention (Fig. 15-7).

REFERENCES

1. Carney AL. Vertebral artery surgery: historical development, basic concepts of brain hemodynamics, and clinical experience of 102 cases. In: Carney, Anderson (eds.). Diagnosis and treatment of brain ischemia: advances in neurology (vol. 30). New York: Raven Press, 1981:249–282
2. Walt AJ. The story of vertebrobasilar surgery. In: Berguer, Bauer (eds.). Vertebrobasilar occlusive disease, New York: Raven Press, 1984:225–230
3. Willis. The cerebral circulation. In: Fishman, Richards (eds.). Circulation of the blood: men and ideas. New York: Oxford University Press, 1964:713–716
4. Smythe AW. A case of successful ligature of the innominate artery. New Orleans J Med 1869;22: 464–469
5. Cate WR, Scott HW. Cerebral ischemia of central origin: relief by subclavian-vertebral artery thromboendarterectomy. Surgery 1959;45:19–31

6. Crawford ES, DeBakey ME, Fields WS. Roentgenographic diagnosis and surgical treatment of basilar artery insufficiency. JAMA 1958;168:509–514
7. Bhattacharji ER, Hutchinson EC, McCall AJ. The Circle of Willis: the incidence of developmental abnormalities in normal and infarcted brains. Brain 1967;90:747–758
8. Williams D, Wilson TG. The diagnosis of major and minor syndromes of basilar insufficiency. Brain 1962;85:741–774

Management of Extracranial Cerebrovascular Disease, edited by Keith D. Calligaro et al.
Lippincott-Raven Publishers, Philadelphia © 1997.

16

Causes and Management of Perioperative Stroke After Carotid Endarterectomy

Glenn R. Jacobowitz, Thomas S. Riles

It is a paradox that the most frequent complication of carotid endarterectomy is stroke: the patients who undergo this operation do so only with the hope that it will provide them protection against stroke. The incidence of perioperative stroke has steadily decreased over the years. This is due, in part, to better selection of patients for surgery, improved operative and anesthetic technique, and better training of surgeons. Many centers report the incidence of perioperative stroke to be less than 3%.[1–3] Nevertheless, it is the fear of perioperative stroke that limits the acceptance of carotid endarterectomy as the treatment of choice for carotid bifurcation disease.

It is generally accepted that there is a close relationship between the technical performance of carotid endarterectomy and failure of the procedure, manifested as perioperative stroke or in some cases, silent occlusion of the operated artery. For years surgeons have used perioperative stroke rates to support or criticize particular techniques (local versus general anesthesia, patch closure versus primary closure, routine shunting versus selective or no shunting, intraoperative EEG monitoring versus stump pressure measurements). We now know that experienced surgeons can achieve excellent results and low complication rates using any one of a variety of techniques.[4–11] Furthermore, it is clear that no single technique has entirely eliminated the risk of perioperative stroke.

Despite years of experience with carotid endarterectomy and hundreds of presentations and publications on technique and operative results, perioperative stroke still remains the primary cause of morbidity and death with this operation. In the recent North American Symptomatic Carotid Endarterectomy Trial (NASCET), 1.8% of the operated patients had a major perioperative stroke, and an additional 3.7% had a minor cerebrovascular event perioperatively. The combined rate of all perioperative stroke and death was 5.8%.[12] In the Veterans Administration asymptomatic carotid stenosis study, the perioperative stroke rate was 2.4%, and the combined stroke and mortality rate was 4.3%.[13] Unfortunately, few of the discussions of carotid surgery have focused on the cause of the perioperative strokes. It has often been difficult to know if a perioperative stroke was caused by a failure of the surgical technique or an unrelated event.

An understanding of the probable cause of a perioperative stroke is important both as a basis on which to prevent such poor outcomes, and as the foundation on which to formulate therapeutic plans once such an event occurs. In this chapter we outline the causes of perioperative stroke after carotid endarterectomy as well as diagnostic and therapeutic plans.

CAUSES OF PERIOPERATIVE STROKE

At our institution, most carotid endarterectomies have been performed in the awake patient, and it has often been possible to correlate the onset of operative strokes with the specific events of the procedure such as carotid dissection, clamping, and declamping. For those patients who developed postoperative strokes, efforts were

TABLE 16-1. *Mechanisms of perioperative stroke*

Mechanism	Number of patients
I. Cerebral ischemia during surgery	10
a. difficulty placing shunt	5
b. hypotension—shunt in place	1
c. bradycardia—no shunt	1
d. occlusion of contralateral ICA, stroke contralateral	3
II. Postoperative thrombosis and embolism	25
a. immediate postoperative thrombus	15
b. delayed postoperative embolus—no thrombus	10
III. Intracranial hemorrhage	12
IV. Strokes from other mechanisms—surgery related	14
a. thrombectomy of occluded ICA	3
1. hemorrhage or reperfusion injury	(1)
2. thrombosis	(1)
3. carotid-cavernous sinus fistula	(1)
b. strokes related to other complications	3
1. wound infection with cervical hemorrhage	(1)
2. suture disruption with cervical hemorrhage	(1)
3. global anoxia, premature extubation	(1)
c. strokes in other vascular territories	4
1. occipital	(2)
2. brain stem	(1)
3. contralateral hemisphere	(1)
d. strokes from sources unrelated to reconstructed carotid	4
1. atheroemboli from aortic arch	(1)
2. cardiac embolus	(1)
3. cerebral angiography	(1)
4. cardiac surgery	(1)
V. Intraoperative embolism	2
1. carotid dissection	(1)
2. carotid declamping	(1)
VI. Unknown	3
Total	66

(From Riles TS, Imparato AM, Jacobowitz GR, Lamparello PJ, Giangola G, Adelman MA, Landis R. The cause of perioperative stroke after carotid endarterectomy. J Vasc Surg 1994; 19:209)

made whenever possible to determine the cause of the stroke. In some instances, this was by rapid reexploration of the carotid artery. In others, it was by means of arteriography, noninvasive testing, and CT scans of the head. These efforts led to a determination of the mechanism of the stroke in the majority of the patients. In all but a few, the data eliminated many possibilities, leaving a most probable cause. Over the years, information regarding perioperative stroke and other bad outcomes has been carefully recorded. In more recent years this data has been maintained as part of a computerized file of all patients undergoing carotid surgery.

In a recent review of our own experience with perioperative strokes over a 27-year period, we identified more than 20 mechanisms that led to neurologic injury.[14] Excluding those strokes that were unrelated to the carotid surgery, attributed instead to other medical conditions, surgeries, or procedures, most perioperative strokes could be grouped into several broad categories:

1. Stroke resulting from inadequate cerebral perfusion or embolization during the carotid endarterectomy
2. Stroke due to embolization of fresh thrombus or thrombotic occlusion after restoration of flow in the carotid artery
3. Stroke due to intracerebral hemorrhage resulting from a reperfusion injury to the brain (Table 16-1).

These three mechanisms accounted for 51 of 66 (77%) strokes. Postendarterectomy thrombosis accounted for half of these events (26 of 51). In recent years this mechanism has become the major cause of perioperative stroke—with improved cerebral monitoring and more frequent use of shunts, strokes due to ischemia during carotid clamping have become rare (Fig. 16-1).

The major groups of perioperative stroke are discussed in separate sections with specific observations and recommendations for prevention.

Inadequate Cerebral Perfusion or Embolization During Carotid Endarterectomy

Over the years we have favored regional anesthesia and selective shunting.[15] In the awake patient shunts have been used for those who show signs of ischemia with test clamping (*i.e.,* loss of consciousness, aphasia, extremity weakness, confusion, or slowing of mentation). Patients undergoing general anesthesia were routinely shunted. By observing the neurologic status of the awake patient, we have been able to determine the onset of temporary and permanent ischemic events and relate these to the specific steps of the operation during which they occur.

Ten patients suffered perioperative strokes related to ischemia during the endarterectomy. Five strokes were related to difficulty with placement of the shunt in patients who were clearly shunt dependent. We have learned from these cases and others with successful outcomes that a host of potential problems may arise with shunt placement, such as dissection of the arterial wall, finding of a proximal plaque, diffi-

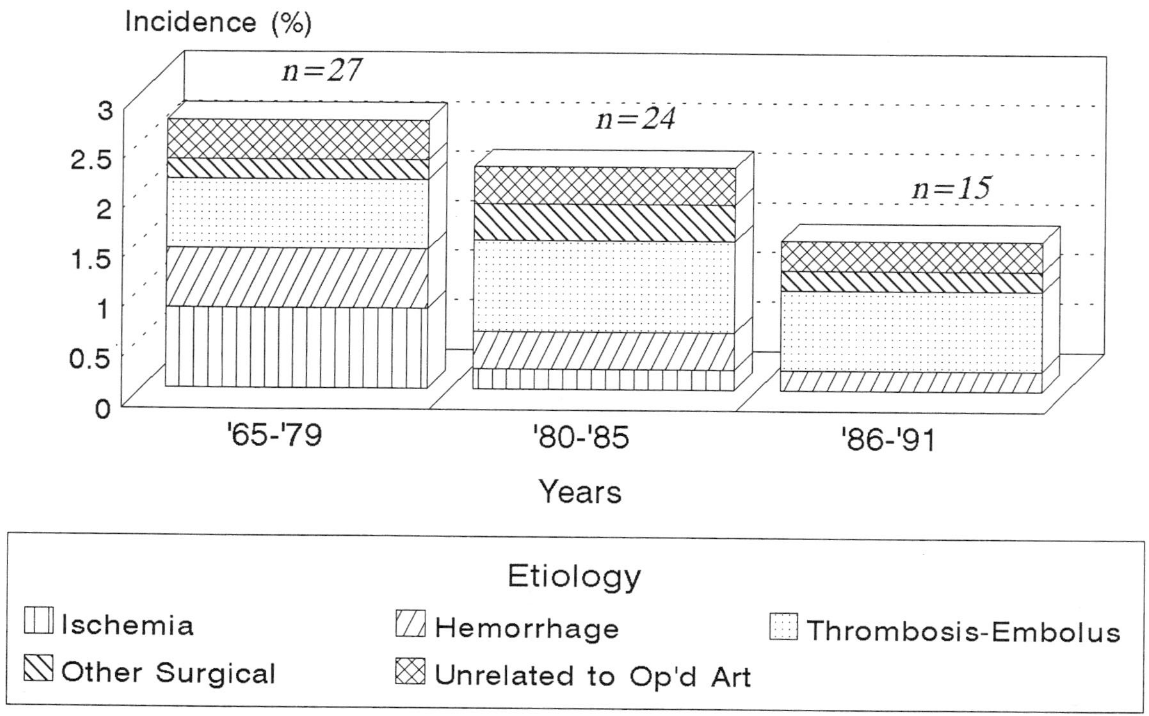

FIG. 16-1. Cause of perioperative stroke 1965 to 1991. (From Riles TS, Imparato AM, Jacobowitz GR, Lamparello PJ, Giangola G, Adelman MA, Landis R. The cause of perioperative stroke after carotid endarterectomy. J Vasc Surg 1994;19:208)

culty securing a shunt, or dislodgement of the shunt. Each must be anticipated and alternative plans prepared for the management of specific problems.

One patient developed hypotension while the shunt was in place. The ischemic event was due to inadequate cerebral perfusion during hypotension. Another patient tolerated clamping without a shunt and was stable during the endarterectomy until he developed bradycardia and then cerebral ischemia. It appears that the brain was well-perfused via collateral flow as long as there was adequate cardiac output. The bradycardia resulted in a reduction of cerebral blood flow and subsequent brain ischemia.

The three remaining strokes during clamping occurred in the contralateral hemisphere in patients with an occlusion of the contralateral internal carotid artery. Under these circumstances, the operated artery is often the major blood supply to both hemispheres. We learned from these experiences that it is sometimes difficult to monitor ischemia in the contralateral hemisphere, particularly if the patient has already had a stroke referable to that side. Having identified this as a high-risk situation, we have liberalized our indications for intra-arterial shunting in the patient with contralateral occlusion to include any patient with a preoperative neurologic deficit or recent cerebral infarction by CT scan. Whereas only 29% of patients with contralateral occlusion were shunted before 1985, in more recent years this has risen to 53%. There has been a decrease in the perioperative stroke rate in patients with contralateral occlusion to 0.7%, as compared to an earlier rate of 6.7%.[16]

Overall the incidence of perioperative stroke due to cerebral ischemia has decreased since the early years of carotid surgery (see Fig. 16-1). Only one such case has occurred during the last 10 years. Although some patients are identifiable as being high risk for cerebral ischemia, we have learned that until the carotid artery is occluded, it is impossible to be certain that an individual patient has adequate collateral circulation to maintain cerebral perfusion. When shunts are used, extra exposure is advised. Meticulous surgical technique must be used when placing an intra-arterial shunt. Once the shunt is in place and functioning properly, it is important that normal cardiac output is maintained for adequate cerebral perfusion.

Embolization of plaque material during dissection of the carotid bulb or at the moment of releasing the clamp is often cited as a cause of perioperative stroke.[17,18] In our series we found these events to be rare (2 of 66). These mechanisms were readily identified in awake patients demonstrating intraoperative mental status changes associated with specific intraoperative steps. We believe it is important to do minimal dissection of the carotid bulb until the distal clamp is placed to avoid this complication.

Postoperative Thrombosis and Embolism

This mechanism was responsible for 26 of the strokes after routine carotid endarterectomy. This group includes two subgroups: immediate postoperative internal carotid thrombosis with embolization and postoperative embolization without evidence of arterial occlusion. Both subgroups are part of a common mechanism—a technical imperfection at the endarterectomy site. Presumably the only difference is the amount of thrombus that forms at the site of flow disturbance.

Postoperative Thrombosis

This mechanism accounted for 16 strokes. Most occurred immediately postoperatively, while the patient was in the recovery room. By coincidence, almost all of these patients had tolerated carotid clamping under cervical block anesthesia. It is presumed, therefore, that the stroke was not due to the obstruction of blood flow by the thrombus, but rather from embolization of thrombus that was forming prior to occlusion.

On reexploration, the technical defect was usually identified at a point of platelet aggregation. Defects noted included clamp injuries, kinks in redundant vessels, ledges at the end of the endarterectomy, stenosis at the closure of the arteriotomy, and rough endarterectomy surfaces. In several cases, no specific defect was identified. One patient had a siphon stenosis that might have been associated with the thrombosis.

Some authors have used intraoperative Duplex scanning and angiography to assess immediately technical adequacy of carotid endarterectomy.[19,20] When flow abnormalities were found, reexploration revealed technical defects, including intimal flaps, platelet aggregation, and stricture. Residual flow disturbances correlated with an increased incidence of perioperative thrombosis and stroke.[20]

In reviewing our own data on patients with intraluminal thrombosis, we have concluded that most of the technical defects were preventable. As our experience has increased, greater emphasis has been placed on the reconstruction of the carotid artery after endarterectomy. Every effort is made to leave a conduit that will be free of turbulent flow. We rely on patch angioplasty, and frequently a plication of the internal or common carotid artery is used to eliminate redundancy that occurs once a rigid plaque is removed from a curved or elongated internal carotid artery. We do not routinely use intraoperative angiography or Duplex scanning to evaluate technical adequacy. Although some have found this useful, this is most likely unnecessary, as our use of long arteriotomies, plication, and patch closure has reduced the incidence of postoperative thrombosis to a level that renders these techniques of little value for routine cases. However, if we encounter a very small carotid artery, a very high plaque, or any unusual circumstances, we do not hesitate to obtain an intraoperative arteriogram to assess the repair.

Delayed Embolization Without Evidence of Thrombosis

Whereas the stroke mechanism of postoperative thrombosis is quite clear, the exact pathophysiology of this subgroup remains a question. Ten patients had a stroke during their recovery phase. Most of the strokes were mild and ipsilateral to the carotid endarterectomy and generally occurred later than those associated with complete thrombosis. Three occurred while the patient was still in the recovery room. Seven occurred later in the recovery period: 1 on postoperative day 1, 3 on postoperative day 2, 1 on postoperative day 3, and 2 on postoperative day 4. Angiogram or duplex scan ruled out thrombosis of the internal and common carotid artery but occasionally showed a defect that could have been the source of the embolus. CT scans, when obtained, showed no intracranial hemorrhage. The exact cause of the stroke was often unknown. The most likely explanation is that the source of the embolus was small, probably related to a minor technical defect, and neither the defect nor residual source of the embolus was evident on duplex scan or angiogram. It appears that without evidence of thrombosis, medical management consisting mainly of supportive care, is sufficient. Anticoagulation was not used, and most patients did not have recurrence of symptoms.

Intracerebral Hemorrhage or Reperfusion Injury

This complication occurred in 13 patients and was almost always related to reopening of a severely stenotic carotid artery. The intracerebral hemorrhages occurred at various points in the postoperative course, from day 1 to 10, and with no warning signs. Other risk factors included severe intraoperative and postoperative hypertension, while previous stroke did not appear to play a role.[21] High-grade stenosis has been the only identifiable preoperative risk factor for intracranial hemorrhage. The occurrence of intracranial hemorrhage is totally unpredictable and its mechanism of action is poorly understood. It is likely that the blood–brain barrier may be overcome by rapid increases in cerebral blood flow that occur after carotid endarterectomy.[22] Severe hypertension may exacerbate this mechanism. However, intracerebral hemorrhage does not occur in the vast majority of patients with high-grade stenoses or severe intraoperative and postoperative hypertension. For reasons not entirely clear, this complication fortunately is occurring less frequently in our own series. There has been only one intracranial hemorrhage in the last 1,000 operations.

Strokes from Other Mechanisms

Other strokes have a variety of causes. Three patients sustained strokes as a result of attempted thrombectomy of occluded internal arteries, a practice that is rarely indicated. Thrombectomy is known to be associated with a high perioperative stroke rate.[23,24] Occasionally it is still used when there is evidence that the thrombosis is of acute onset, particularly when patients have had continued transient ischemic attacks after the occlusion or have a known occlusion in the contralateral carotid artery as well. We have had the occasion to do this in less than 20 patients in our series. All have been unusual cases with complicated presentations and high-risk anatomic situations. Among the strokes following thrombectomy, one was due to a reperfusion injury, one was due to rethrombosis of the artery, and the third was related to a carotid–cavernous sinus fistula.

Two patients had strokes due to asphyxia secondary to cervical hemorrhage from disrupted suture lines. One patient sustained global anoxia following premature extubation. Four patients had strokes in territories other than the operated carotid. Another 4 patients had strokes from sources unrelated to the reconstructed carotid artery, including a cardiac embolus, aortic arch embolus (multiple emboli to the brain and other organs), a cerebral angiogram, and one stroke during subsequent coronary surgery.

THERAPEUTIC PLANS FOR PERIOPERATIVE STROKE

Once a perioperative stroke has occurred, the surgeon must assess the patient, the nature and timing of the neurologic deficit, and he must then initiate a diagnostic and therapeutic plan based on the most likely causes. Unless there is clear evidence that the stroke occurred during the dissection or at the moment of restoration of blood flow, one should not assume this to be the cause of the stroke. If one readily concludes this to be the mechanism of the stroke, there is a tendency not to consider other possibilities that may require emergency reoperation or other therapies. Although embolization to the cerebral circulation usually occurs with strokes due to technical problems at the site of the endarterectomy, the difference between this and embolization during the procedure is that with the former, the process may continue until the technical problem is repaired.

If the problem was not related to clamp ischemia (a shunt was used or the patient was properly monitored during the clamping of the carotid), the two most likely causes for the postoperative stroke are thrombus formation at the site of the endarterectomy or reperfusion injury. Inasmuch as the therapeutic goals are quite different, it is extremely important to differentiate between these two mechanisms as quickly as possible. If the stroke is due to thrombus formation within the carotid artery, the surgical goal is to return to the operating room and remove the thrombus as quickly as possible and at the same time to repair the underlying defect that led to the thrombosis. If the patient has hemorrhaged into the brain, it may be important to consider evacuation of the hemorrhage or placement of an intraventricular shunt to prevent hydrocephalus.

We have on occasion noted some subtle differences between patients who had postoperative ischemic strokes and those who had hemorrhagic strokes. The patients with intracranial hemorrhage often are hypertensive and the stroke may be heralded by a seizure, particularly if it is a cortical bleed. This observation, however, is not sufficiently reliable to make a correct diagnosis. The definitive tests to diagnose carotid thrombosis and intracranial hemorrhage are an angiogram and a CT scan or MRI. These tests, however, often require considerable time to arrange and perform. If the patient is thrombosing his carotid artery or embolizing from thrombus at the site of the endarterectomy, the ultimate outcome may be determined by the length of time it takes to correct the underlying problem.

If the patient is in the recovery room when the stroke occurs, our first response is to make plans for immediate return to the operating room. Generally this requires a few minutes to set up. While these arrangements are being made, we can often obtain an emergency Duplex scan. The Duplex scan has been extremely helpful to determine whether the artery has intraluminal thrombus, or is open with obstruction. If the artery is found to be widely patent, and we have clinical suspicion that the patient is having an intracranial bleed, we may postpone the return to the operating room and obtain a CT scan. If, on the other hand, there is evidence of a flow defect, the patient is returned to the operating room as soon as possible. If the Duplex scanner is not available, the patient is taken to the operating room for reexploration of the artery. Although the patient may be suffering a bleed, we feel it is most important to be certain that the surgical repair is not the cause, since the diagnosis and correction of a technical problem is the best chance for recovery for the patient. In the operating room an angiogram can be performed. More commonly, the artery is simply opened and examined for intraluminal thrombus and technical defects.

If thrombus is found, it is very helpful to "read the clot" to determine the cause of the thrombus formation. Usually the point where platelets are aggregated is the site of technical defect. The common causes of platelet aggregation and thrombosis (retained plaque, ledges where the plaque was transected, kinking or narrowing of the internal carotid artery, rough endarterectomy surface, clamp injury) must be repaired. If a patch was not used, it should certainly be used for the secondary closure.

If the artery is completely thrombosed, we will usually try to restore flow by simply extracting the clot or using a Fogarty catheter. It is important that the catheter is not passed more than 8–10 cm, the length of the extracranial carotid artery. A catheter passed into the siphon portion of the carotid may lead to a carotid–cavernous sinus fistula. If there is any doubt about complete removal of the clot, an intraoperative angiogram using 2–3 cc of contrast is necessary to visualize the distal internal carotid artery. The angiogram should be performed before restoration of flow through a rubber catheter approximately the same size as the internal carotid artery. It is important that the catheter is not securely fixed to the internal carotid. If there is a distal obstruction, intraluminal pressure will increase from the injection of the contrast dye. If the catheter is not secured, it will simply disengage. One does not wish to "push" thrombus into the intracranial circulation, nor does one wish to rupture the artery due to excessive pressure. If the artery is patent, a few cc of dye will easily flow into the vessel and outline the distal carotid.

Occasionally the question is asked whether it is better to leave an artery thrombosed or to do the thrombectomy in a patient with a fresh stroke. We generally follow the principle that it is better to restore flow, except for the rare occasion when the patient has dense coma. Although there are no studies to answer this question, experience from patients with carotid trauma and neurologic deficits suggest that the individual is more likely to recover from the stroke if flow is restored to the occluded artery.[25,26] The risk of converting a bland stroke into a hemorrhagic stroke in the early minutes or hours after a complete occlusion seems to be minimal.

In spite of the lack of data to prove that reoperation is the best treatment, we continue to treat early neurologic deficits due to thrombosis in this manner for several reasons. First, we feel it is important to prevent any further embolization. Secondly, we hope recovery will be better with an open carotid artery than with one that is occluded. Finally, we think it is important to examine the area of occlusion with the hope that the information will lead to better surgery in the future.

If the patient is a day or two after the carotid surgery and a new neurologic deficit occurs, the diagnostic and therapeutic options may be quite different. The patient may be in a regular hospital room, it may be the middle of the night, or in some cases a patient may already be home. Thrombosis of the carotid artery may still be the cause, but the longer the interval between the surgery and the new stroke, the more likely that the stroke may be due to intracerebral hemorrhage. Because of this, and also because the operating room is not immediately available, we rely upon the Duplex scan and the CT scan to guide us in treatment. If intraluminal thrombus is found, plans are made for reexploration. With these delayed neurologic deficits, the surgeon must determine which resources are available and which will most expeditiously lead to the correct diagnosis and therapy.

Although postoperative intracranial hemorrhage is a very rare complication, it is one of the most devastating for carotid surgery. It generally occurs in patients with severe stenosis and a preoperative neurologic deficit.[14] The operation is often uncomplicated and void of technical errors. Although these patients are often noted to be hypertensive at the onset of the neurologic event, it is never clear if the hypertension contributed to the bleed, or if it is the result of the bleed. Early evaluation of the carotid artery by Duplex scan, arteriogram or reexploration will show unobstructed flow. The CT scan of the head will confirm the diagnosis.

For patients with small intracranial hemorrhages, there is little to offer in the way of therapy other than careful blood-pressure control and general supportive measures. For major bleeds there are critical decisions to be made. It is advisable to enlist the aid of a neurosurgeon early, in the event that cranial surgery may be necessary. For patients with massive bleeds into the parenchyma of the brain, evacuation of the hematoma may be a life-saving procedure. In some cases, the hemorrhage may mainly involve the ventricle. Since bleeding into the ventricles may lead to obstruction, increased intraventricular pressure, and worsening of the neurologic deficit, a temporary intraventricular shunt may prove critical to the recovery of the patient.

CONCLUSION

Much has been written regarding patient risk factors for stroke, such as age, general health, history of previous neurologic deficit, and contralateral carotid occlusion.[2,3] In our experience, preexisting factors have become less important as the operative experience has grown. Whereas contralateral occlusion has been related to increased perioperative stroke rates in the past, this has not been a factor in recent years. This appears to be due to an increased use of cerebral protection via intraarterial shunts, and may in part account for the overall decrease in the incidence of perioperative stroke shown in Figure 16-1. Most strokes can be traced to technical mishaps occurring during placement of a shunt, endarterectomy, or carotid reconstruction. We find that these events occur randomly and are no more prevalent among the aged, patients with prior neurologic deficits, women, or patients with associated mental illness than in the general population undergoing carotid endarterectomy.

The majority of perioperative strokes associated with carotid endarterectomy are directly related to the technical aspects of the operation. Vascular surgeons should be equipped with a variety of techniques to manage the various problems which may be encountered. The focus should be on

A method for ensuring that the patient is receiving adequate cerebral perfusion during carotid clamping

Careful reconstruction of the endarterectomized carotid artery to provide unobstructed and nonturbulent flow once the clamps are removed.

Since strokes may occur for a variety of reasons in patients with atherosclerotic disease and associated medical problems, there will always be a small risk of stroke for these patients during the operation and recovery period. Furthermore, because of the difficulty in being absolutely certain that a carotid bifurcation lesion is the source of neurologic symptoms, it is inevitable that some patients will be misdiagnosed, have successful removal of the carotid plaque, but continue to have neurologic symptoms on the basis of another mechanism (*e.g.,* intracranial disease, arch atheroemboli). Although there is little the surgeon can do to prevent these unrelated causes for stroke, it is possible to prevent most of the other reasons for perioperative stroke. If we can solve the problems of cerebral ischemia at the time of carotid clamping, postoperative thrombosis and embolization, and intracerebral hemorrhage and reperfusion injury, it will be possible to perform carotid surgery with less than a 1% risk of perioperative stroke.

Finally, it is important for the vascular surgeon to have a predetermined therapeutic plan for the postoperative carotid patient with a new neurologic deficit. The patients' best chance for recovery requires such a plan, which must be implemented rapidly and have clear objectives and alternatives, all of which are based on an understanding of the possible causes of perioperative stroke.

REFERENCES

1. Till JS, Toole JF, Howard VJ, et al. Declining morbidity and mortality of carotid endarterectomy: The Wake Forest University Medical Center experience. Stroke 1987;18:823–829
2. Lees CD, Hertzer NR. Postoperative stroke and late neurologic complications after carotid endarterectomy. Arch Surg 1981;116:1561–1568
3. Kirshner DL, O'Brien MS, Ricotta JJ. Risk factors in a community experience with carotid endarterectomy. J Vasc Surg 1989;10:178–86
4. Callow AD, Matsumoto G, Baker D, et al. Protection of the high risk carotid endarterectomy patient by continuous electroencephalography. J Cardiovasc Surg 1978;19:55–64
5. Whitney DG, Kahn EM, Estes JW, Jones CE. Carotid artery surgery without a temporary indwelling shunt, 1917 consecutive procedures. Arch Surg 1980;115:1393–1399
6. Baker WH, Dorner DB, Barnes RW. Carotid endarterectomy: is an indwelling shunt necessary? Surg 1977;82:321–326
7. Rich NM, Hobson RW II. Carotid endarterectomy under regional anesthesia. Am Surg 1975;41:253

8. Moore WS, Yee JM, Hall AD. Collateral cerebral blood pressure: an index of tolerance to temporary carotid occlusion. Arch Surg 1973;106:520
9. Sundt TM, Houser O, Sharbrough F, et al. Carotid endarterectomy: results, complications and monitoring techniques. Adv Neurol 1977;16:97–119
10. Lord RSA, Raj TB, Stary DL, et al. Comparison of saphenous vein patch, polytetrafluoroethylene patch and direct arteriotomy closure after carotid endarterectomy. Part I. Perioperative results. J Vasc Surg 1989;9:521–529
11. Eikelboom BC, Ackerstaff RGA, Hoeneveld H, et al. Benefits of carotid patching: a randomized study. J Vasc Surg 1988;7:240–247
12. North American Symptomatic Carotid Endarterectomy Trial (NASCET). Beneficial effect of carotid endarterectomy in symptomatic patients with high-grade stenosis. N Engl J Med 1991;325:445–453
13. Towne JB, Weiss DG, Hobson RW II. First phase report of cooperative Veterans Administration asymptomatic carotid stenosis study—operative morbidity and mortality. J Vasc Surg 1990;11(2): 252–259
14. Riles TS, Imparato AM, Jacobowitz GR, Lamparello PJ, Giangola G, Adelman MA, Landis R. The cause of perioperative stroke after carotid endarterectomy. J Vasc Surg 1994;19:206–216
15. Imparato AM, Ramirez A, Riles TS, Mintzer R. Cerebral protection in carotid surgery. Arch Surg 1982;117:1073–1118
16. Adelman MA, Jacobowitz GR, Riles TS, Imparato AM, Lamparello PJ, Baumann FG, Landis R. Carotid endarterectomy in the presence of a contralateral occlusion: a review of 315 cases over a 27-year experience. Cardiovasc Surg 1995;3:307–312
17. Hertzer NM, Beven EG, Greenstreet RL, Humphries AW. Internal carotid artery back pressure, intraoperative shunting, ulcerated atheromata, and the incidence of stroke during carotid endarterectomy. Surgery 1978;83:306–312
18. Perdue GL. Management of postendarterectomy neurologic deficits. Arch Surg 1982;117:1079–1081
19. Sandmann WK, Kniemeyer HW, Peronneau P, et al. Improvement of carotid artery reconstruction using intraoperative Doppler spectrum histogram (DSH). Stroke 1984;15(1):190
20. Bandyk DF, Kaebnick HW, Adams MB, Towne JB. Turbulence occurring after carotid bifurcation endarterectomy: a harbinger of residual and recurrent carotid stenosis. J Vasc Surg 1988;7:261–274
21. Pomposelli FB, Lamparello PJ, Riles TS, et al. Intracranial hemorrhage after carotid endarterectomy. J Vasc Surg 1988;7:240–247
22. Sundt TM, Jr, Sharbrough FW, Piepgras DG, et al. Correlation of cerebral blood flow and electroencephalographic changes during carotid endarterectomy with results of surgery and hemodynamics of cerebral ischemia. Mayo Clin Proc 1981;56:533
23. Rushton FW, Kurkora JS. Surgical management of the occluded carotid artery. Surgery 1984;96: 845–852
24. Toole JF, Janeway R, Choi K, et al. Transient ischemic attacks due to atherosclerosis. A prospective study of 160 patients. Arch Neurol 1975;25:413–517
25. Weaver FA, Yellin AE, Wagner WH, Brooks SH, Weaver AA, Milford MA. The role of arterial reconstruction in penetrating carotid injuries. Arch Surg 1988;123:1106–1111
26. Richardson R, Obeid FN, Richardson JD, Hoyt DB, Wisner DH, Gomez GA, Johansen K, McSwain NE, Jr, Weigelt JA, Blaisdell FW. Neurologic consequences of cerebrovascular injury. J Trauma 1992;32:755–760

Management of Extracranial Cerebrovascular Disease, edited by Keith D. Calligaro et al.
Lippincott-Raven Publishers, Philadelphia © 1997.

17

Management of Extracranial Carotid Artery Fibromuscular Disease and Spontaneous Dissection

Elliot L. Chaikof, Robert B. Smith III

FIBROMUSCULAR DYSPLASIA OF THE CAROTID ARTERY

Despite a 30-year history of case reports and collected retrospective reviews, our understanding of the management of extracranial arterial fibromuscular dysplasia (FMD) remains incomplete. The rarity of the process and the sole reliance on angiographic findings to diagnose and categorize FMD have limited clinical decision making. We suspect that in the coming years widespread use of ever-improving imaging modalities will present the vascular surgeon with an increasing pool of such patients. The challenge for all of us will be to continue a careful examination of this nonatheromatous, noninflammatory process. Ultimately, we must base clinical recommendations on an understanding of the disease progression and our ability to alter this process.

For the most part, extracranial fibromuscular disease consists of two primary pathologic subtypes—intimal and medial fibroplasia.[1] Intimal fibroplasia is the less common of the two and is typically associated with either an isolated web or a smooth tubular stenosis of the internal carotid artery. Webs appear to be more common among older patients, while long stenoses typically occur in the young adult. Elongation, kinking, or coiling of the carotid artery may also be noted. This variety of FMD appears to be predominantly a localized arteriopathy, and the occurrence of simultaneous lesions, whether aneurysmal or fibrodysplastic, is unusual. Several authors have suggested that a highly stenotic web may represent a lesion that is associated with a greater risk for subsequent stroke. Medial fibroplasia has the angiographic appearance of the classic "string-of-beads" stenoses. It most often involves a 2- to 6-cm segment of internal carotid artery adjacent to the second and third cervical vertebrae and spares the origins and proximal portions of the carotid. The artery is often elongated, and kinking is noted in approximately 5% of patients. Reviews have documented bilateral disease in 35% to 85% of patients.

The incidence of medial fibroplasia in most carotid arteriographic studies has ranged between 0.25% and 0.68%. It presents commonly in females, infrequently in African Americans, and most patients presenting with extracranial FMD are diagnosed at a later age than those with renovascular dysplasia. Notably, approximately 20 to 50% of patients may have associated atherosclerotic disease of the carotid bulb.[2,3] Thirty-nine percent of the patients treated by graded intraluminal dilation (GID) in a series reported by Collins et al[2] and 20% of those reported by Effeney et al[3] also required a concomitant carotid bifurcation endarterectomy. Although most cases of medial fibroplasia occur as isolated findings, this process should be considered a systemic arteriopathy. In approximately 10 to 20% of patients who present with a carotid dissection, contralateral fibromuscular disease is present. Coexistent carotid and vertebral fibrodysplasia occurs in approximately 20% of patients. Additionally, carotid fibromuscular disease associated with intracranial and, on rare occasions, extracranial aneurysms has been observed. Certainly, the most common site for either simultaneous or subsequent development of fibrodysplasia is the renal artery. Concomitant renovascular and extracranial fibromuscular disease has been noted in 25 to 50% of patients.

Conventional arteriography remains the sole means for definitively diagnosing carotid fibrodysplasia (Fig. 17-1). The presence of FMD in any one of the extracranial vessels should prompt a thorough four-vessel cerebral angiogram, including examination of the intracranial vessels to detect possible sites of aneurysmal disease. In addition, renal arteriography should be performed owing to the proclivity to concomitant disease.

Though radiographic findings are pathognomonic for medial fibroplasia, a differential diagnosis should always be considered when the diagnoses of intimal fi-

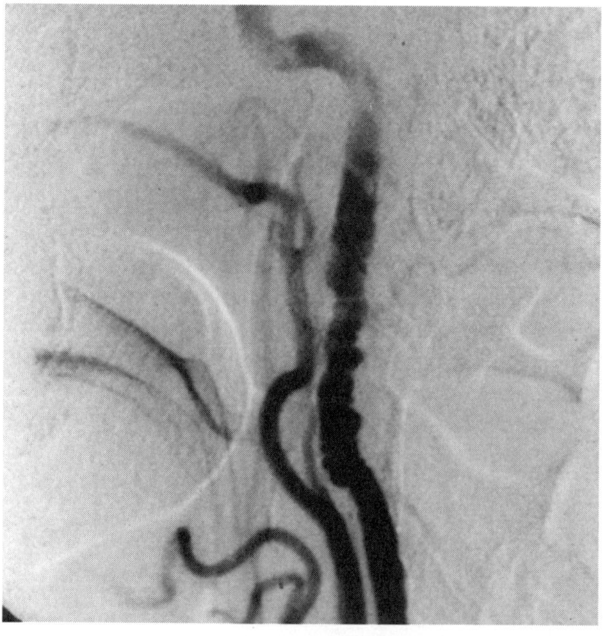

FIG. 17-1. Classic angiographic "string-of-beads" appearance for medial internal carotid artery fibromuscular dysplasia.

broplasia or medial hyperplasia are entertained. These lesions may be confused with arteriosclerotic plaques, inflammatory processes such as Takayasu's arteritis, and vascular lesions of neurofibromatosis or Ehlers-Danlos syndrome. Arteriosclerotic lesions can usually be distinguished by their eccentric appearance and location at the level of the carotid bifurcation. In Takayasu's arteritis, the aorta is usually involved and the large arteries are stenotic at their origin. The associated stigmata of Ehlers-Danlos syndrome and neurofibromatosis should aid in identifying these entities.

Recent reports of concurrent fibromuscular disease in the superficial temporal artery imply that biopsy may be helpful to confirm the diagnosis in patients who present with either a carotid dissection or multiple intracranial aneurysms of the internal carotid artery and no other evidence of systemic FMD. This information would have important prognostic implications and may aid in obtaining a more precise disease classification.

In reported surgical series, as in our experience, the spectrum of symptoms is similar to that of patients with atherosclerosis undergoing carotid endarterectomy—amaurosis fugax, transient ischemic attacks, nonfocal cerebral ischemia, and stroke. Suggested etiologies of symptoms have included both impaired perfusion as a consequence of multiple stenoses or embolic debris originating from aneurysmal cul de sacs. Alternatively, symptoms may originate following dissection of either the vertebral or internal carotid artery. Headaches, vertigo, and tinnitus have also been observed in association with extracranial arterial fibroplasia. It has been suggested that the occurrence of headaches is related to the release of vasoactive substances, such as serotonin or thromboxane A2, from aggregating platelets. In many cases, however, the angiographic finding of carotid FMD is only incidental, with no symptomatic correlation.

The assumption that patients with carotid FMD have a prognosis and natural history similar to patients with atherosclerosis is unproved. Repeat angiography has rarely been documented in patients with carotid FMD, and the incidence of progressive disease has not been clarified. Only 15 patients with carotid FMD undergoing serial angiography have previously been described in the literature. Of these, progressive FMD was observed in 5 and a new lesion in 2. Of 8 patients followed at Emory, only one developed a new lesion of FMD in the contralateral vessel, and atherosclerotic stenosis evolved in one other. The significance of angiographic progression is uncertain as these changes were not correlated with new clinical symptoms. Similarly, in a series of 79 patients reported by Corrin and colleagues[4] from the Mayo Clinic, carotid FMD was an incidental finding in the majority, and only three had or developed ischemic symptoms during a mean follow-up period of 5 years. This is in direct contrast to renovascular FMD, where progression is much more common. In one report, progression of renal FMD was documented in 35% of patients after a 3-year observation period.

The presumption that recurrent symptoms or cerebral infarction will inevitably occur in the patient with symptomatic carotid FMD remains an open question. In a review from the Emory University Hospital of 35 nonoperated patients with carotid FMD, all but 7 of whom were symptomatic, none had a stroke during an average follow-up period of 91 months.[5] Only 2 patients had persistent symptoms of nonfocal cerebral ischemia. In our experience, even patients with symptoms of focal ischemia will probably have spontaneous cessation of these symptoms on antiplatelet therapy. Similar findings have been observed by others.[6] This is not to say that carotid FMD cannot cause cerebral infarction, but the incidence is probably very low. Certainly, there seems little need to intervene surgically in the asymptomatic patient with carotid or vertebral FMD. However, in those patients who remain symptomatic despite antiplatelet therapy, a variety of techniques have been advocated, including arterial resection, bypass with saphenous vein, excision of fibromuscular tissue with patch grafting, and graduated internal dilation (GID). GID has become the standard surgical approach and good results have been reported with its application from several centers. Experience with balloon angioplasty is growing, but the risks of secondary embolization or arterial wall trauma are not well defined.

SPONTANEOUS DISSECTING HEMATOMA OF THE INTERNAL CAROTID ARTERY

Dissecting hematomas of the extracranial internal carotid artery are rare yet potentially devastating causes of cerebral ischemia. The term spontaneous implies the occurrence of internal carotid dissection without recognizable traumatic antecedent, although not infrequently spontaneous dissections are observed in association with fibromuscular dysplasia, Erdheim's cystic medial necrosis, and arteriosclerosis.[7–9] Since the original description by Anderson and Schecler in 1959,[10] over 200 cases have been reported, with the largest series from Ehrenfeld and Wylie,[11] Fisher et al,[12] and Bogousslavsky et al.[13] Blunt and penetrating cervical trauma and acceleration–deceleration cervical injuries are well recognized causes of arterial dissection but are excluded from this consideration. Likewise excluded are dissecting aneurysms of the ascending and transverse aorta, which may extend into the proximal carotid system and, rarely, into the internal carotid artery. Whether dissection of the extracranial internal carotid artery is ever clearly spontaneous remains controversial. As emphasized by Trosch et al,[14] antecedent trauma may be trivial and either not recalled or too embarrassing to disclose. Such trauma as coughing, vigorous nose blowing, shaving, brushing teeth, head turning while leading a parade, neck flexion while scolding a child, and "head banging" during punk rock dancing have been recorded prior to "spontaneous" carotid dissections. In the majority of patients, however, the etiology is unknown. Males and females appear to be afflicted at similar rates, with the mean age at diagnosis being 46 years (range 11 to 74 years). Both internal carotids appear to be affected with similar frequency.[13]

Presenting clinical manifestations of internal carotid dissection include focal cerebral neurologic deficits—whether transient or permanent—in over 80% of cases, but it appears that the regional extent of neurologic complaints in this condition is often greater than that attributable to atherosclerotic embolization. Thus, many patients present with signs of both retinal ischemia and contralateral hemiparesis or hemihypesthesia, in addition to multiple cranial nerve palsies.

Noteworthy physical symptoms and signs of carotid dissection may include the rapid onset of severe hemicrania; Horner syndrome; Raeder trigeminal syndrome; scalp hyperalgesia; dysgeusia; central sixth, seventh, and eighth cranial nerve palsy; as well as contralateral focal sensory and motor deficits. These neurologic features may occur singly or in variable combinations or may be preceded by transient cerebral ischemia in about 20% of patients.[13] Dysgeusia is thought to result from involvement of the chorda tympani branch of the seventh cranial nerve. Importantly, the evolution of a Horner oculosympathetic palsy may occur asynchronously or may be incomplete. The acute onset of ipsilateral head and facial pain in the frontal, parietal, or periorbital area may be followed in 24 to 72 hours by the development of one or more features of Horner syndrome, with anhydrosis most frequently absent. The headaches are typically nonthrobbing and fluctuating in intensity; they frequently require 2 to 6 months to resolve completely. During this interval, rarely is there complete relief of the cephalalgia. Other complaints include pulsatile or machinery vascular tinnitus.[11,12,15,16]

Physical findings of carotid dissection vary enormously. The multiplicity of neurologic findings mentioned above—in addition to tenderness over the carotid bulb, carotidynia, and an evolving cervical bruit—are strongly suggestive of the diagnosis. The origin of the internal carotid dissecting hematoma is usually 2 to 3 cm distal to the carotid bulb. Through the usually vertically oriented intimal rent, the hematoma pulsates deep into the tunica media, creating a subadventitial cleavage plane.[11,12] The entire arterial circumference is rarely involved; however, thrombosis of the false channel severely compromises the true lumen, leading either to markedly reduced flow or to secondary complete thrombosis. The dissection seldom extends beyond the base of the skull, but cavernous sinus extension has been reported. On rare occasions, reentry of the hematoma into the true lumen may occur acutely, restoring arterial flow.

The experience of Ehrenfeld and Wylie in 10 patients with dissecting aneurysms has provided the best description of the typical gross pathology.[11] Consistent in their experience was a sharp transition between the normal color and size of the internal carotid artery and the dark-blue discoloration and moderate cylindrical dilatation produced by the dissection. Only 4 patients of their series experienced termination of the dissection at a level easily visualized from the cervical incision, whereas the other 6 experienced dissections beyond the limits of surgical accessibility. Three patients had an arteriotomy performed, and each demonstrated the short vertical intimal rent marking the origin of the dissection. Microscopically, the typical features included organizing hematoma in the deeper layers of the tunica media with reduction of elastic tissue and fragmentation of internal elastic laminae. Smooth-muscle cells were widely separated and diminished in number. Mucopolysaccharide stains demonstrated the deposition of mucoid material indicative of degenerative changes. Atherosclerosis was consistently absent.[11]

In 1972, Ojemann et al[17] suggested that the long stenotic segment of extracranial

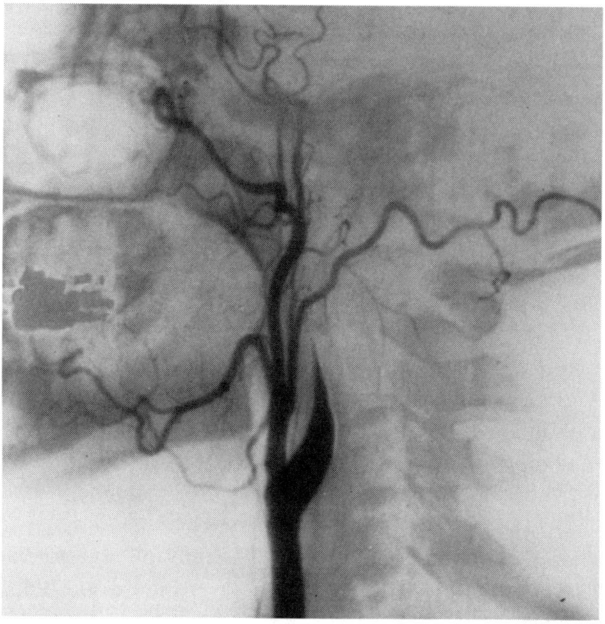

FIG. 17-2. Angiographic appearance of spontaneous dissection of the internal carotid artery.

internal carotid artery visualized angiographically ("string sign") might be a reliable indicator of carotid dissection (Figs. 17-2 and 17-3). Adopting this radiographic feature, radiologists became convinced that spontaneous carotid dissection was clearly not as rare as previously suspected. Typically, the angiogram of the carotid dissection reveals an irregular, extremely narrow column of contrast beginning slightly above the carotid bulb with a gradual taper ending at the base of the skull. Usually there is little or no evidence of atherosclerotic plaque. These radiographic features are highly suggestive of carotid dissection, but the "string sign" may also occur with other types of vascular disease such as atherosclerosis, fibromuscular dysplasia, arteritis, moya moya, and vasospasm.[12] Although the degree of stenosis is usually high, the length of the angiographic stenotic segment can be variable. Occasionally a small cul-de-sac projecting cephalad and posteriorly is identified and is thought to represent the residual lumen at the origin of the intimal tear. If spontaneous organization of the false channel hematoma develops, retraction of the intima occurs at variable rates, producing scalloped or undulating angiographic margins of the recanalizing carotid artery walls. Pseudoaneurysm formation has been noted on long-term follow-up of the recanalized carotid artery due to the focal injury in the arterial wall (Fig. 17-4). Bilateral and recurrent carotid dissections are extremely rare.[12,13] Magnetic resonance imaging (MRI) may supplant conventional arteriography in the diagnosis of the spontaneous dissection because of its ability to detect clearly the intramural hematoma (Fig. 17-5).

Early experience with this condition resulted in a variety of urgent attempts to re-

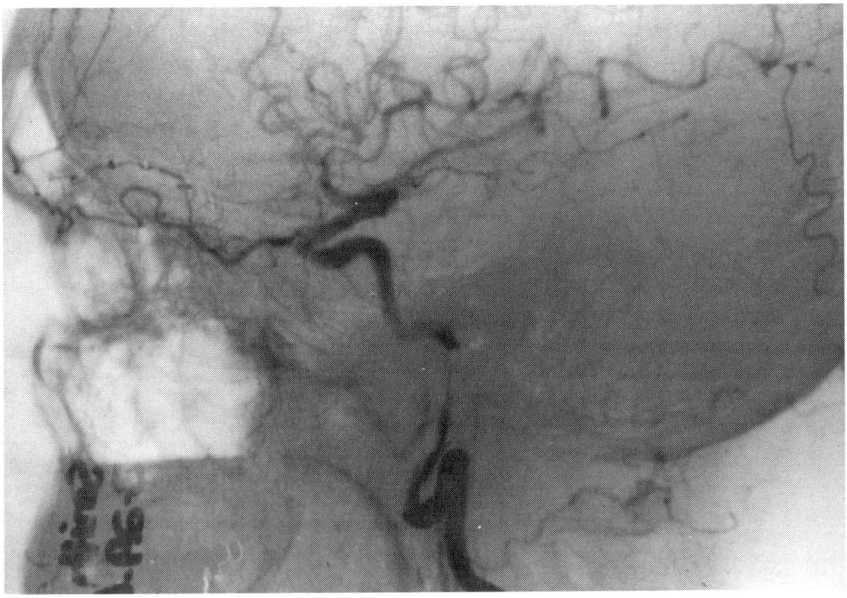

FIG. 17-3. "String sign" is apparent in this angiogram of an internal carotid artery dissection.

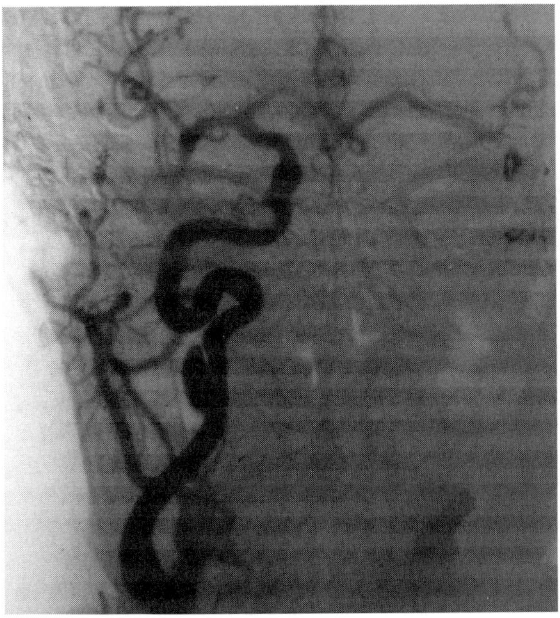

FIG. 17-4. A localized pseudoaneurysm of a recanalized internal carotid artery is noted.

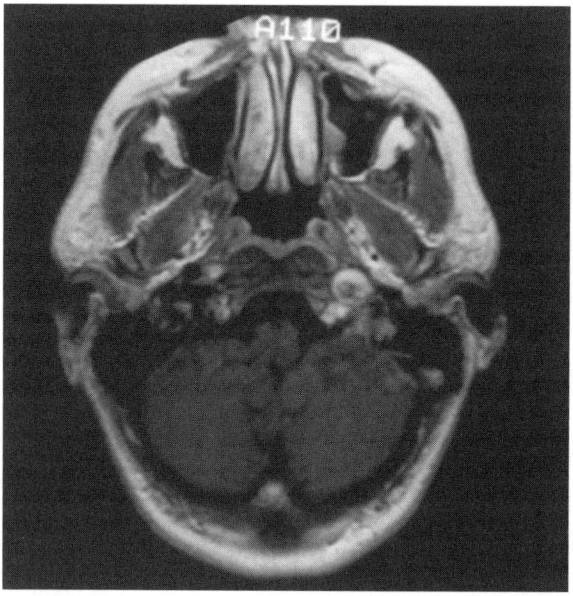

FIG. 17-5. An intramural hematoma in the right internal carotid artery, as visualized by MRI, unambiguously confirms the presence of a carotid dissection.

store cerebral arterial flow. These included resection of the involved segment with saphenous vein interposition grafting, dilation, balloon catheter thrombectomy, or ligation of the internal carotid artery, provided a stump pressure of greater than 65 torr was identified.[11] The majority of these operations were unsuccessful owing to technical difficulties with exposure of the distal point of dissection, the presence of residual thrombus with cerebral embolic potential, or progression of frank stroke as a result of acute revascularization of a bland cerebral infarct. In 1976, taking a new approach, Ehrenfeld and Wylie[11] described experience with 7 patients in whom the carotid artery was not disturbed surgically. Of these patients, 3 underwent cervical exploration only and 4 were managed nonoperatively. Surprisingly, none of the patients had further progression of neurologic symptoms with up to 3 years follow-up. Repeat arteriography was obtained in 6 of these patients from 2 to 16 months following the original arteriogram. One carotid had progressed to total occlusion, whereas the remaining 5 had increased to essentially normal caliber. Others have since reported favorable results with nonoperative therapy;[18] however, the optimum therapeutic protocol is presently unknown. One of the larger, more contemporary clinical series of 30 spontaneous carotid dissection and stroke patients was reported by Bogousslavsky et al.[13] This group represented 2.5% of stroke patients admitted to their unit. Bogousslavsky emphasizes that acute carotid dissection is frequently followed by severe, permanent neurologic impairment or even death: 7 (23%) expired within 7 days of the neurologic event and 11 of 23 survivors (43%) had severe physical limitations or required total custodial care. Maximal functional recovery was achieved within 6 months by the survivors. Of the 23 survivors, 13 (57%) demonstrated recanalization of the carotid artery, which usually occurred within 30 days of the acute dissection. The authors concluded that carotid thrombosis and distal cerebral embolization account for the larger hemispheric infarctions and that early heparin anticoagulation may favorably influence clinical outcome by maintaining carotid patency and preventing luminal thrombosis until natural clot retraction can occur. They also cautioned against heparin therapy whenever the dissection extends intracranially, because of commonly associated subarachnoid hemorrhage. Although the exact role of heparin, warfarin, and antiplatelet drugs is uncertain, a consensus of the recent literature suggests that the initial approach should be nonsurgical.[13] In the absence of massive cerebral infarction or intracranial hemorrhage, systemic heparinization should be initiated and, theoretically, may facilitate resolution of the dissecting hematoma and minimize the threat of distal cerebral embolization. It has been suggested that a minimum of 3 weeks of heparin therapy is necessary;[19] however, continuing heparinization and subsequent warfarin (Coumadin) therapy until there is recanalization—as determined by duplex carotid scanning or arteriography—is a logical approach.[18] Operative intervention is reserved for medical failures. Persistence of transient ischemic neurologic events with failure of recanalization may necessitate graft replacement of the disease carotid artery or ligation, preferably preceded by extracranial–intracranial bypass. Bilateral extracranial carotid dissections may require extracranial–intracranial bypass grafting for low-flow symptoms that endanger the brain. Very rarely, the spontaneous dissection originates in the common carotid artery, permitting reconstruction by subclavian-carotid bypass to preserve ipsilateral cerebral perfusion.[20]

REFERENCES

1. Chaikof EL, Smith RB III. Pathology of carotid and vertebral arterial fibrodysplasia. In: Ernst CB, Stanley JC (eds.), Current therapy in vascular surgery. Philadelphia: Mosby Year Book, Inc., 1994
2. Collins GJ, Jr, Rich NM, Clagett GP, Spebar MJ, Salander JM. Fibromuscular dysplasia of the internal carotid arteries: clinical experience and follow-up. Ann Surg 1981;194:89–96
3. Effeney DJ, Ehrenfeld WK, Stoney RJ, Wylie EJ. Why operate on carotid fibromuscular dysplasia? Arch Surg 1980;115:1261–1265
4. Corrin LS, Sandok BA, Houser OW. Cerebral ischemic events in patients with carotid artery fibromuscular dysplasia. Arch Neurol 1981;38:616–618
5. Stewart MT, Moritz MW, Smith RB III, Fulenwider JT, Perdue GD. The natural history of carotid fibromuscular dysplasia. J Vasc Surg 1986;3:305–310
6. Wesen CA, Elliott BM. Fibromuscular dysplasia of the carotid arteries. Am J Surg 1986;151:448–451
7. Mettinger KL, Ericson K. Fibromuscular dysplasia and the brain: observations on angiographic, clinical and genetic characteristics. Stroke 1982;13:46
8. Boström K, Liliequist B. Primary dissecting aneurysm of the extracranial part of the internal carotid and vertebral arteries: report of three cases. Neurology 1967;17:179
9. Lukon MG, Ascherl GF, Carrell JW. Spontaneous dissecting aneurysms of extracranial internal carotid artery. Clin Neurosurg 1979;26:353
10. Anderson R, Schechter M. A case of spontaneous dissecting aneurysms of the internal carotid artery. J Neurol Neurosurg Psychiatry 1959;22:195
11. Ehrenfeld WK, Wylie EJ. Spontaneous dissection of the internal carotid artery. Arch Surg 1976;111: 1294
12. Fisher CM, Ojemann RF, Roberson GH. Spontaneous dissection of cervicocerebral arteries. Can J Neurol Sci 1978;5:9

13. Bogousslavsky J, Despland P, Regli F. Spontaneous carotid dissection with acute stroke. Arch Neurol 1987;44:137
14. Trosch R, Hasbani M, Brass L. "Bottoms up" dissection (letter). N Engl J Med 1989;320:1564
15. Waespe W, Niesper J, Imhof H-G. Lower cranial nerve palsies due to internal carotid dissection. Stroke 1988;19:1561
16. Maitland CG, Black JL, Smith WA. Abducens nerve palsy due to spontaneous dissection of the internal carotid artery. Arch Neurol 1983;40:448
17. Ojemann RD, Fisher CM, Rich JC. Spontaneous dissecting aneurysm of the internal carotid artery. Stroke 1972;3:434
18. Gee W, Kaupp HA, McDonald KM. Spontaneous dissection of internal carotid arteries: spontaneous resolution documented by serial ocular pneumoplethysmography and angiography. Arch Surg 1980; 115:944
19. McNeill DH, Dreisbach J, Marsden RJ. Spontaneous dissection of the internal carotid artery: its conservative management with heparin sodium. Arch Neurol 1980;37:54
20. Graham JM, Miller T, Stinnett DM. Spontaneous dissection of the common carotid artery: case report and review of the literature. J Vasc Surg 1988;7:811

Management of Extracranial Cerebrovascular Disease, edited by Keith D. Calligaro et al.
Lippincott-Raven Publishers, Philadelphia © 1997.

18

Do Tandem Lesions, Contralateral Occlusion, or String Sign Increase the Risk of Elective Carotid Endarterectomy?

Bruce A. Perler

Since its introduction more than four decades ago, carotid endarterectomy (CEA) has become the most frequently performed peripheral vascular operation in this country.[1] It has also been one of our more controversial operations. Specifically, the indications for, and safety and efficacy of the procedure have been intensely scrutinized and challenged by some over the years.[2–4] However, several recently completed randomized prospective clinical trials, involving both symptomatic and asymptomatic patients, have more firmly established the appropriate role of this surgical procedure in the management of cerebrovascular disease.[5–8]

The overall long-term benefit of surgery, compared to the medical management of carotid artery disease, obviously is dependent on the operation being performed with a minimum of complications. While it is widely accepted that perioperative neurologic morbidity is most dependent on the symptomatic presentation of the patient and the technical details of operation, other anatomic factors may also influence results. In fact, several of these anatomic variables continue to stimulate controversy and disagreement among experienced vascular surgeons. It is the purpose of this chapter to examine three of these anatomic issues; namely, tandem lesions, contralateral carotid occlusion, and the carotid string sign.

TANDEM LESIONS

Anatomic Considerations

The internal carotid artery (ICA) includes an extracranial portion that extends to the base of the skull and an intracranial portion that is referred to as the siphon. The carotid siphon includes the petrous segment within the petrous bone; the cavernous segment, which follows the contour of the sphenoid bone and pierces the dura; and the intradural portion that gives rise to the ophthalmic artery prior to the Circle of Willis.[9–10] While atheromatous disease has a clear predilection for the carotid bifurcation, the siphon is also affected in some patients. Unlike carotid bifurcation stenoses, however, atheromatous lesions in the carotid siphon are less often ulcerated, and intraplaque hemorrhage is also relatively infrequent.[11] In one study, for example, 65% of carotid siphon plaques were characterized as smooth angiographically.[9] In another investigation, electron microscopy demonstrated evidence of endothelial damage with attachment of red blood cells and platelets in only 30% of siphon, but in 80% of carotid bifurcation lesions.[12] These morphologic observations have prognostic implications. Specifically, while it is widely accepted that cerebral ischemia secondary to carotid bifurcation disease usually is secondary to embolic phenomena, symptoms due to siphon disease much more often result from flow limitation.[13,14]

Incidence

The term "tandem lesions" specifically refers to the coexistence of atherosclerotic lesions in the cervical ICA and siphon.[15,16] The true incidence of tandem lesions is not precisely defined for several reasons. First, different investigators have characterized a "significant" siphon stenosis by different criteria (vida infra). Secondly, the ICA tapers after passing through the petrous canal, and it has been noted that the lumen of the vessel may be normally reduced by up to 40% when compared to its diameter in the neck.[13] This further confounds an accurate assessment of subtle pathologic lesions at this level. Furthermore, fewer patients are undergoing intracerebral arterial study preoperatively since carotid endarterectomy (CEA) is increasingly being performed based on noninvasive Duplex, magnetic resonance angiography, or limited intraarterial digital subtraction angiography (IA/DSA) studies.

In a report from the University of Washington, carotid siphon lesions were identified angiographically in 84% of 282 ICAs among patients scheduled for CEA. However, 42% of the lesions produced only a 20 to 49% luminal diameter reduction. Only 9% of these lesions were greater than 50% stenotic.[9] In a more recent report, a greater than 50% ipsilateral ICA siphon stenosis was identified in 24 (14%) and a significant contralateral siphon stenosis was noted in 13 (7.6%) of 169 patients with significant carotid bifurcation disease.[13] Borozan et al identified either unilateral or bilateral carotid siphon stenoses in 93 (10.5%) of 885 patients who underwent cerebral angiography over a 5-year period, although these authors included lesions with at least a 20% luminal diameter reduction.[17] These investigations confirm much earlier work by Fisher et al, who noted that while carotid siphon calcification is common, hemodynamically significant stenoses occur infrequently.[18]

Natural History

An accurate delineation of the natural history and prognosis of the patient with significant carotid siphon disease is difficult. Some reports include patients with isolated siphon disease as well as tandem lesions, and in many cases patients who presented with tandem lesions underwent endarterectomy of the extracranial carotid disease. Nevertheless, it is clear that significant atherosclerotic involvement of the carotid siphon is a marker for severe systemic arterial occlusive disease.[19,20] In a study from the Cleveland Clinic, for example, strokes occurred in 10 (15%) of 66 patients with at least a 50% carotid siphon stenosis, including 6 with tandem lesions, during a mean follow-up of 3.9 years. The observed stroke rate for patients 35 years of age and older with siphon disease was 13 times the expected rate for a normal population, and was greatest in patients with tandem lesions.[19] In another study, only one third of 58 patients with a 50% or greater siphon stenosis remained alive and completely asymptomatic, with a mean follow-up of 30 months.[21] Specifically, strokes occurred in 17 (29%) patients and 9 (48%) were fatal.[21] On the other hand, Borozan et al reported a stroke incidence of 10.8% among 93 patients with either unilateral or bilateral siphon stenoses followed for 1 to 62 (mean 22.5) months. This translated into an annual stroke rate of 5%.[17] Based on these observations, the authors concluded that although the risk of stroke in patients with siphon disease was worse than the general population, it was more favorable than in patients with symptomatic carotid bifurcation disease.[17] This relatively favorable prognosis may reflect the fact that patients with only a 20% siphon stenosis were included in the analysis.

The incidence of stroke, as well as the prevalence of coronary artery disease in this population, clearly contributes to a reduced life expectancy. Marzewski et al noted a 60% 5-year survival rate among 66 patients with significant siphon disease compared to an expected rate of 87% in the normal population.[19] In another study, 25 (43%) of 58 patients with significant carotid siphon disease died during a mean follow-up of only 30 months.[21] The overall prognosis of these patients could not be directly correlated with the degree of stenosis, emphasizing that siphon disease, in general, is a marker for systemic atherosclerosis.[21] In fact, coronary artery disease is the most frequent cause of death in this patient population.[17,19,21]

Carotid Endarterectomy

The advisability of CEA in the patient with significant tandem carotid lesions has been debated for nearly 30 years and remains problematic today. Indeed, formerly some felt that CEA was absolutely or relatively contraindicated in patients with significant siphon disease, owing to an anticipated high rate of perioperative neurological complications. Specifically, it was suggested that the presence of significant siphon disease would predispose to early thrombosis of the endarterectomy site.[22–25] In addition, it was felt that residual siphon lesions would be responsible for persistent symptoms in a significant percentage of patients.[11] Several recent studies have addressed these issues (Table 18-1). For example, Roederer et al performed CEA upon 18 patients with a 50% or greater ipsilateral siphon stenoses, and there were no perioperative strokes. Furthermore, recurrent symptoms developed during follow-up in only 11% of patients with severe siphon disease, but also in 11% of a cohort of patients without siphon disease.[9] In another recent report, CEA was performed upon 37 patients with at least a 50% stenosis ipsilateral (n = 24) or contralateral (n = 13) to the endarterectomy, including 8 patients with bilateral siphon lesions. There were no

TABLE 18-1. *CEA/Tandem lesions: Results*

Source (yr)	Patients	Strokes	Deaths
University of Illinois (1982)	14	1 (7.1%)	0 (0%)
University of Washington (1983)	18	0 (0%)	0 (0%)
University of New South Wales (1987)*	24	0 (0%)	NA

*Excluded tandem lesions >80%

perioperative strokes.[13] However, operation was withheld from patients with a greater than 80% siphon stenosis.[13] Schuler et al reported 1 (7.1%) perioperative stroke among 14 patients undergoing CEA with a greater than 50% ipsilateral siphon stenosis versus 4 (5.6%) strokes among 77 patients with no siphon disease or a siphon stenosis less than 50%.[15] Furthermore, the presence of tandem siphon lesions did not adversely influence the long-term relief of symptoms in these patients.[15] The impact of siphon disease may be particularly important in elderly patients. Rosenthal et al performed CEA upon 90 octogenarians, with a perioperative stroke rate of 6%, and all 5 patients who experienced stroke had at least a 75% carotid siphon stenosis.[26] On the other hand, 87% of these patients remained asymptomatic with follow-up extending to 8 years.[26]

Perspective

Experience accumulated over the last decade has clearly demonstrated that CEA may be performed proximal to significant siphon disease with an acceptable rate of perioperative morbidity, although it may be somewhat greater than when performed in the absence of tandem lesions. The presence of siphon disease is a marker of underlying coronary artery disease, so that one may want to perform a pre-operative cardiac evaluation more aggressively than in the patient who presents without significant tandem lesions. Furthermore, even accepting a slightly greater risk of perioperative morbidity in this patient population, the preponderance of evidence available to date suggests that the long-term prognosis of patients with tandem lesions who undergo CEA is superior to those who are managed nonoperatively.[13,15] Clearly, if siphon lesions produce symptoms due to flow reduction, relief of proximal obstructing disease should reduce the likelihood of cerebral hypoperfusion.

CONTRALATERAL CAROTID OCCLUSION

Anatomic Considerations

The safety of CEA performed contralateral to a complete ICA occlusion is another issue that has stimulated considerable debate in the past. Patients who present with this anatomic configuration are not unusual, and may be increasingly seen in the future, at least in part as a result of the somewhat conservative approach towards carotid disease taken by some within the medical community in the recent past. For example, in a prospective study of 73 patients with greater than 80% asymptomatic ICA stenoses followed conservatively, 29% progressed to complete occlusion within 2 years.[27] Perler et al reported that progression to total occlusion had occurred in 28 (64%) of 44 patients with symptomatic carotid disease who had been treated with antiplatelet medications.[28] In many cases, the initial symptoms had resolved and the occlusion was only noted when the patient underwent angiography to evaluate new symptomatology in the contralateral hemisphere.[28] Therefore, it is not unreasonable to speculate that either as a result of the development of new symptomatology, or as more patients are referred for evaluation in light of the recently completed randomized clinical trials, an increasing number of patients will be identified with occlusion of at least one ICA.

Natural History

Just as in patients who present with tandem lesions, the long-term prognosis of patients who have a complete occlusion of at least one ICA is not good. In the Joint Study of Extracranial Occlusive Disease, 32 (33%) of 98 patients who presented with a complete ICA occlusion contralateral to an ICA stenosis and who were managed nonoperatively experienced a stroke during a mean follow-up of just over 4 years. Furthermore, approximately 50% of these strokes were fatal.[29] Other series have documented an incidence of stroke ranging from 7 to 29%, with a mean follow-up ranging from just 16 to 56 months.[30–39]

Carotid Endarterectomy

While the prognosis of patients managed medically has been relatively unfavorable, the results of previous surgical interventions, including thromboendarterectomy of the occluded vessel[40–42] and extracranial–intracranial bypass,[30,43] have been equally disappointing. Therefore, endarterectomy of the stenotic ICA contralateral to the occlusion has evolved as the most appropriate intervention in the majority of these patients. Nevertheless, the results of CEA performed contralateral to an ICA occlusion have been somewhat mixed and continue to stimulate controversy with respect to the overall safety of this approach (Table 18-2).[44–53] A careful analysis of this data should resolve much of this controversy, however. Specifically, while there have been some reports documenting a relatively high rate of perioperative stroke, these studies typically involved a small number of patients and appeared prior to 1980. It is axiomatic that the safety of this procedure in general has improved over the years because of refinements in technical detail, improved methods of cerebral monitoring and protection intraoperatively, and better perioperative anesthetic and medical management of the patient. In fact, over the past decade the reported results of CEA performed contralateral to an ICA occlusion have clearly confirmed the safety and efficacy of this intervention (see Table 18-2). The author's series is representative of this experience.

TABLE 18-2. *CEA/Contralateral occlusion: Results*

Source (yr)	Patients	Strokes	Deaths
	Pre 1980		
Vancouver General (1974)	31	4 (13%)	2 (6%)
Walter Reed (1977)	28	3 (11%)	0 (0%)
Loyola University (1977)	34	3 (9%)	1 (3%)
Boston VA (1979)	37	0 (0%)	1 (3%)
TOTALS	130	10 (7.7%)	4 (3.0%)
	Post 1980		
Southern Illinois University (1984)	53	2 (4%)	1 (2%)
Emory University (1984)	54	3 (6%)	0 (0%)
St. Antonius Hospital (1984)	33	0 (0%)	1 (3%)
New York University (1987)	145	9 (6%)	3 (2%)
New England Medical Center (1991)	63	3 (5%)	0 (0%)
Johns Hopkins (1992)	36	1(3%)	0 (0%)
TOTALS	384	18 (4.7%)	5 (1.6%)

The Johns Hopkins Experience

The results of 205 consecutive CEAs were divided into two groups: Group I included 36 cases performed contralateral to an ICA occlusion and Group II included 169 operations performed contralateral to a patent ICA. There were no significant differences in the mean age (67 versus 66); proportion of males (66 versus 69%); or prevalence of hypertension (56 versus 53%), diabetes mellitus (17 versus 20%), or hyperlipidemia (8 versus 14%) between the two groups. Since carotid artery disease is known to be an excellent marker for coronary artery disease, it was not surprising to find a greater prevalence of coronary disease among the Group I patients who had more severe carotid disease. Specifically, Group I patients had a greater prevalence of exertional angina (56 versus 30%, $p < 0.01$) and previous myocardial infarction (25 versus 12%, $p < 0.05$) than Group II patients. The indications for operation included symptomatic disease in 78% of the patients in each group, respectively. The specific indications included previous stroke (19 versus 22%), TIAs (36 versus 36%), amaurosis fugax (17 versus 12%), nonhemispheric symptoms (6 versus 8%), and asymptomatic stenoses (22 versus 22%). All operations were performed under general anesthesia, and shunts were used in 89% of Group I and 50% of Group II patients.

Perioperative strokes occurred in 1 (2.8%) patient with a contralateral ICA occlusion. However, there were 7 (4.1%) strokes among the 169 patients in whom the contralateral ICA was patent. This difference was not significant. All of the strokes occurred in patients with prior hemispheric symptoms, including 4 (5%) of 73 patients who presented with hemispheric TIAs, and 4 (11%) of 44 patients with a prior stroke. The one stroke in Group I occurred in a shunted patient, but no strokes occurred among 4 Group I patients in whom shunts had not been used. Operative mortality occurred follow 2 (1%) of the 205 procedures, including none of the Group I and 2 (1%)

of the Group II cases. Major cardiac complications occurred in 2 (5.6%) Group I and 9 (5.3%) Group II patients. This difference was not statistically significant.

Perspective

The author's experience is consistent with several other recent studies (see Table 18-2) and confirms that CEA may be performed on patients with a contralateral ICA occlusion with acceptable safety. In fact, unlike the patient population presenting with intracranial tandem disease, the risk does not appear to be greater than among patients without a contralateral ICA occlusion. This data in fact suggests that operative results are far more dependent on symptomatic indications and the technical details of operation than the status of the contralateral carotid circulation. Since intraoperative cerebral ischemia is felt to be the predominant risk factor in this patient population, shunts were used liberally in the Hopkins series. Yet the one patient with a contralateral ICA occlusion who sustained a perioperative stroke had been shunted, while no strokes occurred among 4 patients with ICA occlusions who had not been shunted. It is difficult from a review of previous experience to comment definitely on the role and impact of shunting in this clinical setting, because heterogeneous patient populations are presented and the use of shunts has varied from series to series (see Table 18-2). Nevertheless, it should be noted that the stroke rate was greater in shunted patients with a contralateral ICA occlusion in at least two other large recent series.[51,52] Finally, contralateral ICA occlusion (like tandem disease) is an excellent marker for underlying coronary artery disease. Nevertheless, the author's series, like most other reports over the last two decades, clearly demonstrate that this patient population may undergo CEA with minimal risk of operative mortality (see Table 18-2).

Finally, one must also examine the risk of CEA in this patient population within the context of the natural history of the disease without surgical intervention. The evidence available to date strongly suggests that not only may CEA be performed on patients with a contralateral ICA occlusion safely but, in fact, it substantially improves the long-term prognosis of this patient population. Moore et al reported that only 5 (10%) of 50 patients who underwent CEA contralateral to an ICA occlusion suffered a stroke with an average follow-up of 51 months, and 4 of these strokes occurred contralateral to the side of endarterectomy.[48] In another series including 145 patients who underwent CEA contralateral to an ICA occlusion, stroke-free survival was 88% at 5 years.[51] Mackey et al also reported stroke-free survival rates of 91% at five-year follow-up and 76% at 10-year follow-up in a cohort of 63 patients.[52]

CAROTID STRING SIGN

Anatomic Considerations

The term "string sign" was first used by Ehrenfeld and Wylie nearly 20 years ago to describe the angiographic appearance of an ICA dissection.[54] Extreme narrowing of the entire extracranial internal carotid artery diameter has also been coined the slim

TABLE 18-3. *Carotid String Sign: Etiologies*

Dissection
Radiation arteritis
Congenital hypoplasia
Fibromuscular dysplasia
Subintimal contrast injection
Critical atherosclerotic stenosis

sign,[55] hypoplasia,[55,56] and pseudoocclusion.[57] In fact, a variety of pathologic entities may produce this angiographic appearance (Table 18-3). For the practicing vascular surgeon, however, a critical proximal atherosclerotic stenosis is the most frequently encountered etiology and therefore will be the subject of this discussion. In this situation, partial collapse of the internal carotid lumen occurs distal to the stenosis due to low perfusion pressure. In addition, layering of dense contrast material along the dependent artery wall during angiography may exaggerate the apparent narrowing of the vessel.[57–58]

Diagnosis

Establishing the correct diagnosis in the patient with poor visualization of the cervical ICA is crucial to judging operability. There is general agreement that Duplex scanning is fairly inaccurate in this regard. In three recent reports, for example, angiographically proven string signs were incorrectly predicted to be total occlusions in 25 to 30% of cases by Duplex evaluation.[59–61] ICA flow velocity in some of these cases may be too low to be picked up by this noninvasive technology. Since MRA also requires a minimum flow velocity of 5–10 cm/sec, it is unlikely to be more sensitive than Duplex scanning in this setting.[62] Contrast-enhanced CT scanning may be able to establish the patency of the artery, although it will not provide the information available from a comprehensive arteriogram.

If an arteriogram demonstrates a continuous smooth wisp of dye progressing antegrade into the skull, the diagnosis is most likely a string sign so that CEA is both technically feasible and likely to be successful. The difficulty arises when a continuous stream of dye is not visualized into the skull. It has been suggested that a tapered "stump" of ICA is more suggestive of the string sign, whereas a more abrupt, blunt, stump suggests a true occlusion.[57] In addition, angiographic visualization of the intracranial ICA through collaterals other than the ophthalmic artery is consistent with a string sign.[56,57] At least 10% of ICA occlusions diagnosed angiographically have been noted on later review to be consistent with the string sign.[63] On the other hand, an ascending pharyngeal or other external carotid artery branch may be misinterpreted as an ICA string sign in the patient with a chronically occluded and inoperable ICA. Finally, the true string sign denotes a vessel that is relatively undiseased, albeit quite small, beyond the offending atherosclerotic plaque. In some cases, however, the vessel may be extremely fibrotic and diseased along its entire cervical extent so that endarterectomy is not likely to be satisfactorily completed or successful. While in some cases one may be able to identify this disease presentation on the preoperative arteriogram, typically it can be confirmed only by direct operative exploration. In these cases, proximal ICA ligation may be the most appropriate treatment. In fact, attempted CEA of the diffusely fibrotic vessel may be one explanation for poor results associated with CEA in some patients with a string sign.

Incidence

While the carotid string sign occurs relatively infrequently, it will be encountered from time to time in the practice of most busy vascular surgeons. In one of the earliest studies, the carotid string sign was noted in 13 (3.6%) of 356 patients who underwent arteriography at the Mayo Clinic.[55] These findings were confirmed in a more recent study in which a string sign was noted in 34 (3%) of 1,092 patients undergoing carotid arteriography.[64] Furthermore, 33 (97%) of these patients were symptomatic.[64] Conversely, Ringelstein et al identified a string sign in only 9 (0.6%) of 1,458 patients undergoing Duplex evaluation, which may in part reflect the relative insensitivity of this technology in identifying this low flow phenomenon.[63] Eight (88%) of these patients were symptomatic.[63] In fact, the majority of patients in whom a string sign is identified are symptomatic.[59,61,63,64]

Natural History

Although the long-term prognosis for patients with the carotid string sign is not well-defined, the preponderance of evidence available to date suggests that this angiographic phenomenon represents one point in the evolution from arteriosclerotic stenosis to total occlusion of the ICA (*i.e.,* from operable to inoperable). The severely fibrotic and atrophied vessel that one may encounter at exploration in some cases probably reflects the final preocclusive stage. Although the risk of progression to complete occlusion has not been precisely quantified, when one considers the prognosis of the patient population with a complete ICA occlusion it is difficult to argue against an aggressive surgical approach to the patient with a string sign. In addition to preserving the integrity of the vessel, there is substantial evidence that the patient with a carotid string sign is at increased risk of subsequent cerebral infarction.[29,39,65] The possible mechanisms for stroke in these patients include terminal thrombosis of the ICA with intracerebral propagation, emboli arising from the evolving occlusion, or "stump" emboli transmitted via external carotid collaterals.[64,66–70] On the other hand, since these vessels provide so little cerebral perfusion, infarction due to hypoperfusion is felt to occur relatively infrequently.[64]

Carotid Endarterectomy

Defining the risk of CEA in the patient with a string sign requires an examination of three issues, including the risk of angiography, the risk of perioperative neurologic morbidity, and the likelihood of the vessel remaining patent during long-term follow-up. Optimal angiographic evaluation requires the selective injection of high-dose contrast material and prolonged filming.[64] However, the injection of a large volume of the contrast agent under high pressure may predispose to neurologic complications in some patients with a string sign if there is relatively fresh thrombus within the ICA lumen. In one recent series, for example, 5 (15%) of 34 patients with the string sign developed neurologic complications following angiography, including 3 TIAs and 2 strokes.[64] The use of IA/DSA digital should minimize this risk.

As noted in Table 18-4, while reported clinical experience is largely anecdotal, it is clear that CEA can be performed with a very acceptable rate of operative neurologic morbidity and death.[58,59,62–64,71–73] The keys to minimizing operative risk and maximizing the likelihood of long-term vessel patency include careful scrutiny of the preoperative arteriogram, critical examination of the ICA at operation, as well as assessment of ICA flow immediately after closing the arteriotomy. For example, several workers have noted that failure to visualize the ipsilateral intracerebral circulation is an especially poor prognostic sign.[74,75] The angiogram may also demonstrate a very irregular ICA wall (Fig. 18-1). Typically in these cases one will find an exceptionally small ICA, usually due to extensive fibrotic atrophy rather than hypoperfusion, at operation. In my experience, and that of others, a satisfactory endarterectomy is usually not feasible or likely to result in a patent vessel, so that proximal ligation should be performed.[61,62] In fact, Archie has described six anatomic patterns, including combinations of proximal atherosclerotic disease, diffuse fibrotic disease, and intraluminal thrombus, that one may encounter at operation in the patient with the preoperative diagnosis of the carotid string sign.[62] In my view, however, the crucial issue is whether one is dealing primarily with proximal atherosclerotic plaque and a fairly normal, albeit extremely small, more distal cervical ICA, or a diffusely fibrotic, and most likely preocclusive, vessel. In the latter situation, if endarterectomy is begun but cannot be ended satisfactorily, it is preferable to simply ligate the vessel at operation rather than risk acute postoperative thrombosis with intracerebral clot propagation. On the other hand, the finding of a fresh thrombus within the vessel should not preclude attempting endarterectomy, if technically feasible.[62]

TABLE 18-4. *CEA/String sign: Results*

	Patients	Strokes	Deaths
UMDNJ (1979)	5	0 (0%)	0 (0%)
Stanford (1980)	6	0 (0%)	0 (0%)
University of Pittsburgh (1980)	3	0 (0%)	0 (0%)
University of Michigan (1980)	5	0 (0%)	0 (0%)
Rheinisch-Westfalische (1983)	7	0 (0%)	1 (14%)
NE Deaconess (1989)	25	2 (8%)	1 (4%)
Bowman Gray (1989)	26	1 (4%)	1 (4%)
Wake Medical Center (1994)	16	1 (6.2%)	1 (6.2%)
Totals	93	4 (4.3%)	4(4.3%)

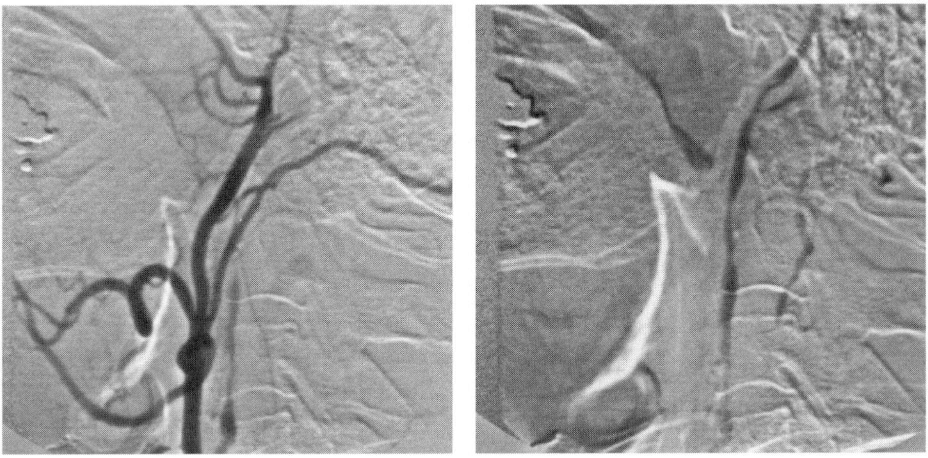

a b

FIG. 18-1. (a) Intraarterial DSA in a patient with a carotid string sign. Note poor visualization of the distal cervical internal carotid artery; (b) Delayed imaging demonstrates opacification of very irregular internal carotid artery lumen.

Finally, it is important to note that a successful clinical outcome in these cases initially does not necessarily correlate with long-term vessel patency. O'Leary et al performed noninvasive testing on 23 patients with a string sign who underwent successful CEA, and the operated ICA was occluded in 4 (17%), with a mean follow-up of 30 months. All of these patients had remained asymptomatic, however.[64] In another study, 5 (31%) of 16 operated vessels were noted to be occluded by Duplex evaluation, with a mean follow-up of 27 months, although none of these patients had developed new symptoms.[62] Poor ICA flow immediately after completion of the endarterectomy portends an increased risk of early postoperative occlusion, so the surgeon should assess ICA flow by Doppler prior to leaving the operating room. In some cases, poor flow reflects extensive distal disease, which may be an indication for ligation, as noted above. On the other hand, a relatively undiseased ICA may not dilate to normal size immediately after endarterectomy of the proximal obstructing plaque. In this situation, the author has found gentle passage of a Fogarty catheter may dilate the distal vessel, as reported by others.[71] Finally, while the appropriate role of patching continues to be studied, it would seem that the patient who undergoes endarterectomy for a string sign is an ideal candidate for patch angioplasty repair.

CONCLUSIONS

Among the patient population affected with atherosclerotic disease at the carotid bifurcation of sufficient severity to warrant surgical intervention, only a small minority will present with the anatomic problems described in this chapter. Tandem lesions, contralateral carotid occlusion, and the string sign have each been considered, at least previously, to substantially increase the risk of neurologic complications of CEA. However, with proper patient selection and attention to technical detail, none of these problems represents prohibitive risks to the safe performance of the operation. Furthermore, those risks must be viewed against the natural history of the underlying disease in these patients. Within that context, in each case carotid bifurcation endarterectomy still offers the optimal prognosis for these patients. Furthermore, although the patient population with tandem lesions or contralateral occlusion has a greater prevalence of significant coronary artery disease, there is no evidence that the risk of cardiac complications is greater than that among patients undergoing CEA in the absence of these associated lesions.

REFERENCES

1. Pokras R, Dykon ML. Dramatic changes in the performance of endarterectomy for disease of the extracranial arteries of the head. Stroke 1988;19:1289–1290
2. Warlow C. Carotid endarterectomy: does it work? Stroke 1984;15:1068–1076
3. Dykon ML. Carotid endarterectomy studies: a glimmering of science. Stroke 1986;17:355–357
4. Winslow CM, Dolomen DH, Chassin MR, Kosecoff J, Merrick NJ, Brook RH. The appropriateness of carotid endarterectomy. N Engl J Med 1988;318:721–727
5. North American Symptomatic Carotid Endarterectomy Trial (NASCET). Beneficial effect of carotid endarterectomy in symptomatic patients with high-grade carotid stenosis. N Engl J Med 1991;325: 445–453
6. European Carotid Surgery Trialists Collaborative Group. MRC European Carotid Surgery Trial: interim results for symptomatic patients with severe (70–99%) or with mild (10–29%) carotid stenosis. Lancet 1991;337:1235–1243
7. Hobson RW II, Weiss DG, Fields WS, et al. Efficacy of carotid endarterectomy for asymptomatic carotid stenosis. N Engl J Med 1993;328:221–227
8. Clinical Advisory: Carotid endarterectomy for patients with asymptomatic internal carotid artery stenosis. September, 1994
9. Roederer GO, Langlois YE, Chan ARW, Chikos PM, Thiele BL, Strandness DE, Jr. Is siphon disease important in predicting outcome of carotid endarterectomy? Arch Surg 1983;118:1177–1181
10. Gibo H, Lenkey C, Rhotan A. Microsurgical anatomy of the supraclinoid portion of the internal carotid artery. J Neurosurg 1981;55:560–574
11. Lord RSA. Relevance of siphon stenosis and intracranial aneurysm to results of carotid endarterectomy. In: Ernst CB, Stanley JC (eds.). Current therapy in vascular surgery (2nd ed). Philadelphia: B.C. Decker, 1991:94–100
12. Saunders FW, Shedden P. The carotid siphon: a scanning electron microscope assessment of its embolic potential. Can J Neurol Sci 1985;12:263–266
13. Lord RSA, Raj TB, Graham AR. Carotid endarterectomy, siphon stenosis, collateral hemispheric pressure, and perioperative cerebral infarction. J Vasc Surg 1987;6:391–397
14. Batjer H, Mickey B, Samson D. Potential roles for early neurorevascularization in patients with acute cerebral ischemia. Neurosurgery 1986;18:283–291
15. Schuler JJ, Flanigan DP, Lim LT, Keifer T, Williams LR, Behrend AJ. The effect of carotid siphon stenosis on stroke rate, death and relief of symptoms following elective carotid endarterectomy. Surgery 1982;92:1058–1067
16. Barnett HJM, Gent M, Sackett DL, et al. A randomized trial of aspirin and sulfinpyrazone in threatened stroke. N Engl J Med 1978;299:53–59
17. Borozan PG, Schuler JJ, LaRosa MP, Ware MS, Flanigan DP. The natural history of isolated carotid siphon stenosis. J Vasc Surg 1984;1:744–749
18. Fisher CM, Gore I, Okabe N, White PD. Atherosclerosis of the carotid and vertebral arteries-extracranial and intracranial. J Neuropath Exp Neurol 1965;24:455–476
19. Marzewski DJ, Furlan AJ, St Louis P, Little JR, Modic MT. Intracranial internal carotid artery stenosis: long-term prognosis. Stroke 1982;13:821–824
20. Thiele BL, Young JV, Chikos PM, Hirsch DE, Strandness DE, Jr. Correlation of arteriographic findings and symptoms in cerebrovascular disease. Neurology 1980;30:1041–1046

21. Craig DR, Meguro K, Watridge C, Robertson JT, Barnett JM, Fox AJ. Intracranial internal carotid artery stenosis. Stroke 1982;13:825–823
22. Bauer RB, Meyer JS, Fields WS, et al. Joint study of extracranial arterial occlusion. Part III. Progress of controlled study of long-term survival in patients with and without operation. JAMA 1969;208: 509–518
23. Day AL, Rhoton AL, Quisling RG. Resolving siphon stenosis following endarterectomy. Stroke 1980;11:278–281
24. Hugenholz H, Elgie RG. Carotid thromboendarterectomy: a reappraisal: criteria for patient selection. J Neurosurg 1959;16:705–730
25. Sundt TM, Sandok BA, Whisnant JP. Carotid endarterectomy: complications and preoperative assessment of risk. Mayo Clin Proc 1975;50:301–306
26. Rosenthal D, Rudderman RH, Jones DH, et al. Carotid endarterectomy in the octogenarian: is it appropriate? J Vasc Surg 1986;3:782–787
27. Monetta GL, Taylor DC, Nicholls SC, et al. Operative versus nonoperative management of asymptomatic high grade internal carotid artery stenosis: improved results with endarterectomy. Stroke 1987;18:1005–1010
28. Perler BA, Burdick JF, Williams GM. Progression to total occlusion is an under-recognized complication of the medical management of carotid disease. J Vasc Surg 1991;14:821–828
29. Fields WS, Lamak N. Joint study of extracranial arterial occlusion X: internal carotid artery occlusion. JAMA 1976;235:2734–2738
30. Barnett HJM. EC-IC Bypass Study Group. Failure of extracranial–intracranial arterial bypass to reduce the risk of ischemic stroke. N Engl J Med 1985;313:1191–1200
31. Cote R, Barnett HJM, Taylor DW. Internal carotid occlusion: a prospective study. Stroke 1983;14: 898–902
32. Nicholls SC, Kohler TR, Bergelin RO, Primozich JF, Lawrence RC, Strandness DE, Jr. Carotid artery occlusion: natural history. J Vasc Surg 1986;4:479–485
33. Burns J, Satiani B, Vasko JS. Long-term survival following total carotid artery occlusion. Cardiovasc Rev Rep 1984;5:903–911
34. Furlan AJ, Wisnant JF, Baker HL. Long-term prognosis after carotid artery occlusion. Neurology 1980;30:986–988
35. Sacquegna T, DeCarolis P, Pazzaglia P, et al. The clinical course and prognosis of carotid artery occlusion. J Neurol Neurosurg Psychiatry 1982;45:1037–1039
36. Persson AV, Griffey EE, Jaxheimer EC, Jewel ER. The natural history of total occlusion of the internal carotid artery. Vasc Diagn 1984;5(3):15–21
37. Norrving B, Nilsson B. Carotid artery occlusion: acute symptomatic and long-term prognosis. Neurol Res 1981;3:229–236
38. Dyken ML, Klatte E, Oldrich JK, Spurgeon C. Complete occlusion of common or internal carotid arteries. Arch Neurol 1974;30:343–346
39. Grillo P, Patterson RH. Occlusion of the carotid artery: prognosis (natural history) and the possibilities of surgical revascularization. Stroke 1975;6:17–20
40. Erickson DL, Long DM, Seljeskog EL, Chou SN, French LA. Carotid endarterectomy for stroke. Minn Med 1970;53:607–610
41. Heyman A, Young WG Jr, Brown IW, Jr. Long-term results of endarterectomy of the internal carotid artery for cerebral ischemia and infarctions. Circulation 1967;36:212–221
42. Toole JF, Janeway R, Choi K, et al. Transient ischemic attacks due to atherosclerosis: a prospective study of 160 patients. Arch Neurol 1975;32:5–12
43. Whisnant JP, Sundt WG Jr, Brown IW, Jr. Long-term mortality and stroke morbidity after superficial temporal artery-middle cerebral artery bypass operation. Mayo Clin Proc 1985;60:241–246
44. Chung WB. Long-term results of carotid artery surgery for cerebrovascular insufficiency. Am J Surg 1974;128:262–268
45. Anderson CA, Rich NM, Collins GJ, McDaniel PT, Boone SC. Unilateral internal carotid occlusion: special considerations. Stroke 1977;8:669–671
46. Baker WH, Dorner DB, Barnes RW. Carotid endarterectomy: is an indwelling shunt necessary? Surgery 1977;82:321–326
47. Phillips MR, Johnson WC, Scott RM, Vollman RW, Levine H, Nasbeth DC. Carotid endarterectomy in the presence of contralateral carotid occlusion: the role of EEG and intraluminal shunting. Arch Surg 1979;114:1232–1239
48. Moore DJ, Modi JR, Finch WT, Sumner DS. Influence of the contralateral carotid artery on neurologic complications following carotid endarterectomy. J Vasc Surg 1984;1:409–414

49. Sachs SM, Fulenwider JT, Smith RB III, Darden WA, Salam AA, Perdue GD. Does internal carotid occlusion influence neurologic fate of carotid endarterectomy? Surgery 1984;96:839–844
50. Hammacher ER, Eikelboom BC, Bast TJ, DeGeest R, Vermeulen FEE. Surgical treatment of patients with a carotid artery occlusion and a contralateral stenosis. J Cardiovasc Surg 1984;25:513–517
51. Friedman SG, Riles TS, Lamparello PJ, Imparato AM, Sukwa MP. Surgical therapy for the patient with internal carotid artery occlusion and contralateral stenosis. J Vasc Surg 1987;5:856–861
52. MacKey WC, O'Donnell TF Jr, Callow AD. Carotid endarterectomy contralateral to an occluded carotid artery: perioperative risk and late results. J Vasc Surg 1991;11:778–785
53. Perler BA, Burdick JF, Williams GM. Does contralateral carotid artery occlusion increase the risk of carotid endarterectomy? A ten year experience. J Vasc Surg 1992;16:347–353
54. Ehrenfeld WK, Wylie ES. Spontaneous dissection of the internal carotid artery. Arch Surg 1976;111: 1294–1301
55. Houser OW, Sundt TM, Holman CB, Sandok BA, Burton RC. Atheromatous disease of the carotid artery. J Neurosurg 1974;41:321–331
56. Lippman HH, Sundt TM, Holman CB. The poststenotic carotid string sign: spurious internal carotid hypoplasia. Mayo Clin Proc 1970;45:762–767
57. Ammar AD, Turrentine MW, Fatha SJ. The importance of arteriographic interpretation in occlusion or pseudo-occlusion of the carotid artery. Surg Gynecol Obstet 1988;167:119–123
58. Sekhar LN, Heros RC, Lotz PR, Rosenbaum AE. Atheromatous pseudo-occlusion of the internal carotid artery. J Neurosurg 1980;52:782–789
59. Fredericks RK, Thomas TD, Lefkowitz DS, Troost BT. Implications of the angiographic string sign in carotid atherosclerosis. Stroke 1990;21:476–479
60. O'Leary DH, Gibbons GW, Pinel DF. Limitations of noninvasive testing in assessing the "occluded" carotid artery. Am J Neuroradiol 1983;4:159–163
61. Curl GR, Ricotta JJ. The carotid string sign: differential diagnosis and management. In: Veith FJ (ed). Current critical problems in vascular surgery (vol 6) St. Louis: Quality Medical Publishing, 1994:269–279
62. Archie JP, Jr. Carotid endarterectomy when the distal internal carotid artery is small or poorly visualized. J Vasc Surg 1994;19:23–31
63. Ringelstein EB, Berg-Dammer E, Zeumer H. The so-called atheromatous pseudoocclusion of the internal carotid artery: a diagnostic and therapeutic challenge. Neuroradiology 1983;25:147–155
64. O'Leary DH, Mattle H, Potter JE. Atheromatous pseudo-occlusion of the internal carotid artery. Stroke 1989;20:1168–1173
65. Rushton FW, Kukora JS. Surgical management of the occluded carotid artery. Surgery 1984;96: 845–853
66. Einsiedel-Lechtape H. Secondary emboli: a fragment sequela of complete extracranial internal carotid occlusion. Neuroradiology 1978;16:96–100
67. Barnett HJM, Peerless SJ, Kaufman JCE. "Stump" of internal carotid artery: a source of further cerebral embolic ischemia. Stroke 1978;9:448–456
68. Ringelstein EB, Zeumer H, Angelou D. The pathogenesis of strokes from internal carotid artery occlusion: diagnostic and therapeutic implications. Stroke 1983;14:867–875
69. Finkelstein S, Kleinman GM, Cuneo R, Baruger R. Delayed stroke following carotid occlusion. Neurology 1980;30:84–88
70. Bogousslavsky J, Regli F, Hungerbubler JP, Chrzanowski R. Transient ischemic attacks and external carotid artery. Stroke 1978;12:629–630
71. Countee RW, Vijayanathan T. Reconstitution of "totally" occluded internal carotid arteries: angiographic and technical considerations. J Neurosurg 1979;50:747–752
72. Mehigan JT, Olcott C IV. The carotid "string" sign: differential diagnosis and management. Am J Surg 1980;140:137–143
73. Gabrielsen TO, Seeger JF, Knake JF, Burke DP, Stilwill EW. The nearly occluded internal carotid artery: a diagnostic trap. Neuroradiology 1981;138:611–618
74. Shucart WA, Garrido E. Reopening some occluded carotid arteries. J Neurosurg 1976;45:442–446
75. Kish GF, Adkins PC, Slovin AJ. The totally occluded internal carotid artery: indications for surgery. Am J Surg 1977;134:288–292

Management of Extracranial Cerebrovascular Disease, edited by Keith D. Calligaro et al.
Lippincott-Raven Publishers, Philadelphia © 1997.

19

Carotid Body Tumors: Diagnosis and Management

Christopher J. Kwolek, David C. Brewster

NATURAL HISTORY

Carotid body tumors (CBT) are uncommon neoplasms and are the only pathologic process known to involve the carotid body.[1] The carotid body is a 3–4 mm structure arising within the adventitial layer on the posterior aspect of the carotid bifurcation. Its blood supply arises primarily from the external carotid artery but branches from the superior thyroid, occipital, subclavian, vertebral, and thyrocervical arteries may also play an important role when planning operative resection.[2] These highly vascular structures function to regulate heart rate, blood pressure, and respiration in response to alterations in the chemical composition of the bloodstream. The carotid body receptors respond to decreased O_2, increased CO_2, increased acidity, and increased temperature by increasing sympathetic activity, leading to an increase in heart rate, blood pressure, respiratory function, and increased cortical activity in the brain.[3] Such tumors are sometimes referred to as chemodectomas, or, more accurately, carotid paragangliomas. Patients with CBT can also present with multiple paragangliomas at other sites such as the jugular bulb, aortic arch, vagus nerve, the abdominal aorta, and in the retroperitoneum. In addition, an increased incidence of CBT has been noted in patients with relative hypoxia (*i.e.,* individuals with cyanotic heart disease or those living at high altitudes).[1]

CBT are slow growing neoplasms. Nonetheless, relentless enlargement is to be expected, eventually leading to encasement of the carotid vessels and adjacent cranial nerves. Thus, elective resection of even small tumors is recommended when the diagnosis is first made. Although most CBTs are benign, the criteria for malignancy are controversial and the reported rates of malignant characteristics range from 6 to 30%. While true metastases are only present in 5–10% of patients, the possibility of malignant change is an additional factor favoring early surgical resection.[4]

While most tumors are unilateral (95%), bilateral tumors do occur and their incidence approaches 30% in patients with a family history of CBT.[5,6] These tumors appear to be inherited in an autosomal dominant fashion in the familial form. Despite their origin from neural crest cells, these tumors are rarely functional (*i.e.,* secrete catecholamines). However, preoperative catecholamine screening is advisable in patients with possible symptoms of catecholamine excess such as significant hypertension, headaches, palpitations and diaphoresis. This is particularly true in patients with bilateral tumors or a family history. These patients will tend to have paragangliomas at other sites as well.[1]

DIAGNOSIS

Most CBTs present as a painless, asymptomatic neck mass in the region of the carotid bifurcation, just below the angle of the mandible. Symptoms may develop due to pressure on the adjacent cranial nerves or local structures, leading to neck or ear pain, dysphagia, hoarseness, tinnitus, or dizziness. Approximately 10% of patients will present with cranial nerve deficits; thus, a thorough preoperative neurologic examination, including indirect laryngoscopy, should be part of the initial evaluation.

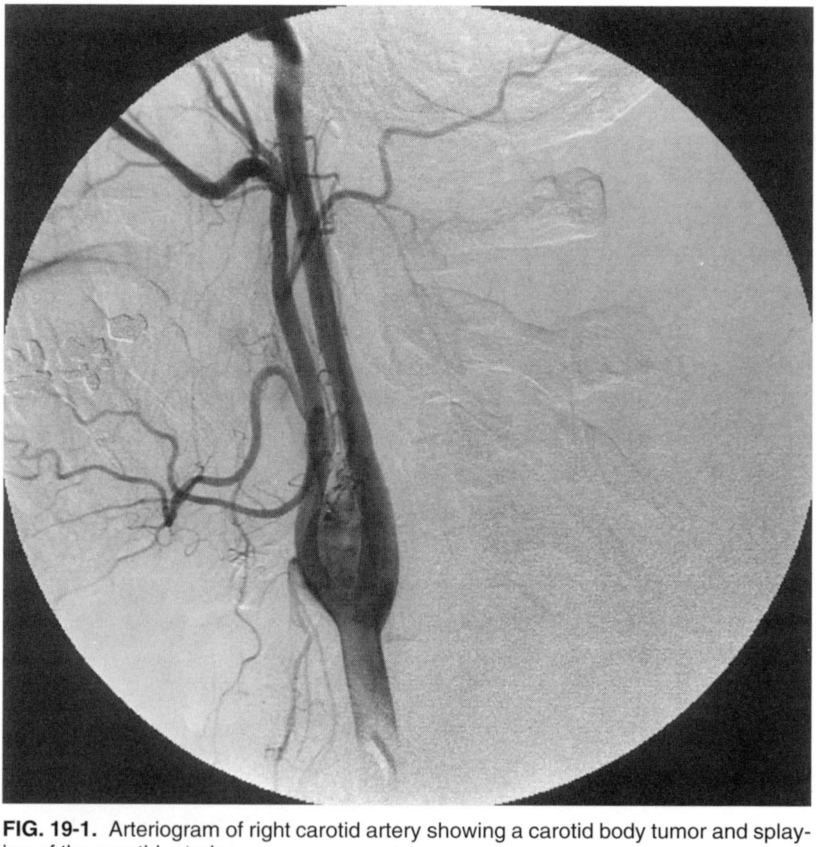

FIG. 19-1. Arteriogram of right carotid artery showing a carotid body tumor and splaying of the carotid arteries.

On physical examination, CBTs are usually felt to be pulsatile, owing to transmitted pulsations from the carotid vessels, but not expansile. This is in contrast to carotid aneurysms, which are both pulsatile and expansile. In addition, it is often said that patients with a CBT will have a non-tender mass that can be moved from side to side but not up and down. Approximately 25% of these patients will also have a carotid bruit.[1]

The differential diagnosis for CBT includes carotid aneurysm, metastatic tumors, benign enlargement of cervical lymph nodes from a variety of causes, salivary gland tumors, and branchiogenic cysts.

Arteriography remains the mainstay of definitive diagnosis, but Duplex scanning is often a useful initial step that can delineate a hypervascular mass in the carotid bifurcation and suggest the correct diagnosis. Characteristic arteriographic features are the splaying apart of the internal and external carotid arteries by a strikingly vascular mass with a rich blood supply arising from the external carotid artery (Fig. 19-1). Arteriography is also useful in planning surgical resection by delineating blood supply, showing coexistent atherosclerotic disease, and evaluating the adequacy of the collateral cerebral circulation.[7] Bilateral arteriography should be performed to rule out bilateral CBT and identify any additional cervical paraganglioma. CT or MRI scans can be useful to further delineate the upper extent of the mass (Fig. 19-2). Whether MRI offers any unique advantages over other imaging modalities is not clearly established at present. Needle and open biopsy should obviously be avoided owing to the potential hazard of bleeding complications.

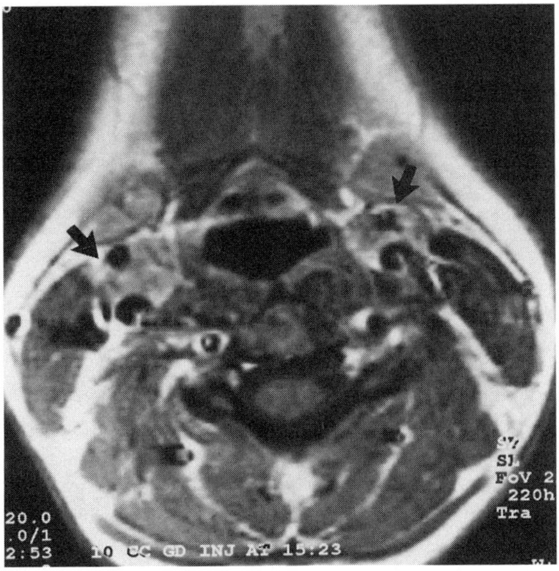

FIG. 19-2. Cervical MRI scan showing bilateral CBTs adjacent to the larynx.

SURGICAL TREATMENT

It is well recognized that resection of CBT is often difficult because of the tumor's extreme vascularity, the danger of arterial injury owing to the tumor's intimate adherence to the vessel wall, and the hazard of injury to regional cranial nerves (VII, IX, X, XI, XII), which are often in close proximity to or involved with large tumors. In addition, most surgeons have had limited experience with resection of CBT because of their relative rarity. Despite these challenges, innovations in operative techniques and recognition of certain general principles allow successful resection in almost all cases in contemporary practice.

The difficulty of surgical resection is usually related to tumor size and the gross relationship with the carotid vessels. Shamblin and associates[2] originally classified these tumors into three types based on this anatomic relationship. This was reemphasized recently in Hallett's large series of cases from the Mayo Clinic.[8] Type I tumors, accounting for approximately 25% of cases, are small localized neoplasms that are easily dissected with minimal involvement of the vessel wall. Type II tumors com-

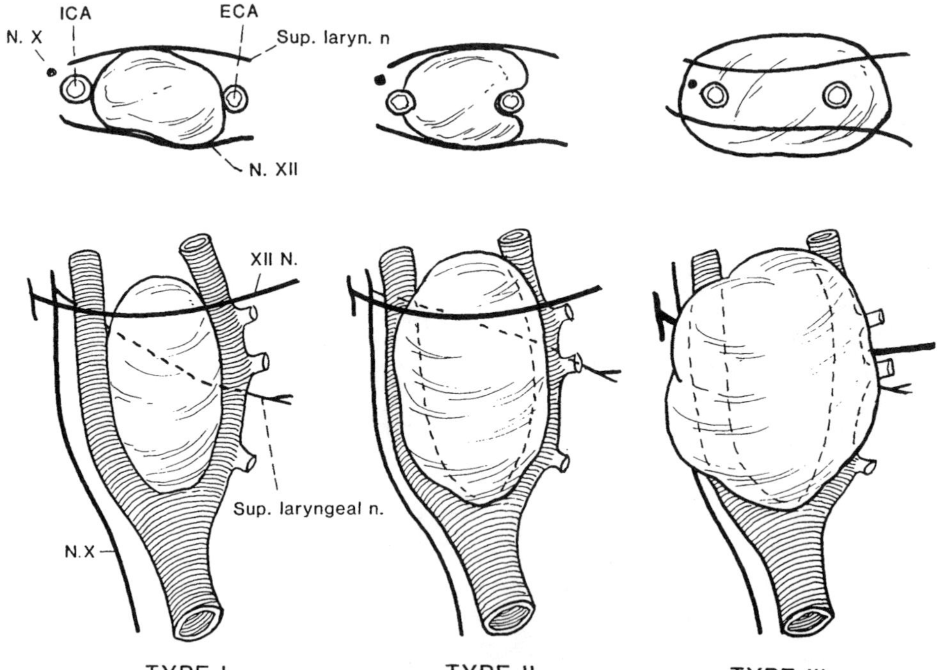

FIG. 19-3. Shamblin classification for carotid body tumors. Type I tumors are localized and easily resected. Type II tumors are adherent and partially surround the vessels. Type III tumors encase the vessels. (From Hallett JW et al. Trends in neurovascular complications of surgical management for carotid body and cervical paragangliomas: a fifty-year experience with 153 tumors. J Vasc Surg 1988;7:284–291)

prise approximately 50% of cases. These tumors are larger, more adherent, and partially surround the adventitia of the blood vessels, making removal more difficult. Type III CBT are large, often 4–5 cm in diameter, and are characterized by dense adherence to the vessel wall (Fig. 19-3). These tumors may completely encase carotid branches or the cranial nerves.[9] Such lesions may be extremely difficult to manage surgically. They account for approximately 25% of cases and are associated with most of the complications attributable to surgical treatment.

Several perioperative techniques have been found to be useful in the surgical management of CBT. Nasotracheal intubation for general anesthesia is often preferable, allowing greater upward displacement of the floor of the mouth and easier retraction and dissection beneath the mandible. For large tumors or those with known high extension, mandibular subluxation may also be helpful. A standard oblique incision along the anterior border of the sternocleidomastoid muscle is generally employed, although for large tumors a modified T-radical neck incision may provide better exposure (Fig. 19-4). Cranial nerve injury is best avoided by initial identification and gentle mobilization of major nerves off the surface of the tumor. Hallett described three zones of tumor dissection. Zone I includes the common carotid artery, the bifurcation, and the vagus nerve. Zone II involves the external carotid artery, the superior laryngeal nerve, the hypoglossal nerve, and the marginal mandibular branch of

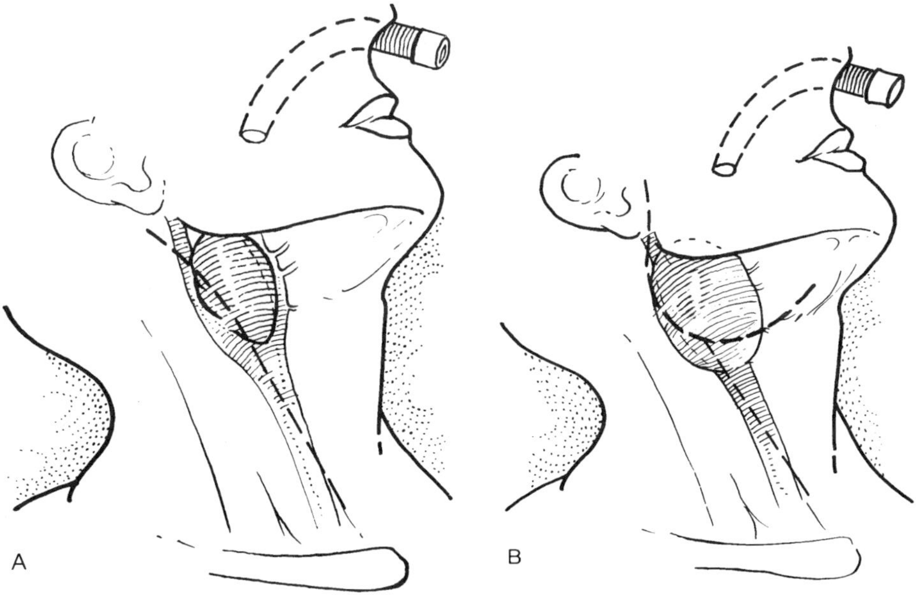

FIG. 19-4. Neck incisions for resection of carotid body tumors. Nasotracheal intubation allows greater displacement of the floor of the mouth. A. Incision for small tumor, Shamblin type I. B. Incision for larger tumors, Shamblin types II and III. (From Hallett JW et al. Trends in neurovascular complications of surgical management for carotid body and cervical paragangliomas: a fifty-year experience with 153 tumors. J Vasc Surg 1988;7:284–291)

the facial nerve. Zone III includes the internal carotid artery, the hypoglossal nerve, and the marginal mandibular branch of the facial nerve. Most serious neurovascular injuries occur when dissecting in Zone III. Standard steps in the dissection of a CBT are shown in Fig. 19-5.[9] In addition, bipolar cautery is very helpful in minimizing blood loss during dissection and reduces the chance of thermal or electrical injury to adjacent nerves.

For large tumors, brief carotid artery clamping following low-dose heparin administration may be useful to minimize bleeding during the course of operative dissection. A saphenous vein donor site should be prepared in case vessel injury occurs or the vessel is so encased that resection is required. In this case, a saphenous vein

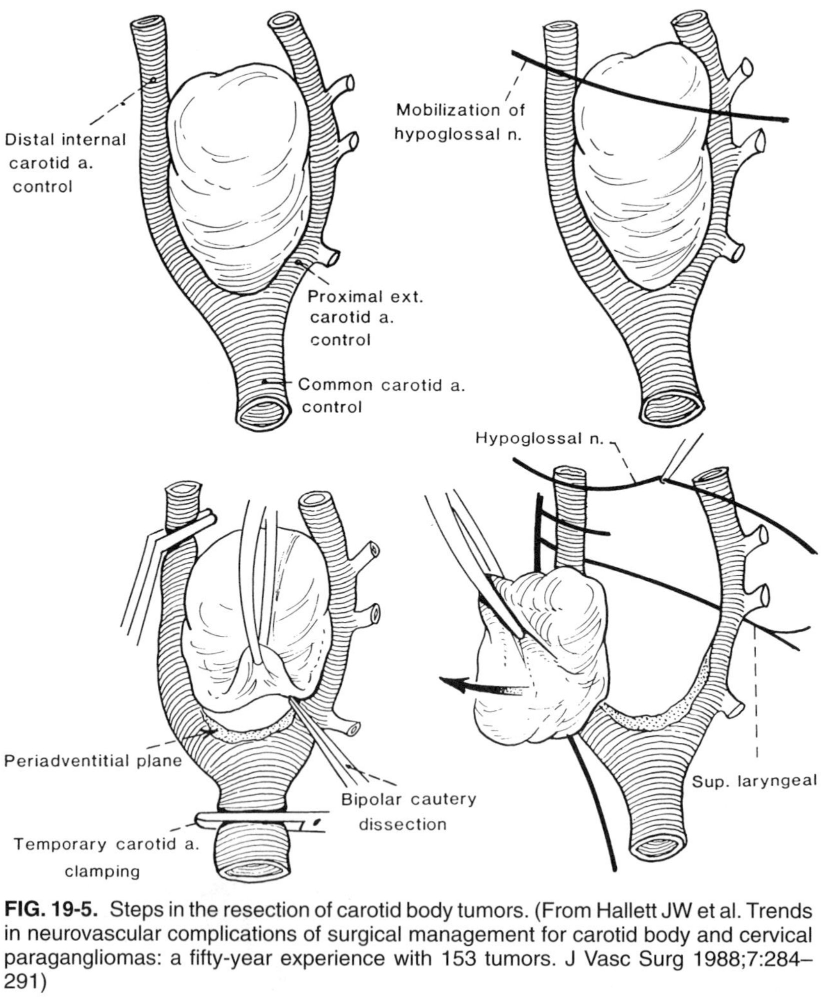

FIG. 19-5. Steps in the resection of carotid body tumors. (From Hallett JW et al. Trends in neurovascular complications of surgical management for carotid body and cervical paragangliomas: a fifty-year experience with 153 tumors. J Vasc Surg 1988;7:284–291)

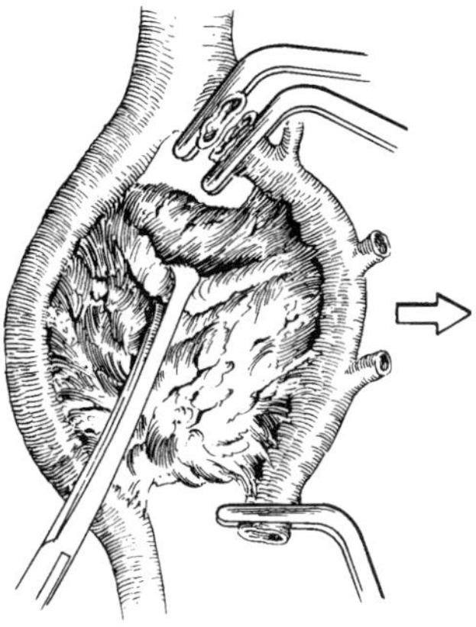

FIG. 19-6. Resection of the external carotid artery to reduce bleeding during removal of a CBT. (From Krupski WC et al. Cervical chemodectoma: technical considerations and management options. Am J Surg 1982;144:215–220)

graft can be inserted over a shunt. Intraoperative EEG monitoring is frequently helpful to detect hemispheric ischemia and the need for shunting, should problems occur with carotid blood flow during resection. In recent series, patching or replacement of the internal carotid artery is required in approximately 25% of cases, while lateral repair of the vessel is required in another 10%.[9] Extremely large tumors may require resection of the encased external carotid artery to reduce blood loss and facilitate removal of the tumor from the internal carotid artery (Fig. 19-6).[3]

Although controversial, preoperative tumor embolization by arteriographic transcatheter obliteration of feeding vessels, usually arising from the external carotid artery, may be helpful in reducing the vascularity and size of the tumor, thus facilitating resection. Gel foam, spring coils, and polyvinyl alcohol beads have all been used to occlude the feeding vessels.[7,10] The procedure is somewhat complex, however, and has the potential for significant neurologic complications of its own. Thus, it should only be performed by experienced interventional radiologists. In addition, embolization is probably not necessary or particularly helpful for small (type I or II) tumors. It can be quite helpful in our experience and in that of several other groups for large (4 or 5 cm) CBT. Embolization should not be regarded as definitive treatment, however, as the tumor will reacquire a blood supply from other collateral pathways and continued enlargement can be anticipated. Similarly, other alternative therapies such as chemotherapy and radiation have not proven useful in the management of these tumors.

Results of Surgical Treatment

Early reports for the surgical treatment of CBTs had extremely high rates of morbidity and mortality. Most of these complications were related to cranial nerve injury and ligation or injury of the carotid vessels. The technical challenges of surgical extirpation of CBT may lead to excessive blood loss, stroke, or other neurologic deficits and significant postoperative disability associated with cranial nerve dysfunction. With improvements in surgical technique and the management of carotid artery injuries, most modern series report significantly diminished perioperative mortality and stroke rates. This is illustrated by the series from the Mayo Clinic detailing trends over a 50-year period. In the most recent decade of their experience, there is no perioperative mortality and only a 2.7% stroke rate.[8] However, postoperative cranial nerve injury continues to be the major cause of postoperative morbidity. In over 40% of cases, there was evidence of postoperative cranial nerve problems. Approximately half of these will be temporary and the other half permanent.[11] The vagus, hypoglossal, and glossopharyngeal nerves are at greatest risk; however, injuries to the sympathetic chain and branches of the facial nerves have also been described. Several other contemporary series, including our own, have documented similar satisfactory perioperative and long-term results.[3,7] Thus, although the incidence of permanent cranial nerve dysfunction is still approximately 20% when operating on large tumors (*i.e.,* those greater than 4–5 cm) an aggressive approach to the surgical management of CBT is justified.

REFERENCES

1. Cottrell ED, Smith LL. Management of uncommon lesions affecting the extracranial vessels. In: Rutherford RB, ed. Vascular Surgery. 4th ed. Philadelphia: W.B. Saunders Co, 1995:1622–26
2. Shamblin WR, ReMine WH, Sheps SG, Harrison EG. Carotid body tumor (chemodectoma): clinicopathologic analysis of ninety cases. Am J Surg 1971;122:732–739
3. Krupski WC, Effeney DJ, Ehrenfield WK, Stoney RJ. Cervical Chemodectoma: technical considerations and management options. Am J Surg 1982;144:215–220
4. Meyer FB, Sundt TM, Pearson BW. Carotid body tumors: a subject review and suggested surgical approach. J Neurosurg 1986;64:377–385
5. Smith RF. Carotid body tumors. In: Stanley JC, Ernst CB, eds. Current therapy in vascular surgery. 2nd ed. Philadelphia: B.C. Decker Inc, 1991:166–169
6. Ridge BA, Brewster DC, Darling RC, Cambria RP, LaMuraglia GM, Abbott WM. Familial carotid body tumors: incidence and implications. Ann Vasc Surg 1993;7:190–194
7. LaMuraglia GM, Fabian RL, Brewster DC, et al. The current surgical management of carotid body paragangliomas. J Vasc Surg 1992;15:1038–1045
8. Hallett JW, Nora JD, Hollier LH, Cherry KJ, Pairolero PC. Trends in neurovascular complications of surgical management for carotid body and cervical paragangliomas: a fifty-year experience with 153 tumors. J Vasc Surg 1988;7:284–291
9. Hallett JW. Carotid body tumor resection. In: Bergan JJ, Yao JST, eds. Techniques in arterial surgery. 1st ed. Philadelphia: W.B. Saunders Co, 1990:214–222
10. Smith RF, Shetty PC, Reddy DJ. Surgical treatment of carotid paragangliomas presenting unusual technical difficulties. J Vasc Surg 1988;7:631–637
11. Nora JD, Hallett JW, O'Brien PC, et al. Surgical resection of carotid body tumors: long-term survival, recurrence, and metastasis. Mayo Clin Proc 1988;63:348–352

Index

Note: Page numbers followed by an *f* indicate figures; those followed by a *t* indicate tables.

M

N

O

P

T